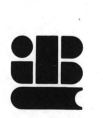

A publication of the
Association of American Medical Colleges

Continuing Education for the Health Professions

Developing, Managing,
and Evaluating Programs
for Maximum Impact
on Patient Care

Joseph S. Green, PH.D.
Sarina J. Grosswald, M.ED.
Emanuel Suter, M.D.
David B. Walthall III, M.D.
EDITORS

Continuing Education for the Health Professions

Jossey-Bass Publishers
San Francisco • Washington • London • 1984

CONTINUING EDUCATION FOR THE HEALTH PROFESSIONS
Developing, Managing, and Evaluating Programs
for Maximum Impact on Patient Care
    by Joseph S. Green, Sarina J. Grosswald, Emanual Suter,
    David B. Walthall III, Editors

Copyright © 1984 by: Association of American
                      Medical Colleges
                      One Dupont Circle, Suite 200
                      Washington, D.C. 20036

                      Jossey-Bass Inc., Publishers
                      433 California Street
                      San Francisco, California 94104

                      Jossey-Bass Limited
                      28 Banner Street
                      London EC1Y 8QE

Library of Congress Cataloging in Publication Data
Main entry under title:

Continuing education for the health professions.

    (Association of American Medical Colleges series in
academic medicine) (The Jossey-Bass higher education
series)
    Includes bibliographies and index.
    1. Medicine—Study and teaching (Continuing education)
2. Medical personnel.   I. Green, Joseph S.   II. Series.
III. Series: Jossey-Bass higher education series.
[DNLM: 1. Health occupations—Education.   2. Education,
Continuing.   W 18 C7628]
R845.C63   1984   610'.7'154   83-49261
ISBN 0-87589-604-9

Manufactured in the United States of America

The paper in this book meets the guidelines for
permanence and durability of the Committee on
Production Guidelines for Book Longevity of the
Council on Library Resources.

JACKET DESIGN BY WILLI BAUM
FIRST EDITION

Code 8417

The Jossey-Bass
Higher Education Series

Association of American Medical Colleges
Series in Academic Medicine
JOHN A. D. COOPER, *Editor*

Contents

Part One: How Adults Learn

Contents

Foreword

Over the last decade significant developments in the evolution of
continuing education for physicians and other health professionals
have taken place, along with increasing public concern for what
used to be the almost exclusive domain of the professional. One
cause for these trends is the tendency, justified or not, to link continuing education to the quality assurance of health care. One result
is that continuing education is becoming mandatory for most health
professionals. Another is that investments of private and public resources in continuing education are increasing. This emergent public awareness of continuing education has been accompanied by a
demand for greater accountability to assure professionals that their
investment of time and other resources in continuing education is
worthwhile and to assure the public that the professions make every
effort to maintain the competence of their memberships.

     The trend toward institutionalizing continuing education
has been particularly evident in the Veterans Administration (VA)
health care system. In 1973 Congress authorized the establishment of

regional medical education centers to provide continuing education to health professionals employed in the VA system. Putting such an educational component to use created the need for a mechanism for internal quality control and accountability—a mechanism that would be responsive to the needs of the health professionals, the veteran beneficiaries, and the public.

In the private sector, particularly in medicine, the concept of mandated continuing education for relicensure, medical and specialty society membership, board recertification, and maintenance of hospital privileges called for a more broadly based accreditation system than the one pioneered in the 1960s by the American Medical Association. The result was the establishment in 1976 of the Liaison Committee for Continuing Medical Education, subsequently the Accreditation Council for Continuing Medical Education, jointly sponsored by seven organizations: the American Board of Medical Specialties, the American Hospital Association, the American Medical Association, the Association of American Medical Colleges, the Association of Hospital Medical Education, the Federation of State Medical Boards, and the Council of Medical Specialty Societies.

It became evident that the quality assurance demands of both the Veterans Administration continuing education system and the Accreditation Council for Continuing Medical Education could best be met if the principles underlying quality continuing education were more clearly defined and translated into a set of workable criteria and standards. The availability of such criteria would permit the establishment of procedures for assessing the quality of programs and of organizations or institutions responsible for them. To meet this need, the Veterans Administration and the Association of American Medical Colleges initiated a joint project to study the theoretical and experiential foundations of continuing education and to develop a set of criteria for quality continuing education. It was agreed that the project also should develop materials that would aid those responsible for developing programs in accordance with the criteria developed for quality assurance.

The project was funded through a grant (EMI-78-002-01) by the Veterans Administration to the Association of American Medical Colleges. This collaborative effort of the Veterans Administration and a professional organization is not unique in the history of the

VA. VA medical centers and medical schools and other health profession schools have a long established tradition of affiliation for furthering high-quality patient care for veterans and opening Veterans Administration health care resources to professional education and biomedical research.

This book represents one of the outcomes of the project. Its intent is to share the results of this study with those responsible for continuing education of health professionals in the Veterans Administration health care system and in the private sector. Through this effort, a tradition of successful collaboration between the private sector and a federal agency is maintained for the benefit of our veterans and the wider public.

February 1984   John A. D. Cooper, M.D., Ph.D.
                                               President of the Association of
                                               American Medical Colleges
                                               Washington, D.C.

                                               Donald L. Custis, M.D.
                                               Chief Medical Director
                                               Veterans Administration
                                               Washington, D.C.

Preface

Very few continuing education professionals in the health fields have formal training in education or management; their backgrounds are almost wholly in the health sciences. But as more and more health disciplines and state licensing agencies mandate continuing education, more and more health professionals find themselves involved in helping their colleagues continue their learning. Until now, a major roadblock to that effort has been the paucity of publications dealing with continuing education *in the health professions.* Health professionals need information directed specifically to them—written in their vernacular and with their realities in mind. This volume is the first publication that puts together into a handy reference the kinds of continuing education information vital to busy practitioners.

Continuing Education for the Health Professions provides the most comprehensive and integrated treatment to date of learning theory, adult education, and management principles. It is designed to aid everyone who has responsibility for planning and implementing continuing education activities. Primarily, it is intended for those involved in continuing education in all health profession schools, including medicine, dentistry, nursing, pharmacy, allied health, and public health. It will equally benefit deans or vice-presidents of academic health science centers and education directors of hospitals, professional organizations, and other nonprofit or for-profit enterprises that offer continuing education opportunities. Because it contains both the theoretical foundations for developing appropriate continuing education activities *and* practical applications, it will also serve as a resource for graduate programs in adult learning and educational administration, for training programs in business and industry, and for health professionals wanting to develop skills and programs for self-directed learning. In addition, it will aid those responsible for quality assurance programs, such as accreditors of continuing education.

This book grew out of a project that was established jointly by the Association of American Medical Colleges (AAMC) and the Veterans Administration (VA). The mandate of the project—the Continuing Education Systems Project (CESP)—was to define what constituted quality in continuing education for the health professions—and then *to translate* the definition into guidelines for the everyday practice of continuing education. In this book, seventeen individual contributors present critical information from their training and experience in education, health, and management to assist others in solving problems related to the practice of continuing education. The result is a conceptual model of continuing education and a set of criteria that define the educational and management tasks necessary for developing, implementing, and evaluating quality continuing education. (These criteria are called *quality elements* within this work and are described in the first chapter and in the Appendix.)

Overview of Contents

The introduction describes the Continuing Education Systems Project, detailing the realities of continuing education in the health professions that dictated a need to define explicitly the model and quality elements. The two chapters in Part One outline the theo-

retical perspectives that are the underpinnings of the entire book. A
description is provided of the research in learning theory that serves
as the foundation for defining quality continuing education. Generalizations about how adults and adult health professionals learn
are described, along with the theoretical contributions of motivation
theory toward the understanding of learning. It is from these bodies
of knowledge that a definition of quality continuing education
emerges.

The role of continuing education in serving the health professions is the focus of Part Two. An in-depth study of the
information-seeking behaviors of a group of Michigan family physicians describes the sources they use and their criteria for selecting
these sources. A treatise on the history of continuing medical education illustrates the evolution of continuing education from "repair
shops" for those who had received inadequate medical education to
today's emphasis on relevant continuing education for improving
the practice behaviors of physicians. The last chapter in Part Two
describes the health professional, client of the program that provides
continuing education (referred to as the *provider unit*), and the provider unit, facilitator of learning for the health professional. The
traditional roles of provider units are contrasted with a proposed
new role.

Part Three of the book deals with the development of continuing education. The gestalt of and rationale for a systematic approach to educational development is provided as an overview.
Descriptions of that process are detailed in chapters addressing needs
assessment, design of education activities for groups of learners,
evaluation, and facilitation of self-directed learning for individual
health professionals.

Part Four focuses on decision making in the continuing education provider unit by giving a description and rationale for a
strategic management approach to leadership. It analyzes the continuing education management process and proposes four functions
of managing the provider unit that can be used as a foundation for
developing a management information system. Methods are discussed for identifying the critical information needs that would
allow a manager to develop quality continuing education. Two
systems are described for assuring the quality of all activities of a

continuing education provider unit and for assuring the quality of its *most important activity*—the educational development process. The last chapter returns to the Continuing Education Systems Project and shows how provider units can and have used the quality elements to improve their continuing education. The Epilogue suggests additional resource materials for interested readers and sums up strategies that can strengthen the continued learning of health professionals.

How to Use This Book

A major aim of this book is to enable people involved in continuing education to increase their responsiveness to the practice-related needs of the health professionals they serve. A great deal of attention is paid to the principles of adult learning—making education practical and responsive to the real-world needs of health care professionals. Although reading the book from the first chapter to the end is certainly valuable, an alternative approach is also possible. Because Chapter One explains the context from which the model and the quality elements emerged, it is best to begin at the beginning. Next, however, readers will do well to go to Chapter Sixteen, which tells how different organizations involved with the project improved their processes by focusing on certain quality elements. Readers could then go through the list of quality elements, noting and reading in detail about those that are most relevant for their professional responsibilities and that are thus most likely to serve as catalysts for bringing about needed change. In order to make the book more responsive to those professional responsibilities, it is suggested that readers be selective as to which chapters then become the focus of their attention. For example, for readers who have responsibilities in designing and evaluating learning activities, Chapters Seven through Eleven offer the most practical assistance. For managers of continuing education organizations, the utmost concern would probably be related to establishing management information systems or quality control mechanisms, which are discussed in Chapters Twelve through Fifteen.

Acknowledgments

The Continuing Education Systems Project (CESP) final report lists all the groups and individuals who contributed to the development of the quality elements and other aspects of the project. The initial idea of addressing in a single project the quality assurance needs of both the VA's Regional Medical Education Centers and the AAMC relative to its membership in the Liaison Committee for Continuing Medical Education is credited to William D. Mayer, M.D., then assistant chief medical director for academic affairs in the VA. Dr. Mayer and John D. Chase, M.D., then chief medical director of the VA, were instrumental in the development of the project. Their respective successors, Donald L. Custis, M.D., and David Worthen, M.D., and John A. D. Cooper, M.D., president of AAMC, have all been equally supportive of the entire effort. The individuals who served as chairpersons of the two steering committees to the project, John D. Chase, M.D., and Alan B. Knox, Ed.D., deserve special acknowledgment for their ideas, suggestions, and continuing support for both the project and the book. Similar recognition goes to Barbara Pryor, former special assistant to the chief medical director of the VA.

Special thanks must also go to those who assisted directly in the completion of this manuscript and who generously agreed to read and comment on it; their criticism and suggestions were of great value to the editors. Thanks for this assistance goes to Richard M. Caplan, M.D., John D. Chase, M.D., Roy Lindahl, D.D.S., Robert Raszkowski, M.D., Barbara Redman, R.N., Ph.D., Howard Sparks, Ed.D., Robert Sparks, M.D., Cheryl Walthall, R.N., Francis A. Zacharewicz, M.D., and Carter Zeleznik, Ph.D.

Grateful acknowledgment is made to the extremely competent support staff handling the word processor and the many details involved in preparing the manuscript through its many revisions. Special thanks go to Jeanne Lonsdale and Katherine Ramsay at AAMC for their endless patience and outstanding effort. The help and assistance of Cathy Farrell at the Continuing Education Center of the VA Medical Center in Washington, D.C., and of Sally Oesterling at the AAMC office are also acknowledged.

Finally, we would like to take this opportunity to thank our families and friends who shared in the joys and pains of developing this book.

It is not possible to list all individuals who in one way or another furthered the work of CESP. The staff of CESP and the editors of this book deeply appreciate all of these, named or unnamed, contributors.

February 1984   Joseph S. Green, Ph.D.
                                                   Laguna Niguel, California

                                                   Sarina J. Grosswald, M.Ed.
                                                   Washington, D.C.

                                                   Emanuel Suter, M.D.
                                                   Washington, D.C.

                                                   David B. Walthall III, M.D.
                                                   Washington, D.C.

Contributors

Joseph S. Green is currently assistant clinical professor, Department of Medical Education, University of Southern California School of Medicine. He is also employed in private business and as a private consultant. He was director of the Continuing Education Systems Project at the Association of American Medical Colleges (AAMC) in Washington, D.C., between April 1980 and September 1981. Green also served as the coordinator of Educational Design and Evaluation and codirector of the Veterans Administration's InterWest Regional Medical Education Center in Salt Lake City, Utah, between 1975 and 1979. He received his B.A. degree (1968) from the University of California at Santa Barbara in sociology, his M.Ed. degree (1972) from the University of Illinois in educational psychology, and his Ph.D. degree (1975) from the University of Illinois in educational psychology and adult learning.

Green's main professional activities have been in continuing professional education in the health fields. He has been involved in research, teaching, program development and evaluation, administration, and accreditation. He is currently the AAMC representative on the Accreditation Council for Continuing Medical Education. In 1979 Green was awarded the first annual Ben Wells, M.D., Memorial Award for excellence in the advancement of quality continuing health education in the Veterans Administration (VA) and the federal training officer's annual Distinguished Service Award for professional contribution to the design of a continuing education quality assurance and assessment program. His publications include "Comparative Analysis of the Program Development Process in Six Professions" (1977, with F. C. Pennington), "Pathways for Impact Evaluation" (1980, with P. L. Walsh), "Regionalized Continuing Medical Education: Building Multi-Institutional Support" (1981), and "Continuing Education of Health Professionals: Proposal for a Definition of Quality" (1981, with others).

Green has served as consultant to several medical schools, the VA health care system, the National Hospice Association, and the National Council on Foundations. He has also taught various courses on aspects of the program development process in continuing health professions education.

Sarina J. Grosswald is administrator of the division of Educational Resources Development at the American College of Obstetricians and Gynecologists in Washington, D.C. She received her B.A. degree in English (1973) from the University of North Carolina at Chapel Hill, and her M.Ed. in educational media and instructional design (1977) from the University of North Carolina.

Grosswald's primary area of interest has been professional education in the health fields, including undergraduate and continuing education for national and international projects.

While serving as instructional designer and project director for the Continuing Education Systems Project at the Association of American Medical Colleges from 1981 to 1983, Grosswald coordinated the development of instructional materials that describe a systematic approach to design and evaluation of continuing education.

Between 1976 and 1981, at the University of North Carolina Office of Medical Studies, Grosswald designed and produced instructional materials utilizing a variety of media. Her publications include *Writing Self-Instruction* (1979) and *Hypertension: A Study*

Resource for Medical Schools, as well as numerous patient and professional educational materials.

Emanuel Suter, M.D., is the former director of the Division of Educational Resources and Programs at the Association of American Medical Colleges in Washington, D.C. He was born in Basel, Switzerland, and received the M.D. degree (1942) from the medical faculty of the University of Basel. He then was engaged in biomedical research at the pharmacological laboratories of Sandoz Pharmaceuticals, Inc. (1943 to 1945) and at the Institute of Hygiene of the University of Basel (1945 to 1949). In January 1949 he joined the Laboratory of Pathology of Dr. René Dubos at the Rockefeller Institute for Medical Research in New York City and subsequently taught bacteriology and immunology in an integrated course of the basic medical sciences at Harvard Medical School (1952 to 1956). After serving at the University of Florida College of Medicine in Gainesville as the first chairman of the Department of Microbiology (1956 to 1964) and then as dean of the college (1964 to 1972), he joined the staff of the Association of American Medical Colleges. He directed and codirected several projects in the area of international medical education, educational resources development, and continuing education, among them the Continuing Education Systems Project. Dr. Suter is the author of numerous original research publications and reviews in bacteriology, immunology, and educational development. Since January 1984 he has served as a consultant in medical education to the New Jersey Department of Higher Education.

David B. Walthall III, M.D., has been the medical director of the Veterans Administration, Department of Medicine and Surgery, Continuing Education Center in Washington, D.C., since 1980. He received the B.A. degree (1957) in psychology and the M.D. degree (1961) from the University of Virginia. Walthall practiced family medicine in Dublin, Virginia, from 1963 until 1973. He served as associate professor of family practice and assistant dean for continuing medical education at the Medical College of Virginia from 1973 to 1977. From 1977 to 1980, he was chief of the Continuing Education Division and acting director of the Continuing Education Service for the central office of the Veterans Administration's Department of Medicine and Surgery.

Dr. Walthall has been actively involved in Medical Quality Assurance at the hospital, state, and national level and served as president of the American Heart Association, Virginia Affiliate. He is a Charter Diplomate of the American Academy of Family Physicians.

David M. E. Allan, M.D., is a consultant in continuing education, La Jolla, California.

Donald L. Cordes, Ph.D., is associate director of the Continuing Education Center, Veterans Administration Medical Center, Washington, D.C.

Linda K. Gunzburger, Ph.D., is codirector of the Division of Continuing Medical Education, Loyola University of Chicago, Stritch School of Medicine, Chicago.

Alan B. Knox, Ed.D., is professor of education at the University of Wisconsin at Madison.

Kenneth Lawrence, M.F.A., is instructional design officer in the Continuing Education Center, Veterans Administration Medical Center, Washington, D.C.

Harold G. Levine, M.P.A., is professor of preventive medicine and community health and special assistant in medical education in the Office of Educational Development, University of Texas Medical Branch, Galveston.

J. Morris McInnes, Ph.D., is head of the Accounting, Planning, and Control Group, Sloan School of Management, Massachusetts Institute of Technology, Cambridge, Massachusetts.

Robert P. Means, Ph.D., is associate director of programming at the Regional Medical Education Center, Veterans Administration Medical Center, Brecksville, Ohio.

Donald E. Moore, Jr., Ph.D., is director of Continuing Medical Education, Eastern Virginia Medical Authority, Norfolk.

Floyd C. Pennington, Ph.D., is vice-president for education in the National Arthritis Foundation, Atlanta, Georgia.

Gregg R. Seppala, M.S., is chief of the Professional Support Group, Continuing Education Center, Washington Veterans Administration Medical Center, Washington, D.C.

Patrick L. Walsh, Ph.D., is codirector of the InterWest Regional Medical Education Center, Veterans Administration Medical Center, Salt Lake City, Utah.

Carter Zelenik, Ph.D., is associate director of the Offices of Medical Education, Jefferson Medical College, Philadelphia, Pennsylvania.

Continuing Education for the Health Professions

Developing, Managing, and Evaluating Programs for Maximum Impact on Patient Care

You have done so by your own seeking, in your own way, through thought, through meditation, through knowledge, through enlightenment. You have learned nothing through teachings.
                                                                    HERMAN HESSE

I am always wanting to learn, although I may not always be ready to be taught.
                                                                    WINSTON CHURCHILL

1

Introduction:
Defining Quality
for Continuing Education

Emanuel Suter, Joseph S. Green
Sarina J. Grosswald, Kenneth A. Lawrence
David B. Walthall III, Carter Zeleznik

This chapter presents the context for the Continuing Education Systems Project (CESP) and provides a rationale for this book. It is suggested that all readers start with this chapter since the conceptual model of continuing education (CE) and the list of quality elements (QEs) are provided herein. The reader is encouraged to read the Appendix at the conclusion of this book, which provides an in-depth discussion of each of the QEs, and Chapter Sixteen, which discusses how to apply the quality elements to the operations of a CE provider unit.—Editors

Continuing education (CE) for health professionals can be defined as processes aimed at improving health care outcomes through learning, either by individual efforts or as part of activities,

1

products, and services developed by CE provider units. Learning may result in the maintenance or enhancement of professional competence and performance or in health care organizational effectiveness and efficiency (Suter and others, 1981). Thus, in today's health care milieu, many people consider continuing education of health professionals to be a vehicle for changing not only an individual professional's behavior but also the functioning of the health care system.

Contextual Realities and External Pressures

Irrespective of the highly disparate views people hold of the purposes and the value of CE, common sense and observation indicate that health professionals who have been away from formal training for significant lengths of time practice their professions quite differently than they did when their professional education was still in progress or recently completed (Caplan, 1983). Though some change can be attributed to situational factors, some must reasonably be attributed to the effects of CE (Goldfinger, 1982).

With the explosive expansion of knowledge and the technological development of the past half century, the major emphasis in the substance of continuing education has been on knowledge and technical skills, often at the expense of other competencies of health professionals. These other competencies relate to how health care is rendered and include, for instance, interpersonal skills, attitudes, and values. This imbalance in emphasis may be exerting a limiting effect. For example, achieving any real impact on health care cost containment is likely to require not only the application of new knowledge and technology but also an attitudinal change by health professionals. Similarly, effective responses to increasing demands for geriatric care may depend as much on reordering of values and attitudes regarding the elderly patient and chronic impairment as on the transfer of new knowledge and technology into that care.

A further dimension is added to continuing education, as to all education, by the rapid development of electronic technology for information management. The strides in technology have raised the quantity and quality of information available to the public and have increased the demands that physicians and other health professionals have access to the latest information and use it.

The pressures on the health professions and their continuing education systems are great. These pressures become apparent in exchanges between patients and health professionals, in the activities of consumer groups, and in legislative and fiscal actions of state and federal governments. One manifestation of these pressures is the introduction of mandated continuing education for many health professions, which has been spearheaded by professional groups, regulatory agencies, and state governments. As a consequence, there is not only greater need for continuing education opportunities in the various professions but also increasing demand for public accountability of the continuing education process.

For many reasons, the existing continuing education system for the health professions is not well equipped to respond to the pressures and demands made upon it. Some of the resulting shortcomings and the issues currently confronting CE are discussed in this and in following chapters.

CE as Educational Continuum. Undergraduate, graduate, and continuing education of health professionals constitute a continuum, particularly in dentistry and medicine; nearly every graduate in these fields enrolls in graduate education programs before becoming a practitioner. A student's progress through this continuum from preprofessional to professional status should be accompanied by a shift in control over professional learning from the institution to the individual. This transition represents a significant change in the relationship between the learner and the institution, for during preparatory professional education, the institution's input far outweighs the individual's (Keller, 1979). While a student in medicine, nursing, or any other health profession has a personal goal of becoming a physician, nurse, or other health professional, the faculty sets the specific objectives and the conditions for reaching that goal. The faculty usually prescribes a curriculum or, as in some institutions recently, identifies the objectives that students must reach in their own way. Often the curriculum provides motivational stimuli; examinations and the expectation of obtaining a degree or a certificate are among the strongest of these. The educational cycle is dominated by institutions that decide on learning needs and objectives, frequently prescribe instructional methods (usually lectures), and determine and design evaluations (Eldridge, 1982). Finally, the application of learned knowledge and skills to the patient care process occurs under close institutional supervision.

In summary, the passage from learning in preparation for a profession to learning as a professional entails a transition from an institutional to an individual impetus for learning. This is not an all-or-none or an instant phenomenon but rather a gradual maturing of the professional as a learner. While preparatory education permits but does not depend on individual initiative, professional or continuing education depends on or should depend on self-motivated learning.

In CE, as institutional influence decreases, individual professionals are expected to assume primary control over identifying their personal learning needs, setting their own learning goals and objectives, choosing learning approaches, selecting methods of evaluation, and—the ultimate goal—applying their acquired competencies to practice. However, this premise is not always realized. Many professionals do not easily make the transition from dependent to independent learning; they continue to depend heavily on institutions to direct their learning. Likewise, the faculty charged with assisting professionals in their continuing education fail to recognize that different approaches are needed in CE from those used in preprofessional education. Rather than assume new functions as facilitators and information brokers, the faculty continue in their traditional roles as instructors and content experts (Matheson and Cooper, 1982).

Educational institutions and their faculties, students, and graduates, must translate the concept of the educational continuum into programmatic realities. This means that students, through the acquisition of knowledge, skills, and experience, should increasingly gain independence in their approaches to learning. By precept and educational design, students should be prepared for independent, self–directed, and lifelong learning. They need to acquire skills, attitudes, and habits that will help them continually assess their performance and their professional needs as well as to plan and implement the necessary learning activities.

Various Issues in CE. When the goals of continuing education are matched to its present practices, substantial incongruities become apparent. The discrepancy between expectations and ability to deliver causes many of the problems hampering continuing education today.

The *increasing demand* for continuing education opportunities, brought about by the expanding role of technological change and by the relatively recent introduction of mandated CE for many health professions, represents a major burden to the individual professional and the educational system alike. While mandated continuing education may have merit in certain professions and under some circumstances, it has a tendency to overload the system and to hinder learning. Overloading any system often results in the erosion of standards of quality; quantity may take priority over quality, and flaws in the system may grow into deficiencies under such stress (Driver and Streufert, 1969). In addition, approaches to CE that rely on institutionally controlled activities may conflict with the premise of individualized CE.

Many people claim that there is *little proof of any impact* of continuing education on patient care (Cooper, 1977), and that attempts to measure the impact are not scientifically sound (Bertram and Brooks–Bertram, 1977). If this once was true, it is no longer. Recent experience in several health fields has shown that the lack of demonstrable impact is due to the design of the educational experience or its evaluation rather than to a failure of CE per se. It appears that the more general the learning objectives of a given educational activity, the more difficult it is to assess and evaluate impact, possibly due to "contamination" from uncontrollable sources of information (Goldfinger, 1982). By contrast, the use of limited, clearly circumscribed objectives can result in measurable impact on a specified area of competence, performance, or even care outcome (Stein, 1981). It appears that the demands for demonstrating a causal relationship between instruction and practice behavior are more stringently placed on CE than they are on the preparatory phase of health professions education. Rarely is a health professional school required to justify the quality of its educational program in terms of demonstrable performance of its graduates. Rather, the judgment of institutional quality relies on assessing input to and process of the educational program.

Most institutions or organizations that serve as sponsors or providers of CE activities for groups or disciplines of health professionals have organized *continuing education provider units* (defined later in this chapter). In many units, especially in small organizations, the person in charge is likely to have little previous experience in adult and continuing education. Because financial support from the parent organization is often insignificant or absent, many CE provider units operate with marginal resources and depend heavily on income generated from enrollment fees. This reality forces CE provider units to plan programs aimed at attracting large numbers of participants, frequently at the expense of assessing and attending to the needs of individual professionals. This reality also prevents or stifles innovative approaches to CE planning and research.

High expectations that continuing education will work as a panacea for health care deficiencies are another cause of disappointments in CE. Public authorities may make unwarranted assumptions about the effectiveness of CE in assuring health care professionals' competency and performance, without regard to the many other factors that relate to the situation. The long-term consequences are disappointment and unjustified discontent with CE.

Because of the diversity of CE activities and settings it is difficult to arrive at a generalizable *definition of quality*. In simple terms, quality can be defined as four attributes—relevancy, accessibility, efficiency, and effectiveness (Williamson, 1977). When medical practitioners, directors of medical CE provider units, and individuals responsible for accreditation were asked what continuing education for physicians should be like in order to satisfy these four attributes, a statement summarized in the following list emerged (Association of American Medical Colleges, 1981). Accordingly, a CE provider unit should:

- have institutional commitment and support
- document its mission and goals
- provide programs that are authentic and professionally satisfying
- identify needs from multiple perspectives
- have qualified staff and faculty
- provide organized programs that meet the needs of a discipline, area, or region

- provide activities, products, and services that are congruent with adult learning principles
- involve the learner or a subset of learners in the planning process of activities
- use identified needs for choosing and developing objectives
- carry out comprehensive evaluation of content and process
- use evaluation results for program planning
- be administratively well organized and have good management for faculty and other resource utilization

Although these attributes of quality were developed with physicians in mind, it seems justified to extrapolate to other health professionals. Even if this is done, however, the attributes are too vague to be operationally helpful.

These are some of the issues that confront both the professional as a learner and those responsible for sponsoring CE activities, products, and services. They represent a complex web of conceptual, social, educational, managerial, and economic variables that influence CE. These variables must be considered in the search for a definition of quality for the CE process.

Analysis of the Multiple Factors Affecting CE. In 1976 the Association of American Medical Colleges recognized the need for a more systematic, focused approach to CE for the health professions in general and for medicine in particular. With the guidance of an Ad Hoc Committee on Continuing Medical Education, an analysis of the multiple factors affecting continuing medical education (CME) was undertaken to identify potential intervention points. With the assistance of expert consultants, a computerized simulation model based on systems dynamics was developed (Forrester, 1961). The model identified key variables affecting the impact of CME on physicians' capabilities and on the quality of care delivered. It described the relationships of selected variables in qualitative and quantitative terms (Pugh-Roberts Associates, 1978). The major variables of the model were:

- physicians' knowledge and skills, as well as actual performance in utilizing knowledge and skills

- volume and characteristics of several types of CME
- physicians' characteristics that influence CME effectiveness
- physicians' outputs in terms of percentage of cases referred and percentage of cases with correct diagnosis and treatment
- patients' knowledge and skills, and actual performance in following treatment plan
- patients' outputs in terms of percentage of cases with follow-through as directed
- cases with satisfactory outcome in terms of percentage of cases with correct diagnosis, treatment, and patient follow-through

Once the model structure had been developed and the quantitative relationships had been established, the model was represented in the simulation language DYNAMO (Pugh, 1976). Projections could then be made that allowed estimates of the impact over a simulated twenty-year period of specific variables and influences ("what if" questions) on physician competencies and performance and on the outcomes of their actions. The results of each simulation reflected the consequences of the relationships and assumptions originally incorporated in the model. The validity of the model was established on the basis of a literature search, expert opinions, sensitivity and reasonableness tests of the model's results over a broad range of assumptions, and consistency of those results with published ones.

After conducting a number of initial policy analysis simulations, four suggestions for enhancing the impact of CME on physician performance were derived. Accordingly, CME should encourage physicians to become involved in design and implementation of CE activities, acquire self-evaluation and self-directed learning skills, become lifelong learners, and enhance their skills in relating to patients and their efforts to assure appropriate follow-through by patients.

The systems dynamics model suggested strategies for dealing with some of these issues. The outcome of the simulations indicated that new approaches to continuing education had to be sought and tried in order to realize the impact CE could have on the quality of health care rendered. How could these new approaches be accomplished? There was a need to go beyond developing recommendations, as had already been done (Ad Hoc Committee on Continuing Medical Education, 1980). The most logical next steps were to examine the theoretical and conceptual foundations of continuing education, incorporate them into a general model of continuing education, and translate them into process descriptions or guidelines.

Continuing Education Systems Project (CESP)

In a special report, a committee on CE of the Association of American Medical Colleges (AAMC) called for "leadership in developing and applying adult learning principles to continuing medical education" (Ad Hoc Committee on Continuing Medical Education, 1980, p. 154). The interest for quality assurance of continuing education for the health professions was widespread, involving most health professions and both the private sector and federal agencies. In particular, the Veterans Administration (VA) had a mandated commitment to the continuing education of health professionals after Congress had given it the authority in 1973 (PL 92-541) to establish Regional Medical Education Centers (RMECs) for the purpose of providing continuing education to the health care professionals in the VA health care system.

CESP originated as a joint project of the VA and the AAMC. The VA had a need to develop a quality assurance process for the RMEC continuing education system, while the AAMC, as a member organization of the Liaison Committee for Continuing Medical Education (now the Accreditation Council for Continuing Medical Education), was intent on building a sound foundation for the accreditation process in the private sector. The effort of the project was supported over a five-year period by a grant from the Veterans Administration. Although the development of CESP relied predominantly on the experience with CE for physicians, it was assumed that the concepts and general principles developed and the specific criteria derived from them would be equally applicable to CE for all health professions. This assumption seemed justified on the grounds that sound educational principles apply to all professional education. This was later proven to be valid when other health professional groups became involved in the project (for examples, see Chapter Sixteen).

Assumptions, Goals, and Objectives. The CESP was undertaken with the assumptions that CE of health professionals can lead to improvement of patient care; the quality of the CE process can make a difference on its impact; there are generally accepted adult learning concepts that can enhance learning when applied to CE; presently, these concepts, together with modern educational and information management technologies, are not applied systematically to CE of health professionals; and there is increasing interest and desire among health professionals and CE providers to apply these concepts and technologies. It became clear that a general process model of CE based on contemporary theory and concepts of learning was needed, from which guidelines could be developed to aid those in charge of programs and quality assurance.

The overall goals of CESP, therefore, were to improve the quality of CE for health professionals by defining and describing quality CE and by assisting CE providers and accrediting organizations to assure quality CE. To reach this goal, the project identified the following objectives: (1) after a review of the theoretical and experiential foundations of CE, develop a conceptual model of CE and a list of elements or criteria called quality elements for applying the model to CE practice; (2) develop specifications for an information management and reporting system in support of quality CE; (3) produce materials and learning packages that will assist CE providers in applying the model's concepts into CE practice; and (4) pilot test the criteria, the management system, and the learning materials in various CE settings.

Project Development Process. The appointment of two steering committees secured broadly based input into the project. One committee, chaired by Alan B. Knox, professor of adult education at the University of Illinois at Urbana and later the University of Wisconsin at Madison, was representative of the professional education constituency. The other committee, chaired by John Chase, former chief medical director of the VA, had representation from various parts of the VA health care system. Both committees provided overall direction to the project. Two working groups, the Adult Learning Working Group and the Systems Working Group, were assigned the tasks of reviewing both the theoretical aspects of adult learning and the general and specific systems theories that lead to the development of a conceptual process model of continuing education for health professionals and a corresponding set of criteria for quality CE. Finally, several multidisciplinary ad hoc advisory groups were convened to provide expert and real-world review and suggestions during various phases of project development. Drafts of project products, such as the quality elements, learning packages, and other documents, were widely circulated for review and criticism to assess their validity, usefulness, and accuracy.

Conceptual Model for Continuing Education

The prescriptive model of CE as shown in Figure 1 was developed by the CESP to identify and demonstrate the relationships among what was asserted to be the six key domains of CE, namely, the health care setting, new knowledge and technology, the health professional and the learning process, the CE provider unit, and educational quality assurance.

Setting of CE. The delivery of health care depends to varying degrees on three major sources of input—the patient, the care system or care setting, and the health professional—that represent the interacting parts of a complex but flexible health care system (Senior, 1977). Competence and performance of the health professional and of the patient, in conjunction with the condition and performance of the care system, collectively determine the outcome of the intervention (health care). As the figure shows, by influencing competence and performance of the health professional, CE should function as a change agent of one of the components. Modifiers similarly can have an impact on the other two components—the patient and the system. As shown in Chapter Eight on needs assessment, for any identified problem or concern in the delivery of health care, explicit or implicit analysis of the situation must identify which of the health care components requires modification for the desired improvement to occur. Continuing education can only address concerns that can be improved or eliminated through education aimed at improving the competence of the health professional. However, as Brown (1977) points out, when one attempts to eliminate deficiencies identified through the audit process, all three com-

Figure 1. Continuing Education of Health Professionals.

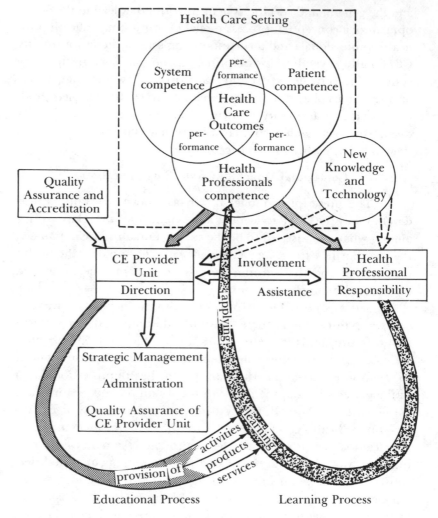

Source: Adapted from Suter and others, 1981, p. 696.

ponents of the health care setting must be considered; otherwise, efforts may be wasted. Therefore, the CE provider should assess the relationship of the system and patients to the educational activities offered and refer noneducational concerns to the appropriate office or department.

New Knowledge and Technology. New knowledge and technology are powerful modifiers of health care outcome. Most often, they are introduced into the system through the health professional. Traditionally, a major purpose of CE has been to familiarize the health professional with new knowledge and technology. This will remain so as long as discoveries are being made and knowledge is expanding. It is equally important, however, that CE address health care deficiencies that originate from a lack of applying or from misapplication of existing knowledge and technology. Such deficiencies might stem, for instance, from attitudinal problems, failing memory, or inability to apply effectively the existing knowledge and technology. The model suggests that new knowledge and technology, together with information about performance insufficiencies of health professionals, provide major inputs into CE.

Health Professional and Learning Process. The learning process loop of the model indicates that changes through learning represent the major function of CE. The driving force is motivation, rooted in the health professional's sense of responsibility. CE can only be successful and lead to the desired result if the health professional is ready to learn and to apply the new competencies in the health care setting. The learning and change of behavior are the goals of CE. They are stimulated and sustained by motivation of the health professionals and are initiated by their willingness to assume responsibility. The outcome of CE depends on the skills of the health professionals to engage in meaningful learning and on the nature of support given by the CE provider unit.

CE Provider Unit. The term *continuing education provider unit* is used to identify that administrative unit that assumes the responsibility and authority for providing continuing education opportunities for health professionals. A parent organization of a CE provider unit may be, among others, a health professions school, a health care organization (hospital, long-term care center, health maintenance organization, or a special service organization), a professional or specialty society, or a board of directors. In the case of a health professional school, the CE provider unit caters predominantly to professionals in practice or in employment outside the institution, while professional organizations assume responsibility for their membership, and the health care organizations concern themselves with their professional staff and employees. A CE provider unit may be a very small administrative unit working part-time, or it may include a large and highly specialized staff.

Educational Process. The model clearly illustrates that the health professional as an adult learner is the focal point of the system. The competencies brought to health care by the professionals, the performance of the professionals, and the potential influence of the learning process are the components of the feedback loop depicted in Figure 1. The CE provider unit's role is to facilitate and support the learning process initiated and undertaken by the health professional. The educational or CE process consists of activities, products, and services placed at the disposal of the health professional. Through the strategic management process, unit administration, and quality assurance process, the CE provider unit leadership provides important management and control functions, critical in the development and implementation of quality CE (see Chapter Twelve).

Depending on the setting and the developmental stage of the CE provider unit, the structure of the CE provider unit will differ (Moore, 1982). Some variables that account for differences relate to organizational context, external relationships, and program performance and leadership styles (Lawrence and Lorsch, 1967).

While management theories usually address larger organizations, it is appropriate for even the smaller organization, such as a CE provider unit, to include sound management as an important component of its working process. Even the individual professional engaged in self-directed learning as a "self-provider" can benefit from using a systematic approach to the planning of CE activities.

The CESP model suggests that CE represents a partnership between health professionals and the CE provider unit. A wide spectrum of interactions between health professionals and CE provider units can be observed, ranging from complete independence and self-directedness to nearly total dependence of professionals on the CE provider unit for their CE activities (for further discussion, see Chapter Six). Whatever the balance between the two, the ultimate goal—the application of modified competencies into the health care process—remains the responsibility of the professional.

Educational Quality Assurance. Quality assurance should address all the CE domains of the model. Within the health care system, various modalities of quality assurance exist that may yield data to serve both the initiation and the completion of the CE process in the form of either needs identification or evaluation. The health professional, on an individual or collective basis, may become engaged in self-assessment activities. The CE provider unit itself is responsible for internal quality assurance of its operation and is usually also subject to outside accreditation requirements. Finally, the health professionals themselves have to conform to professional standards promulgated by their professional organizations, state licensing agencies, and the health care organizations.

Implication of CE Model. This model suggests a number of concepts that, if realized, can have a significant impact on continuing education for the health professions and ultimately on health care. These concepts and suggestions address educational approaches and management strategies for the continuing education provider unit.

The concepts and principles expressed in the model provide a basis for identifying criteria of quality for continuing education for the health professions. Accordingly, a primary condition is that CE become an integral component of the health care setting. To this end, the documentation of health care–related problems and concerns and the identification of new knowledge and technology with a potential for impact on health care assume high priority. Equally important is the preparation of health professionals for their role in CE, because CE can have an impact only on and through the individual professional. Whether the impact is manifested as a renewal of self-confidence, professional competence, or performance in the care situation, improvement of perceived or measured health care outcomes is the ultimate goal of CE. The role of the CE provider unit is to maximize the transformation of the potential state-of-the-art of health care into actual health care practice. The CE provider unit is most likely to accomplish this goal by serving as a facilitator of the individual health professional's learning process and by assisting professionals in applying new information in the health care setting.

The accomplishment of these tasks requires leadership and management capability of the CE provider unit in support of individual and institutional educational activities. The CE provider unit should also provide a link between the learning process and the broader scientific and socioeconomic contexts of health care. Finally, internal and external quality assessment of the CE process should assure the health professional and the public that CE is both effective and efficient and serves their common interest.

Quality Elements

The application of the model to CE practice requires the interpretation of the concepts in the form of discrete and specific actions to be taken by the CE provider unit. These actions have been expressed in the form of quality elements that describe quality CE in behavioral terms (Suter and others, 1981). The quality elements, as presented in the Appendix at the end of this chapter, are organized in five major categories, each composed of several quality attributes. The categories represent the CE provider unit's major functions, namely, setting directions, organizing the unit, administering the unit, providing educational projects and services, and providing educational assistance. The attributes are equivalent to the major critical requirements for the provision of quality CE. The quality elements interpret in behavioral terms the concepts and principles expressed within the model.

The quality elements grouped in these attributes and categories were developed through an extensive group process involving educators, health professionals, administrators, and many professional groups. From an originally larger number, 141 elements were selected to represent all critical aspects of CE provider unit responsibility. The quality elements, each described in detail in the Appendix at the end of the book, can be summarized in five categories, as follows:

Setting Direction for CE Provider Unit. The first category addresses policy and procedural issues concerning the relationship between the CE provider unit, large or small, and its parent institution or organization, be it a professional school, professional society, hospital, health care organization, or any other organization designating a subunit to assume responsibility for a CE program (in this context, *project* refers to the organized delivery of an activity, product, or service; *program* refers to the overall activities of the CE provider unit). The category includes the relationship to other organizations and to the setting in which the unit operates. In later chapters, the importance of these internal and external relationships for the success of the CE provider unit will become fully apparent.

Organizing CE Provider Unit. The second category refers to the internal organization and functioning of the CE provider unit. Emphasis is on the functional necessities rather than organizational formalities. Some of the functions described are formulating plans and policies, providing resources, setting operational standards, and developing a support structure for providing educational activities, products, and services.

Providing CE Activities and Products. The third category covers the tasks that constitute the educational process, including detecting and analyzing needs, establishing priorities for action, setting objectives, selecting educational approaches, implementing activities, and evaluating impact.

Providing Educational Assistance and Services. The fourth category focuses on important functions of some CE provider units. They include facilitating acceptance of responsibility for CE by the health professional, developing self-directed learning habits, and applying acquired competencies to the patient care situation. This category also addresses the assistance given by a CE provider unit to other organizations.

Administering CE Provider Unit. The fifth category addresses the day-to-day tasks of directing and supporting the work of the CE provider unit.

The list of quality elements presented in this chapter's Appendix represents a revision of the listing published earlier (Suter and others, 1981). This revision is the result of experience in applying the elements, combined with opinions of experts in the field obtained from a validation study. The fact that the quality elements underwent a planned review and revision after their first publication highlights an important concept regarding the intention and use of the quality elements. Although the quality elements have been carefully formulated and are all considered essential for quality CE, potential users may need to adapt them to their specific setting and use. Some CE provider units may have the objectives and resources to consider all quality elements for implementation in their operation, while others will have to establish priorities by identifying and concentrating on those elements that in their judgment will have the greatest impact. However, exclusion of any quality element from consideration should be justified. In many instances, the quality elements may serve as a point of departure for debate and developmental efforts by those involved in CE as learners, CE providers, or regulators. Chapter Sixteen discusses the process of selecting and applying quality elements and describes the specific efforts of several CE provider units.

Summary

In the following chapters of this book, the points and issues raised in the foregoing will reappear in one guise or another. There are seven recurring themes that address functioning of the CE provider unit. As the conceptual model shows, they are interrelated and contribute significantly to the quality of the CE process. Accordingly, the CE provider unit should (1) bring CE in close relationship to the practice setting; (2) support assumption of responsibility for learning by the health professional; (3) provide visionary strategic leadership; (4) support the learning and change processes through provision of activities, products, and services; (5) foster application of new competencies to the patient care process; (6) apply adult learning principles and learning theory to the provision of activities, products, and services; and (7) have adequate management in support of quality CE. These themes cover and go beyond the specific factors recently listed by Sanazaro (1983) as contributory to the improvement of physicians' performance or to enhancing the effectiveness of continuing medical education in changing physicians' behavior.

The success of CE depends significantly on the constructive interaction among the professionals, their working environment, and the CE provider unit. The seven themes or mandates to the CE provider unit clearly emphasize this interdependence.

The organization of the book follows closely the evolution of the Continuing Education Systems Project. The first section describes the conceptual and historic framework; the second section addresses professional characteristics, motivation, and learning in greater detail. Section three deals with the continuing education provider unit's educational functions. Section four addresses issues of management and quality control and provides some examples of actual use of the quality elements.

Appendix: Quality Elements for Continuing Education for the Health Professions

I. Setting Direction for the CE Provider Unit
   A. Defining the Mission
      1. Determine the general educational needs of the potential audiences
      2. Identify the relevant expectations of the parent organization and significant external groups and individuals
      3. Identify the present or potential capabilities of the CE provider unit, and limitations and constraints affecting it
      4. Define the mission of the CE provider unit, considering what is expected of the unit, its capabilities and limitations, and the applicable constraints
      5. Obtain approval of the mission from external and parent organizations and agreement on the mission within the CE provider unit
      6. Document and publicize the mission statement of the CE provider unit
   B. Eliciting Support for the CE Provider Unit from Its Parent Organization
      7. Encourage the parent organization to recognize CE as a specific function in its mission

Note: This appendix represents a revised listing of the quality elements originally published (Suter and others, 1981). The original numbering system has been retained; any gaps in the numbering system are due to dropped elements.

8. Seek placement for the CE provider unit within the organization, which will enable and facilitate the accomplishment of the CE mission
9. Request designation of a specific person as leader of the CE provider unit, based on capabilities for defining and accomplishing the CE mission
10. Seek authority for the CE provider unit leader, commensurate with delegated responsibility
11. Negotiate the provision of incentives and rewards for faculty and other experts to become involved with the CE provider unit

C. Developing Support for CE in the Health Care Setting
12. Promote the identification of professional problems or concerns by applying health care quality standards
13. Influence the health care setting to select appropriate individuals to participate in CE activities
14. Promote the provision of time, money, other needed resources, and incentives and rewards for health care professionals to engage in CE
15. Encourage the provision of appropriate practice data and other data to contribute to the detection of potential problems and the evaluation of CE impact
16. Encourage the designation of individuals responsible for the collaborative analysis of practice problems and concerns and for receipt of referred noneducational problems
17. Seek coordination of educational activities with any needed noneducational actions or responses
18. Influence the health care setting to provide support for the application of learning to practice

D. Relating to Other Parties External to the CE Provider Unit
19. Identify individuals and groups or organizations external to the CE provider unit whose actions and attitudes can affect the achievement of its mission
20. Establish and maintain appropriate relationships

              with the identified individuals and groups or organizations

21.   Determine the goals of the identified individuals and groups or organizations and consider their implications for the CE provider unit

  E. Adapting the CE Provider Unit

22.   Review the CE provider unit's mission, goals, objectives, structure, policies, plans, and procedures periodically and as needed

23.   Use information from monitoring the CE provider unit as a source of indicators of potential need for change in the CE provider unit

24.   Use information from monitoring the health care and societal environments as a source of indicators for potential change in the CE provider unit

25.   Promote and foster research in CE and the development of improved methods for CE

  F. Satisfying Accountability

26.   Identify to whom and in what context the CE provider unit is accountable

27.   Identify the proposed accountability requirements for the CE provider unit

28.   Negotiate proposed accountability requirements that would cause problems for the CE provider unit

29.   Provide accountability documentation

II. Organizing the CE Provider Unit

  A. Planning

30.   Define the education and management functions needed to accomplish the mission of the CE provider unit

31.   Develop a strategic plan, a long-range plan, and policies and procedures to enable the accomplishment of the mission

32.   Develop a set of goals and objectives that reflect the mission and the strategic plan of the CE provider unit

33.   Negotiate a resolution whenever requirements and constraints placed on the CE provider unit

by its parent organization conflict with the provision of quality CE

34. Prepare activity plans for the CE provider unit, specifying the tasks to be carried out, sequence of work, time lines, expected progress points, and desired objectives to be achieved

35. Select markets according to the capabilities of the CE provider unit

36. Develop overall promotional strategies to reach the selected markets

37. Obtain concurrence on plans from parent organizations and agreement on them within the CE provider unit

B. Developing the Organization of the CE Provider Unit

38. Delineate the tasks necessary to carry out and manage the provision of CE activities, products, and services

39. Organize the CE provider unit to accomplish the tasks with optimal use of resources

40. Establish lines of communication that facilitate accomplishing the tasks

41. Develop the organizational arrangements for involving individuals and groups external to the CE provider unit who can facilitate the accomplishment of its mission

C. Developing the Information System

42. Define the records and documentation essential to support the educational and management functions of the CE provider unit

43. Describe the records and documentation needed by individuals and groups external to the CE provider unit

44. Develop a system to collect, store, and retrieve the relevant data

D. Obtaining Resources

45. Specify the money, people, facilities, materials, and time needed to perform the educational and management functions of the CE provider unit

46.   Identify the potential sources for obtaining the needed resources

47.   Seek commitment for timely availability of resources

48.   Revise activity plans to resolve resource discrepancies without jeopardizing the quality of the CE provider unit's program

49.   Develop and use criteria for recruiting and hiring staff and selecting faculty, based on their ability to contribute to the accomplishment of the CE provider unit's mission

E. Setting Standards

50.   Set standards to assess the accomplishment of the CE provider unit's plans and the implementation of its policies

51.   Set standards for the educational processes and products of the CE provider unit, to assure the use of effective methods consistent with the resources of the unit

III. Providing CE Activities and Products

A. Detecting Problems or Concerns

52.   Use data from the practice setting and the professions as a source for identifying potential problems or concerns

53.   Consider new knowledge and technology and changing social attitudes as sources for identifying potential problems or concerns

55.   Use aggregate data descriptive of populations, health problems, and health care practices as sources for identifying potential problems and concerns

56.   Corroborate detected problems or concerns by using data from more than one source

57.   Involve learner(s) in identifying problems or concerns

B. Analyzing Problems or Concerns

58.   Work with learner(s) and others to identify cause(s) of problems or concerns

58.1.   Classify problems or concerns as educational or noneducational needs

59.   Attribute educational needs to a present or potential gap between desirable and actual knowledge, skills, or attitudes

60.   Refer noneducational needs to those in the health care setting responsible for their solution

C. Identifying Educational Priorities

61.   Obtain an assessment of the severity or impact of the health care problems associated with the identified need

62.   Estimate the health care benefits derived from meeting each identified need

63.   Estimate the relative potential for meeting the identified needs through education

64.   Determine the relative cost of meeting each identified need

65.   Determine resources available to meet each identified need

66.   Ascertain the potential environmental factors that would assist or hinder meeting each identified need

67.   Verify the degree of match between individual learning needs and goals of the learner's health care organization

68.   Assure congruence of identified needs with the mission and goals of the CE provider unit

69.   Obtain consensus on the relative priority of each identified need

70.   Select educational needs that will be addressed

71.   Establish a schedule for the timely accomplishment of priority educational projects

D. Setting Educational Objectives

72.   Define potential audience for educational projects

73.   Obtain involvement of learner(s) to define desirable learning outcomes from identified needs

74.   Establish relevant, achievable, and assessable objectives from identified learning outcomes

E. Selecting Educational Approaches

75.   Determine resources available for educational activity

76.   Ascertain learning style preferences of learner(s) for consideration in selecting educational approaches

77.   Consider the nature of the learning objectives in selecting educational approaches

78.   Determine when and where instruction should take place

79.1.   Determine what educational activities, products, and services would be best to meet the identified objectives

79.2.   Determine whether educational activities or products can be selected from available resources or must be developed

F. Selecting Faculty and Content

80.   Select faculty with appropriate content and CE teaching expertise

81.   Assess or assist learners to assess present knowledge, skills, or attitudes related to established learning objectives

82.   Inform faculty of learning objectives, the nature of the learners, and their entry-level knowledge, skills, and attitudes

83.   Assure the currency and accuracy of content and its relevance to the learning objectives

G. Determining Instructional Strategies

84.   Sequence content in a manner to assist learner(s) in meeting learning objectives

85.   Assure that instruction incorporates sufficient examples of concepts to be learned

86.   Provide opportunities for involvement if content is related to changing attitudes

87.   Provide opportunities for practice if content is

related to the development or maintenance of skills

88.   Provide learner(s) with feedback on performance

H. Implementing Educational Projects

89.   Implement educational projects as designed
90.   Assure that instruction occurs in a manner, time, and place convenient to the learner
91.   Make relevant resources available to learner(s) to assist in meeting objectives

I. Designing Evaluation

92.1.   Identify the individual(s) or organization(s) having an interest in or a need for evaluation
92.2.   Determine evaluation needs
92.3.   Determine the focus of the evaluation
93.1.   Estimate resources required for the evaluation and compare with resources actually available
93.2.   Determine the scope of the evaluation

J. Planning and Conducting Evaluation

94.   Choose evaluation methods that will best meet the identified information needs within the available resources
95.   Develop an evaluation plan
96.   Implement the evaluation plan
97.   Analyze the evaluation data

K. Using Evaluation Results

98.   Provide reports according to the evaluation plan
99.   Use evaluation results to make decisions concerning issues on which the evaluation was focused

IV. Providing Educational Assistance and Services

A. Facilitating the Assumption of Responsibility for Learning

100.   Promote and facilitate the individual's acceptance of responsibility for maintaining and extending professional performance
101.   Encourage the acceptance of health care quality standards as a basis for identifying professional problems or concerns
102.   Assist health care professionals to compare their personal and professional behavior to the health care quality standards

103. Assist health care professionals to use learning as a mechanism for maintaining and extending professional performance
104. Support the development, maintenance, and improvement of individual learning skills
105. Assist learner(s) in identifying their resources for CE

B. Assisting the Health Care Professional in the Learning Process

106. Assist learner(s) in identifying and analyzing their problems or concerns
107. Assist learner(s) in determining their educational priorities
108. Assist learner(s) in setting their educational objectives
109. Assist learner(s) in determining their learning style preferences, for consideration in choosing educational approaches
110. Assist learner(s) in choosing which educational activities, products, or services would best meet their objectives
111. Assist learner(s) in choosing educational activities, products, or services
112. Assist learner(s) in evaluating their learning activities, including the impact of learning on practice

C. Assisting in Applying Learning to Practice

113. Assist learner(s) in identifying potential reinforcements in the practice setting for application of learning
114. Assist learner(s) whenever possible in applying learning to practice

D. Providing Assistance and Services to Other CE Provider Units

114.1. Provide educational consultation services to other CE provider units

V. Administering the CE Provider Unit

A. Managing Staff and Faculty

115.   Ensure that the CE provider unit's plans, poli
cies, procedures, and standards are known
throughout the unit

116.   Assign responsibility and delegate commensurate
authority for carrying out the educational and
management activities of the CE provider unit

117.   Negotiate work obligations, clearly define what is
expected, and communicate the relevant standards

119.   Create and maintain a supportive environment in
the work place

120.   Provide incentives for quality performance

121.   Promote staff and faculty growth and development as a means to fulfill individual goals and
those of the CE provider unit

B. Managing Other Resources

122.   Allocate money, time, facilities, and materials to
assure cost-beneficial and timely accomplishment
of assigned activities

123.   Make resource allocations consistent with the CE
priorities

124.   Monitor resource status and expenditures

125.   Provide resource maintenance and upkeep as
needed

C. Marketing

126.   Implement the CE provider unit's overall promotional strategies to develop specific approaches
for each educational project

127.   Develop a realistic fee structure

128.   Provide sufficient information in promotional
materials for potential learners to make sound
decisions about participation in educational projects of the CE provider unit

129.   Emphasize the quality aspects of CE activities,
products, and services in promotional efforts

D. Managing Information

130.   Implement the CE provider unit's information
system

131. Implement mechanisms for timely analysis and reporting of essential information

132. Protect confidentiality of data and information as required

E. Coordinating Functions

133. Coordinate the management with the educational functions within the CE provider unit

134. Coordinate the management and educational functions of the CE provider unit with those of its parent organization

135. Accommodate the educational activities of the CE provider unit to the requirements of potential learners and the plans of other CE provider units

F. Monitoring and Controlling

136. Implement the standards set for the CE provider unit

137. Use the information obtained from applying the standards to provide the feedback necessary to maintain and improve performance and to anticipate and correct deficiencies in the CE provider unit

References

Ad Hoc Committee on Continuing Medical Education. "Continuing Education of Physicians: Conclusions and Recommendations." *Journal of Medical Education,* 1980, *55* (2), 149–157.

Association of American Medical Colleges. "Approaches Toward Enhancing the Quality of Continuing Education of Health Professionals." Joint session of the Group on Medical Education and the Society of Medical College Directors of Continuing Medical Education, Association of American Medical Colleges annual meeting, Nov. 2, 1981.

Bertram, D. A., and Brooks-Bertram, P. A. "The Evaluation of Continuing Medical Education: A Literature Review." *Health Education Monographs,* 1977, *5* (4), 330–362.

Brown, C. R., Jr. "The Continuing Education Component of the Bi-Cycle Approach to Quality Assurance." In R. H. Egdahl and

P. M. Gertman (Eds.), *Quality Health Care: The Role of Continuing Medical Education.* Germantown, Md.: Aspen Systems Corp., 1977.

Caplan, R. M. "A Fresh Look at Some Bad Ideas in Continuing Medical Education." *Mobius,* 1983, *3* (1), 55–61.

Cooper, J. A. D. "Can CME Be Made Part of a Medical Education Continuum?" In R. H. Egdahl and P. M. Gertman (Eds.), *Quality Health Care: The Role of Continuing Medical Education.* Germantown, Md.: Aspen Systems, 1977.

Driver, M. J., and Streufert, S. "Integrative Complexity: An Approach to Individuals and Groups as Information-Processing Systems." *Administrative Science Quarterly,* 1969, *14* (2), 272–285.

Eldridge, W. D. "Traditional Academic Programs for Human Service Professions: Poor Experiential Training in Self-Evaluation and Accountability." *Performance and Instruction,* 1982, *21* (8), 26–28.

Forrester, J. W. *Industrial Dynamics.* Cambridge, Mass.: M.I.T. Press, 1961.

Goldfinger, S. E. "Continuing Medical Education: The Case for Contamination." *New England Journal of Medicine,* 1982, *306* (9), 540–541.

Keller, M. K. "Motivation and Instructional Design: A Theoretical Perspective." *Journal of Instructional Development,* 1979, *2* (4), 26–34.

Lawrence, P. R., and Lorsch, J. W. "Differentiation and Integration in Complex Organizations." *Administrative Science Quarterly,* 1967, *12* (1), 1–47.

Matheson, N. W., and Cooper, J. A. D. "Academic Information in the Academic Health Sciences Center: Roles for the Library in Information Management." *Journal of Medical Education,* 1982, *57* (10, Part 2), 1–93.

Moore, D. E., Jr. "The Organization and Administration of Continuing Education in Academic Medical Centers." Unpublished doctoral dissertation, University of Illinois at Urbana-Champaign, 1982.

Pugh, A. L., III. *DYNAMO II User's Manual.* 5th ed. Cambridge, Mass.: M.I.T. Press, 1976.

Pugh-Roberts Associates. *An Analysis Tool for Examining Options in Continuing Medical Education: Final Report.* Cambridge, Mass.: Pugh-Roberts Associates, 1978.

Sanazaro, P. J. "Determining Physician's Performance: Continuing Medical Education and other Interacting Variables." *Evaluation and the Health Professions,* 1983, *6* (2), 197–210.

Senior, T. "Toward the Measurement of Competence in Medicine." *Quality Review Bulletin,* 1977, *3* (11), 19–21.

Stein, L. S. "The Effectiveness of Continuing Medical Education: Eight Research Reports." *Journal of Medical Education,* 1981, *56* (2), 103–110.

Suter, E., and others. "Continuing Education of Health Professionals: A Proposal for a Definition of Quality." *Journal of Medical Education,* 1981, *56* (8), 687–707.

Williamson, J. W. *Improving Medical Practice and Health Care: A Bibliographic Guide to Information Management in Quality Assurance and Continuing Education.* Cambridge, Mass.: Ballinger, 1977.

2

Learning Theory, Educational Psychology, and Principles of Adult Development

Floyd C. Pennington
David M. E. Allan
Joseph S. Green

This chapter presents the theoretical foundations for the propositions about learning by health professionals that are made throughout the book. The primary focus is on the theories of educational psychology, learning, and adult development. Generalizations drawn from the literature reviewed in this chapter provided the rationale for the quality elements listed under "Providing Continuing Education (CE) Activities and Materials" and "Providing Educational Assistance and Services" in the Appendix at the end of this book. The chapter includes some practical implications for CE provider units, which are expanded in Chapters Seven through Eleven.
—Editors

Theories about how people learn and knowledge of the characteristics of adults as learners have direct implications on the provision of continuing education. When exploring the nature of learning, one soon recognizes that there is no single theory of learning; rather, there are a number of theories based partially on findings from scientific inquiries and partially on practitioner-based experiential writing. These theories are generalized statements encompassing research-based findings that help explain how learning occurs. Their primary value is to generate further research and suggest ways of enhancing learning. "Principles" attempt to describe relationships between or among relevant learning variables. Educational principles are not precise enough to be considered rigidly defined rules of learning. This chapter presents specific suggestions for improving the process and outcomes of CE based on these theories and principles.

Types of Learning Theories

In the literature on learning, there is little agreement among theorists about the major components of their respective theories. This is because each theory explores slightly different aspects of learning. However, the varying viewpoints do not diminish the value of what can be gained from the theories as one attempts to formulate practical implications for learning among health professionals. In any specialized field of knowledge, a jargon develops to explain the relevant phenomena. Psychologists are no exception. In the paragraphs that follow, four types of learning theories are named and described in terms that are practical to health professionals in education.

Behaviorist. Behaviorists define learning in terms of changed, observable behavior that results from a response to a specific stimulus. The only elements of learning studied by the behaviorists are observable stimuli and observable responses. For example, if a given learning objective were to teach health professionals a new method of recording blood pressures, the pure behaviorists would be concerned primarily with providing a set of instructions on the new method of recording (stimulus) and monitoring the actual changes in the recording behaviors (responses).

With the publication of "Animal Intelligence" in 1898, E. L. Thorndike was the first to define a unit of learning as comprised of a stimulus, an organism, and a response. He described learning as the "connecting" or "bonding" of sense impressions (stimuli) and impulses to action (responses) through the nervous system of the organism. This theory of learning dominated all others for over fifty years. Many of the theories that followed were reactions to Thorndike's ideas (Hilgard and Bower, 1975). Thorndike postulated three "laws of learning":

- *effect:* The connections made between a stimulus and a response are strengthened or weakened, based on the satisfaction or annoyance that occurs with the action.
- *exercise or frequency:* For learning to occur, the repetition of the response must be followed by a reinforcing consequence. Forgetting is caused by disuse over time.
- *readiness:* The strength of the connection is increased if followed by a satisfying state of affairs, and is decreased if followed by an annoying state.

In his discussion of controlling learning, Thorndike (1913) lists five aspects that improve learning: interest in work, interest in improving performance, significance of the lesson to some goal of the student, problem-attitude in which the student is made aware of a need that will be satisfied by learning the lesson, and attentiveness to the work. Thorndike first described the implications of his learning theories for adults in 1928 in his book *Adult Learning.*

Operant learning theory, as espoused by Skinner (1938), focuses on the ways of influencing the desired response through what psychologists such as Pavlov (1927) call conditioning. The questions posed by this theoretical perspective relate to the effects of rewards and punishments on the desired learning behavior. Using the example of recording blood pressures, Skinner would have been concerned with whether providing some system of rewards for the health professional who uses the new blood pressure recording method would increase the chances that the desired learning response would occur or would occur more quickly. The operant theorist also would have been concerned with the effects that different systems of rewards or punishments would have on shaping (or conditioning) the desired behavior.

Neobehaviorist. Like the behaviorists, neobehaviorists are concerned with the observable aspects of stimuli and responses. However, in addition to focusing on observable behavior, the neobehaviorists are concerned with the inner states of mind that affect a desired response. The neobehaviorists are not satisfied with describing learning solely as a function of a stimulus and an observed response. They are interested in the effects on learning from such phenomena as drive, habit, strength, magnitude of incentive, and intensity of the stimulus. Health professionals' learning can be enhanced by understanding and affecting the inner states that occur between the introduction of a set of instructions (stimulus) and the changes in behaviors (response). To put these concerns in terms of the previous example, what effect do the health professional's preexisting habits of recording blood pressure have on shaping new behaviors? Does the motivation of the individual health professional at the time a stimulus is presented affect learning? What effect occurs if one were to manipulate either the magnitude of the reward (such as more money for correct recording behavior) or the intensity of the stimulus (a one-to-one tutorial as compared with a handwritten set of instructions)?

Hull (1943) espouses a neobehavioristic theory of learning that focuses on habit as a central concept. One of Hull's major contributions is his attempt to explain the role of purposes, insights, and other phenomena that are difficult for pure behaviorists to explain. Hull is concerned with the processes that occur between the stimulation and the response. He defines reinforcement as the process of reducing a drive or satisfying a need. Hull indicates that the strength of a habit is increased when the reinforcement (need reduction) occurs within close temporal proximity to the response. He also postulates that the habit is further strengthened by frequently providing reinforcement. Hull believes that without drive there could be no response or reinforcement.

In later attempts to develop more practical implications from Hull's work, N. E. Miller and Dollard (1941) discuss a four-stage analysis of learning. The four stages include (1) drive—students must want something, (2) cue—students must notice something,

(3) response—students must do something, and (4) reward—students must get something they want.

Cognitivist. Cognitive psychologists recognize that behaviors are only evidence of underlying mental processes and the laws that govern them. Tolman (1951) includes in the study of behaviors the purpose and outcome of the actions. He introduces the concept of the achievement of actions as the fundamental unit of psychological study rather than an individual sequence of behaviors.

Gestalt psychology, introduced in America in the 1930s, provides the basis for the cognitive theories of learning. The most accepted and persistent aspects of Gestalt theory are the roles of background and organization in learning, recall, and problem solving. The solution to a problem comes about when the learner understands the relationships of the different elements in the problem and the environment rather than responding to individual, isolated stimuli. The learning solution is then more lasting, and inferences can be transferred to other problem situations. The way in which learners see a problem—their perceptual organization—determines the mode of action for solving the problem. Further, the information is stored in the same form as the original perception so that remembering is a reactivation of those processes that made up the original perception. Over time, and presumably with repeated use and review, these memory traces become a strong, coherent, and well-organized structure that is not forgotten. For example, if the new method of recording blood pressure is considered by the learner in the broad sense of its significance for patient care and its value for communication among health professionals, then the learning will be easier and more enduring than if it is learned mechanically through repetitious drilling.

As Gestalt theory was evolving, Piaget (1952) was attempting to define the stages of development of a child's intelligence. Piaget studied the effect on learning of experience within physical and social environments. Piaget looked at the acquisition of knowledge in a broader sense than perception. He believed that knowledge was not a copy of reality and that to know an object, the learner had to act on it and understand the way the object was constructed. The inference that has been made from Piaget's work is that the environment affects learning and that to change behaviors, education should encourage learner initiative and active interaction with the knowledge to be acquired. In our example, a health professional who wishes to learn a new method of recording blood pressure readings must understand the overall significances of the new method and be involved in applying the new method in a simulated or supervised environment of patient care.

Jerome Bruner was stimulated by the ideas of Piaget. Bruner's (1960) work is based on the educational problems of children, but many of his basic concepts are relevant for adult learning. Bruner believes that discovery is necessary for the real possession of knowledge, for it allows the knowledge to be organized effectively and promotes long-term retention. The process of mastering the knowledge is rewarding in itself, especially when feedback is provided.

In 1960, Miller, Galanter, and Pribram described several theories of cognitive psychology, which postulated that all behaviors are developed in a succession of hierarchical plans that depend upon one's present needs and values. Problem-solving behaviors are similarly structured and organized.

Another cognitive theorist, Ausubel (1968) is concerned with classroom learning and believes that meaningful learning can be achieved by appropriate presentations of material or by discovery learning. The latter, however, is too time-consuming to be a primary teaching method in most classroom settings. Ausubel has drawn attention to the concept that learners may be closed-minded, rejecting new materials or methods before they are presented. Techniques for dealing with this impediment to learning have not yet been well developed.

Among the primary principles, relevant to both the organization and the learner, that can be drawn from cognitive theories is that opportunities for learner initiative and active interaction with the material should be provided. In addition, careful attention must be paid to the method of presentation of new material, and where appropriate, discovery learning should be incorporated.

Humanistic. The humanistic approach to learning is primarily learner-centered, emphasizing the value of individual differences, styles, and approaches to life. Maslow (1954) and Rogers (1969) suggest that all individuals are involved in their own world. Under the label of humanistic psychology—the study of personal growth, development, and motivation—several concepts of learning have emerged.

Human beings are innately curious and have a natural potential for learning. Continual learning, necessary to meet the inner needs of living and working, leads to the adventure of change. Personal growth, rewarded by both the individual and society, must continue. Change is initiated by an attitude of accepting responsibility for oneself to function as an internal change agent (Havelock and others, 1969). The change has to be seen by the individual as desirable, possible, under the individual's control, and consistent with reality and the demands of society. With this more self-centered desire for change, individuals must develop high self-esteem and self-confidence to allow themselves to be exposed to the risk and threat of failure and, at the same time, to use both the failures and the positive learning experiences as the basis for future learning. While in professional school, students learn in order to meet an idealized concept engendered by a role model or by a multitude of internal and external factors. Once out of school, the desire to change swings more to satisfying internal, idealized, and positive self-concepts. Meeting the standards of others plays a less important role.

Rogers (1969) believes that learning takes place when it is integrated with work or is acquired by placing the student in direct confrontation with practical problems. Learning is facilitated when the learners define their own problems, discover their own learning resources, decide their own course of action, and live with the consequences of their decisions. The most lasting and pervasive learning involves feelings as well as the intellect, so learners recognize the learning as their own. The learner can hold onto it or let it go in favor of new knowledge, without needing the permission of some professional or authoritative figure. Self-directed learners are those for whom change is a central fact of life and who are comfortable incorporating new knowledge in their practice setting (see Chapter Eleven).

Prescriptive Theory of Instruction

In attempting to apply the concepts, principles, and laboratory-based theories of learning to the practical task of designing instruction, Gagné (1964) found that all learning was not alike. He defined eight types of learning that are hierarchical in complexity. The lowest level is *signal learning*, when a general response is given to a specific stimulus, such as a dog salivating when food is presented. In *stimulus-response* learning, a precise response is given to a discriminated stimulus. For example, after a bell is paired with food, the dog salivates at the sound of the bell. *Chaining* results when two or more stimulus-responses are connected, as in tying a shoe. The connection of verbal chains, such as reciting the alphabet or counting, is called *verbal association*. In *discrimination learning*, an infinite number of responses are made to many different stimuli that may resemble each other in physical appearance, as colors or shapes. The ability to make a common response to a class of stimuli that may differ widely in physical appearance is *concept learning*, as in classifying a chair or table into the category of furniture. In *rule learning*, two or more concepts are connected. In the highest level of learning, *problem-solving*, two or more rules are combined to result in a new capacity; for example, the learner discovers a relationship among several concepts.

According to Gagné, each level in the hierarchy is dependent on successful learning at the previous levels. He emphasizes that certain conditions, both internal and external, govern the learning situation. Internal conditions are the capabilities already possessed by the learner or developed within the learner during the instructional event; they include the mastery of the lower levels of learning required for the specific event. External conditions are those that can be manipulated during the educational experience, such as practice, feedback, and reinforcement.

Gagné asserts that there are six "time-tested" principles of learning, based on the various learning theories. Three of these six represent external conditions—contiguity, repetition, and reinforcement. Gagné states that the situation to which the learner is expected to respond must be presented contiguously in time with the desired response, the situation and its desired response must be practiced or repeated to assure learning and increase retention, and learning a new act is strengthened when the occurrence of that act is followed by a reward. The internal conditions reflect the presentation of information and the learner's intellectual skills and learning strategies. According to Gagné, factual information must be brought to bear upon an act of learning through printed directions, previously learned materials, or from memory. Intellectual skills for learning must be recalled in order for learning to occur. Directions or verbal cues can be used to assure that the learners use the skills in the new learning situation. In addition, a learning event requires the activation of strategies for learning and remembering. Self-management of the learning situation requires the learners to govern their own behavior in attending, storing, and retrieving information and in organizing solutions to problems.

Another major contribution of Gagné is his concept of the organization of knowledge, based on a hierarchy of subcomponent skills and rules. Gagné and Briggs (1974) addressed the task of designing instructional sequences by means of a typical hierarchy of course, topic, lesson, and component. The major focus of this work is the implications for sequencing of instruction. Suggestions to course designers, such as teaching the basic concepts before progressing to more complex concepts or teaching the central component of an idea before dealing with peripheral issues, came from the work of such instructional psychologists as Gagné and Briggs (1974), Mager (1968), and Merrill (1971). Their contributions came directly from the work of the learning theorists mentioned earlier. (For more detailed descriptions of these practical implications, see Chapter Nine.)

Adults as Learners

In addition to a familiarity with theories of learning, an understanding of adults and the way they learn has significant application to developing effective CE programs. From studies of adult development and learning and from research in the biological, social, and behavioral sciences, there is now a better understanding of how adults learn. From this research and from experience, a different concept has emerged—learning centered around the needs and experiences of the learner. Though these principles may be appropriate for all learners, the concepts have been associated most often with adult learners. Knowles (1980) explains that learning for adults is based on four crucial assumptions about the characteristics of learners: an individual's self-concept moves from dependence to self-directedness, a growing reservoir of experience represents increasing resources and bases for learning, motivation to learn is increasingly oriented to the developmental tasks of social roles, and learning moves toward a focus on immediate application and accordingly shifts from subject to problem orientation.

Learning in adults is continuous, activated by the individual in response to internal or external stimuli. It is connected to the person's physical and psychological maturity and is affected by the learner's current situational role (Faure and others, 1972; Kidd, 1973; Cropley, 1977; Dave, 1976; Feringer, 1978). Learning allows the individual to reduce the unknown aspects of life to a minimum and to develop ways to predict responses, interactions, and one's own situational predicament (Hebb, 1972; Thibodeau, 1979).

Healthy adults continue to learn throughout their life span (Knox, 1977; Tough, 1971, 1978). They are not simply mature children. The internal and external variables that can influence the learning process differ for adults and children since these are derived from social, psychological, developmental, and situational experiences (Knowles, 1970; McClusky, 1970; Houle, 1972; Hart, 1975).

Substantive research on the linkages between learner characteristics and learning outcomes is scant. This is also true of our understanding of how these interactions change over time and the effect of these changes on learning behaviors. However, CE providers can benefit from an understanding of not only the theoretical foundations of learning but also the characteristics of adult learners.

Physiological Characteristics. Adults mature physically in their twenties. Healthy adults experience few major natural physical changes until their late forties when the sensory receptors for vision and hearing and the speed of response of the nervous system decline. Reduction in the response rate in the nervous system results in a drop in the rate at which impulses are transmitted. Thus, as adults age, they generally require more time to learn and respond negatively to time pressures and anxiety-producing learning activities. Impaired sensory input results in the learner taking in reduced or inaccurate information. Negative educational experiences resulting from these physical changes may bring added stress to the learner's efforts to achieve a desired learning outcome (Botwinick, 1967; Riley and others, 1968; Warren and Warren, 1966; McClusky, 1970; Kidd, 1973).

Psychological Factors. Adults maintain descriptions and feelings about themselves that influence their learning behaviors. The descriptions are referred to as self-concept and the feelings as self-esteem. Adults learn best when the learning is congruent with their self-concept (Rubin, 1969; Tough, 1971; Smith, 1976). Furthermore, adults with high self-esteem and a positive self-concept are more likely to be responsive to change (Klopf, Bowman, and Joy, 1969) and to apply new learning in their professional practice.

An essential component of self-concept relevant to learning is the person's previous learning experiences and the values, skills, and strategies gained from those activities. "An adult learns best when he values the role of learner for himself; when he experiences himself as a competent learner; when he possesses the skills and strategies necessary for managing his own learning and for processing information through multiple channels; when he values the status of learner as a worthy one for adults in society; when he can utilize the resources provided by others for himself; and when he values himself as a resource for others" (Brundage and Mackeracher, 1980, p. 101).

Learners react to all experiences as they perceive them, not as someone such as a teacher presents them. Consumption does not equal presentation (Thompson, 1970; Kidd, 1973). The adult learner reacts to a learning experience out of an organized self-concept and perceives the experience as part of an integrated whole. Activities that support and encourage the organization and integration of what is being learned into a person's current situation will strengthen the desired learning outcome (Brim and Wheeler, 1966; Kidd, 1973).

One response to a threat is stress, involving a hormonal reaction that enhances sensory reception and mental functioning and can increase the ability to cope or change (Selye, 1956; Lazarus, 1966; Toffler, 1970). Emotions, stress, and anxiety can all have an effect on learning. For example, most adults enter learning activities in a state of arousal and do not generally require further motivation. Further arousal may cause the learner to withdraw and appear to lack interest (Larson, 1970; Knowles, 1970). Prolonged or excessive stress reduces one's capability to listen and communicate effectively.

Arousal can motivate the adult to learn, as well as to be defensive. Stress and anxiety contribute to both learning and resistance to learning (Knowles, 1970; McClusky, 1970; Kidd, 1973; Combs, 1974). In the presence of excessive information, adults may delete, distort, oversimplify, or overgeneralize (Katz and Kahn, 1970; Toffler, 1970; Bandler and Grinder, 1975; and Cropley, 1977).

Role of Experience. Adults who value their own experiences as rich resources for further learning or those whose experiences are valued by others are better learners (Landvogt, 1970; Combs, 1974; Pine and Boy, 1977; Thibodeau, 1979). "Past experience is stored in memory, organized according to individualized strategies, and is assigned individualized meanings and values. These meanings, values, and strategies will determine how the individual will interpret new experiences and how he will learn. The adult learner needs to be aware of his own meanings, values, and strategies, and of the way he uses these to plan, make decisions, solve problems, assess information, respond to immediate experience, and relate to others" (Brundage and Mackeracher, 1980, p. 98). When past experience can be applied to a current learning task, learning is facilitated; when it is only modestly related to a current learning task, the learner may have problems integrating the new information into experience.

Life is filled with diversity, contradictions, dilemmas, and paradoxes. Past experience may present a paradox in the learning situation. On the one hand, the stability of past experience and the learner's self-concept lead to confidence and a willingness to enter into the process of change. On the other hand, the process of change has the potential for changing the meanings, values, skills, and strategies of past experience and self-concept, thereby temporarily destabilizing both. This lack of stability may lead to loss of confidence and possibly to withdrawal from the process of change, particularly in those with low self-esteem and poor self-concepts.

Past educational experiences influence the professional's responsiveness to new experiences. Success in achieving one's learning objectives is a strong stimulus for subsequent learning efforts. Failure to achieve one's learning objectives becomes a reinforcer for avoiding learning activities.

Learning Styles. Learners have organized ways of focusing on, taking in, and processing information. These are referred to as cognitive style and are believed to remain relatively constant and consistent throughout adulthood (McKenney and Keen, 1974; Kolb and Fry, 1975; McLaren, 1975; Cawley, Miller, and Milligan, 1976). A learning strategy is a preferred way an individual organizes educative experiences. Learning strategies are subject to change throughout adulthood. Neither cognitive style nor learning strategy is related to mental ability. An individual's cognitive style and learning strategy result in a preference for a particular learning style from which that individual is able to learn most efficiently. Learning is carried out not only through formal, logical, or sequential processes but also through interpersonal interactions, modeling, and experimenting.

All health professionals will have their own style for processing information and for learning. As a group, however, health professionals may be more homogeneous in terms of learning style than others in the adult population because of their extensive indoctrination into one major problem-solving strategy, the medical model—history taking, physical, diagnosis, treatment, and follow up. Whether this is true or not, individual health professionals will bring to any learning activity a complex set of experiences and differing levels of proficiency in their health care delivery behaviors (McKenney and Keen, 1974; Cawley, Miller, and Milligan, 1976; Messick and others, 1976; Means, 1979). It is therefore important to take these differences into consideration when planning CE for health professionals.

Health professionals of all types learn by using a wide array of resources. Each learning situation may require some adaptation in strategy to fit the situation or the problem. Health professionals are highly skilled at problem solving by assessing the problem, examining the options, obtaining additional information, and making a decision. However, most professionals use the process unconsciously to make educational decisions and do not know how to systematically develop an educational plan (Means, 1979; see Chapter Four).

Summary

Health professionals progress through career stages that shape their practice and health care delivery behaviors. As one's career develops and the practice setting changes, however, one's learning behaviors may or may not change. Understanding the health professional as a learner requires an understanding of the dynamic interactions within the individual as a person, professional, and learner—none of which may be static.

The learning theories and characteristics of adults discussed in this chapter have significant implications for the development of continuing education for health professionals. To be meaningful, continuing education must focus on the needs of the learners. Participants in CE are individuals who over time have applied what they learned in school, have adapted it to the circumstances that present themselves in day-to-day practice, and have developed specific needs and perspectives for learning as a result of their experiences and their social and psychological development. There are certain realities about health professionals that are relevant for those involved in providing CE activities and services. These characteristics serve as a useful way to summarize the important themes presented in this chapter.

- *Most health professionals are motivated to continue their learning.* Each patient encounter can lead to learning and increase the pool of knowledge and skills called experience. The majority of the practitioners' learning is geared toward enhancing their role as helping professionals. One's motivation to learn can come from comparing current knowledge to what is required to solve a problem. Based on this process, a decision can be made about the extent to which more learning or change is required. Educational experiences that provide opportunities for self-assessment or peer review can help the health professional focus on continuing learning.
- *Health professionals seek knowledge that has immediate and pragmatic application in their current situation.* They want to devote their learning time to problems, opportunities, concerns, tasks, and needs that confront them now. Program planners must recognize and respond to this immediacy by designing continuing education relevant to the learners' needs.
- *Participation in continuing education is strongly influenced by an individual's past experiences.* Programs should be designed

for the learner as an experienced adult and should provide information that is applicable to current practice. If there are significant obstacles to obtaining or applying learning, the learner will be hesitant to participate again. CE planners should include reinforcers in the instructional process and seek to eliminate obstacles that may become barriers to learning.

- *Efforts to improve the conditions of learning can influence the outcomes of continuing education.* The design and implementation of programs involve the manipulation of the external conditions of learning. The activities of the program, the way in which the content is presented, and the number of opportunities provided for using the new information and receiving feedback all influence the participants' learning. The effectiveness of educational activities can be enhanced by incorporating the concepts of adult learning presented in this chapter.

  The internal conditions of learning that the health professional brings to learning experiences, including learning style, past experiences, and motivation, should also be considered by the CE planner. Efforts to influence the internal conditions of learning can be built into the design of programs. Experienced practitioners assimilate new material by modifying it to fit what they already know. Learning experiences should assist the learners in remembering past experiences and should build on their past experience and knowledge.

- *The realities of the practice world require that the health professionals know how to continue learning, to stay abreast of new developments, and to adapt to new environments.* Though there is little existing research to confirm that there is a significant relationship between learning style and learning, it seems logical that learning would be more efficient if it were presented in the form that the individual prefers. Many health professionals have not consciously examined their own learning styles to identify how they learn best. Formal preparatory education of most health professionals does not encourage the student to assume the responsibility for developing a variety of learning strategies. To enhance the learning process, CE planners can assist health professionals in identifying how they learn most efficiently.

- *Continuing education should support health professionals' natural desire to learn.* Health professionals learn in settings where they work alone, work with other professionals, or interact with larger groups. Continuing education providers tend to assume that health professionals require group settings in order for learning to occur. Any situation where the health professional's knowledge does not equal the information required to solve a problem can provide the context for learning.
- *Health professionals should be encouraged to accept the personal responsibility for learning.* CE planners can assist the health professionals by increasing the professionals' awareness of the skills of self-directed learning and by providing the resources for self-evaluation and professional self-improvement (see Chapter Eleven).

References

Ausubel, D. P. *Educational Psychology: A Cognitive View.* New York: Holt, Rinehart and Winston, 1968.

Bandler, R., and Grinder, J. *The Structure of Magic.* Vol. I and II. Palo Alto, Calif.: Science and Behavior Books, 1975.

Botwinick, J. *Cognitive Processes in Maturity and Old Age.* New York: Springer, 1967.

Brim, O. G., Jr., and Wheeler, S. *Socialization After Childhood: Two Essays.* New York: Wiley, 1966.

Brundage, D. H., and Mackeracher, D. *Adult Learning Principles and Their Application to Program Planning.* Toronto, Canada: Ontario Ministry of Education, 1980.

Bruner, J. S. *The Process of Education.* Cambridge, Mass.: Harvard University Press, 1960.

Cawley, R. W. V., Miller, S. A. and Milligan, J. N. "Cognitive Styles and the Adult Learner." *Adult Education,* 1976, *26* (2), 101–116.

Combs, A. W. "Humanistic Approach to Learning in Adults." In R. W. Bortner (Ed.), *Adults as Learners: Proceedings of a Conference Cosponsored by the Gerontology Center of the Institute for the Study of Human Development, Pennsylvania Department of Education and the Region III Adult Education Staff Develop-*

ment Project. University Park: Pennsylvania State University, 1974.

Cropley, A. J. *Lifelong Education: A Psychological Analysis.* Oxford, England: Pergamon Press, 1977.

Dave, R. H. (Ed.). *Foundations of Lifelong Education.* Oxford, England: Pergamon Press, 1976.

Faure, E., and others. *Learning to Be: The World of Education Today and Tomorrow.* Paris: United Nations Educational, Scientific, and Cultural Organization, 1972.

Feringer, R. "The Relation Between Learning Problems of Adults and General Learning Theory." Address to the Adult Education Research Conference, San Antonio, Tex., 1978. (ERIC: ED 152 992)

Gagné, R. M. "Problem Solving." In A. W. Melton (Ed.), *Categories of Human Learning.* New York: Academic Press, 1964.

Gagné, R. M. *The Conditions of Learning.* 2nd ed. New York: Holt, Rinehart and Winston, 1970.

Gagné, R. M., and Briggs, L. J. *Principles of Instructional Design.* New York: Holt, Rinehart and Winston, 1974.

Goldfinger, S. E. "Continuing Medical Education: The Case for Contamination." *New England Journal of Medicine,* 1982, *306* (9), 540–541.

Hart, L. A. *How the Brain Works: A New Understanding of Human Learning, Emotion, and Thinking.* New York: Basic Books, 1975.

Havelock, R. G., and others. *Planning for Innovation.* Ann Arbor: Center for Research on Utilization of Scientific Knowledge, Institute for Social Research, University of Michigan, 1969.

Hebb, D. O. *Textbook of Psychology.* 3rd ed. Philadelphia: Saunders, 1972.

Hilgard, E. R., and Bower, G. H. *Theories of Learning.* Englewood Cliffs, N.J.: Prentice-Hall, 1975.

Houle, C. O. *The Design of Education.* San Francisco: Jossey-Bass, 1972.

Hull, C. L. *Principles of Behavior.* New York: Appleton-Century-Crofts, 1943.

Katz, D., and Kahn, R. L. "Communication: The Flow of Information." In J. H. Campbell and H. W. Hepler (Eds.), *Dimensions in*

Communication: Readings. 2nd ed. Belmont, Calif.: Wadsworth, 1970.

Kidd, J. R. *How Adults Learn.* Rev. ed. New York: Association Press, 1973.

Klopf, G. J., Bowman, G. W., and Joy, A. *A Learning Team: Teacher and Auxiliary.* Washington, D.C.: U.S. Government Printing Office, 1969.

Knowles, M. S. *The Modern Practice of Adult Education: Androgogy Versus Pedagogy.* New York: Association Press, 1970.

Knowles, M. S. *The Modern Practice of Adult Education: From Pedagogy to Androgogy.* Rev. ed. Chicago: Follett, 1980.

Knox, A. B. *Adult Development and Learning: A Handbook on Individual Growth and Competence in the Adult Years.* San Francisco: Jossey-Bass, 1977.

Kolb, D. A., and Fry, R. "Towards an Applied Theory of Experiential Learning." In C. L. Cooper (Ed.), *Theories of Group Processes.* London: Wiley, 1975.

Landvogt, P. L. "A Framework for Exploring the Adult Educator's Commitment Toward the Construct of 'Guided Learning'." Paper presented to the Adult Education Research Conference, Minneapolis, Minn., 1970. (ERIC: ED 036 765)

Larson, C. G. "The Adult Learner: A Review of Recent Research." *American Vocational Journal,* 1970, *45* (6), 67–68.

Lazarus, R. S. *Psychological Stress and the Coping Process.* New York: McGraw-Hill, 1966.

McClusky, H. Y. "An Approach of a Differential Psychology of the Adult Potential." In S. M. Grabowski (Ed.), *Adult Learning and Instruction.* Syracuse, N.Y.: ERIC Clearinghouse on Adult Education and Adult Education Association of the U.S.A., 1970.

McKenney, J. L., and Keen, P. G. W. "How Managers' Minds Work." *Harvard Business Review,* 1974, *52* (3), 79–90.

McLaren, J. A. "Preference for Structure in Adult Learning Situations as a Function of Conceptual Level." Unpublished master's thesis, University of Toronto, 1975.

Mager, R. F. *Developing Attitude Toward Learning.* Palo Alto, Calif.: Fearon, 1968.

Maslow, A. H. *Motivation and Personality.* New York: Harper & Row, 1954.

Means, R. P. *Information-Seeking Behaviors of Michigan Family Physicians.* Unpublished doctoral dissertation, University of Illinois at Urbana-Champaign, 1979.

Merrill, M. D. (Ed.). *Instructional Design: Readings.* Englewood Cliffs, N.J.: Prentice-Hall, 1971.

Messick, S., and others. *Individuality in Learning: Implications of Cognitive Styles and Creativity for Human Development.* San Francisco: Jossey-Bass, 1976.

Miller, G. A., Galanter, E., and Pribram, K. H. *Plans and the Structure of Behavior.* New York: Holt, Rinehart and Winston, 1960.

Miller, N. E., and Dollard, J. *Social Learning and Imitation.* New Haven, Mass.: Yale University Press, 1941.

Pavlov, I. P. *Conditioned Reflexes.* Translated by G. V. Anrep. Oxford, England: Oxford University Press, 1927.

Piaget, J. *The Origins of Intelligence in Children.* New York: International Universities Press, 1952.

Pine, G. J., and Boy, A. V. *Learner-Centered Teaching: A Humanistic View.* Denver, Colo.: Love, 1977.

Riley, M. W., and others. *Aging and Society.* Vol. I, *An Inventory of Research Findings.* New York: Russell Sage Foundation, 1968.

Rogers, C. R. *Freedom to Learn.* Columbus, Ohio: Merrill, 1969.

Rubin, J. L. *A Study on the Continuing Education of Teachers.* Santa Barbara, Calif.: Center for Coordinated Education, University of California, 1969.

Selye, H. *The Stress of Life.* New York: McGraw-Hill, 1956.

Skinner, B. F. *The Behavior of Organisms: An Experimental Analysis.* New York: Appleton-Century-Crofts, 1938.

Smith, R. M. *Learning How to Learn in Adult Education,* Information Series no. 10. De Kalb, Ill.: ERIC Clearinghouse in Career Education, 1976. (ERIC: ED 132 245)

Thibodeau, J. "Adult Performance on Piagetian Tasks: Implications for Education." Paper presented at Adult Education Research Conference, Ann Arbor, Mich., 1979.

Thompson, J. F. "Formal Properties of Instructional Theory for Adults." In S. M. Grabowski (Ed.), *Adult Learning and Instruction.* Syracuse, N.Y.: ERIC Clearinghouse on Adult Education and Adult Education Association of the U.S.A., 1970.

Thorndike, E. L. "Animal Intelligence: An Experimental Study of the Associative Processes in Animals." Monograph Supplement. *Psychological Review*, 1898, *2* (4) (entire issue).

Thorndike, E. L. *Educational Psychology* Vol. 2, *The Psychology of Learning*. New York: Teachers College, 1913.

Thorndike, E. L., and others. *Adult Learning*. New York: Macmillan, 1928.

Toffler, A. *Future Shock*. New York: Random House, 1970.

Tolman, E. C. *Collected Papers in Psychology*. Berkeley: University of California Press, 1951.

Tough, A. *The Adult's Learning Projects*. Toronto, Canada: Ontario Institute for Studies in Education, 1971.

Tough, A. "Major Learning Efforts: Recent Research and Future Directions" *Adult Education*, 1978, *28* (4), 250–263.

Warren, R. M., and Warren, R. P. "A Comparison of Speech Perception in Childhood, Maturity, and Old Age by Means of the Verbal Transformation Effect." *Journal of Verbal Learning and Verbal Behavior*, 1966, *5*, 142–146.

Relationship of Motivation
to Learning

Donald L. Cordes

This chapter reviews and analyzes the often used term motivation,
*with particular emphasis on its relationship to participation in edu-
cation generally and continuing education specifically. The major
theories of motivation are summarized, and several models for applying these theories to continuing education are described. Read
together, Chapters Two and Three suggest practical implications
for CE providers to increase health professionals' participation in
and learning from continuing education.—Editors*

When considering such complex issues surrounding human
behavior as motivation, it is necessary to discuss the relevant contextual factors. To analyze motivation for learning, one must review
the various theories of motivation and learning, with particular
emphasis on similarities and differences among them. This chapter
will build on those learning theories and concepts discussed in
detail in Chapter Two, focusing on the relationships of motivation
to learning. The theories in this chapter have been classified to

highlight the focus on motivation and to facilitate the use of this body of knowledge.

While, in general, technical terms from the literature of psychology are infrequently used by the lay public, the term *motivation*, a very complex concept, is commonly used by scientists and laymen, because the term is as much a part of folklore as it is of scientific research (Bolles, 1967). What are the implications of this confusion, and why is it worth mentioning here? Disagreement and vagueness about the term *motivation* has lead many to pay little attention to the research done in this area. More importantly, most people have a preconceived notion of what motivation is and how it affects learning. Unless an individual is a student of human behavior or learning, much of that preconceived notion is probably based on folklore.

This chapter will focus on the application of motivation theory to the field of continuing education (CE) in the health professions. Practical suggestions regarding the conduct of continuing education will be made from this analysis of motivation and its relationship to learning. Therefore, this chapter should not be seen as the seminal work on motivation but rather as a discussion of the motivational factors involved in health professional behavior regarding CE, with some theoretical background as a basis for suggested applications in the real world of CE for health professionals. It may be necessary to abandon some long-held beliefs regarding learning and motivation in order to apply various research-based insights to the management and development of continuing education. This chapter takes a broad view of the practice of CE by considering both traditional participation in formal CE programs as well as involvement in self-directed, self-managed CE endeavors.

Theoretical Underpinnings

As mentioned, there are multiple meanings for the term *motivation* among the lay public as well as students of human behavior. Motivation, as a concept, has been described as relating to human experiences, human behavior, unconscious processes, free will, inner forces, external stimuli, and goal objects. The common ground is that motivation is a concept that aids in the study of behavior, focusing on the issue of why behavior of a given type and intensity occurs.

The "why" questions of human behavior have their roots in antiquity. Philosophers such as Plato and Aristotle were among the first to record their thoughts and questions about human behavior. Human beings were said to possess rational powers. Therefore, human behavior was thought to be understood when any act could be traced back to its rationale. However, it was possible for nonrational behavior to exist. Feelings, emotions, and passion were all seen as lower-order (nonrational) human behavior.

The notion that human beings have special powers of rationality began to change with the publication of *Origin of Species* by Darwin ([1859], 1951). Darwin suggested that the differences between animal and man were differences of degree that could be explained as the result of a continuous evolutionary process.

Darwin's conception of man opened the door for theories that postulated that behavior simply followed instincts inherent in all animals, including man. McDougall ([1914], 1960) proposed perhaps the most widely accepted theory of instinct. He saw instinct as an innate, inherited psychophysical disposition causing the organism to pay selective attention to, and experience emotional feelings toward, certain objects—the result being an impulse for action. This complex orientation led to much theoretical activity, postulating the existence of increasing numbers of instincts until the concept of instinct got a questionable scientific reputation. As the debate over instinct grew increasingly heated, the seeds had already been planted for a new era in the study of human behavior.

Psychologist Robert S. Woodworth (1918) used the term *motivology* as a name for a new psychological discipline dealing with drives and related psychological variables. Woodworth, often regarded as the founder of motivational psychology, postulated that drives were dynamic functions. This set the stage for a prodigious amount of theorizing and research in the decades that followed. During this era, psychologists Edward Tolman (1932) and, later, Clark Hull (1943) expanded the drive theory, postulating that human behavior was a function of drive, habit, strength, magnitude of incentives, and intensity of stimulus. Their works, perhaps more than those of any others, provided a foundation for a generation of psychological theorists.

More recent research in the area of human behavior can be classified according to the assumptions the researchers make about human beings. Whether man has a free will is a question that cannot be answered empirically. Therefore, researchers who assume that man has a free will conduct studies designed to answer significantly different questions than researchers who assume that man does not have a free will.

Within the views of motivation just described, two major approaches to the study of human behavior can be recognized, the mechanistic approach and organismic approach. These approaches emanate from their respective views of man. Theories following the mechanistic approach depict man as machinelike, with a tendency to be manipulated by the sum total of forces, none of which is in his control. Organismic theories depict man as being able to manipulate various aspects of his environment for his own perceived good.

Mechanistic Approaches. Examples of mechanistic theories are behaviorism and psychoanalytic theory. Behaviorism, as discussed in Chapter Two, describes behavior as the result of a response to a stimulus, with the type and intensity of behavior being determined by the stimulus-response interaction. Psychoanalytic theory, as described by Freud and his followers, depicts humans as being driven by the interaction of subconscious forces and the environment. Since psychoanalytic theory does not focus on learning behavior, it will not be addressed in this chapter.

Skinner (1953), perhaps the most well-known behaviorist, does not see motivation of behavior per se as an issue worthy of study. Motivational questions, therefore, are really questions that can be answered in terms of reinforcements. These reinforcements are commonly referred to as extrinsic motivators.

A group of behavioral theorists, identified in Chapter Two as neobehaviorists, is not as strict in its interpretation of the stimulus-response interplay. Hull (1943), unlike Skinner, was concerned with motivation. He tended to see reinforcement as a reducer of drive stimulus. Drives and the reduction of drives form the central thrust of Hull's work, which represented the first comprehensive conceptualization of motivation. Miller and Dollard (1941), Brown (1961), and Miller (1959) were other drive-reduction theorists who addressed the internal stimulus-response processes that affect behavioral responses.

Organismic Approaches. Organismic approaches include three major theoretical areas: cognitive theories, affective arousal theories, and humanistic theories. Organismic theories describe human beings as interacting with their environments. This interaction changes both the environment and the organism itself as it adapts to the environment.

Cognitive theories start with the assumption that human beings are free to make decisions about meeting their needs. Cognitive theory asserts that people make choices regarding their behavior, based on whether or not the perceived end result would be good for them. Once a desired endpoint has been identified, the individual sets a goal and selects a behavior to achieve the desired endpoint.

Early theoretical work by Tolman (1932) and Lewin (1936) pointed to cognitive thoughts as factors that cause behavior. Both men saw energy sources, whether from environmental tensions in Lewin's view or internal needs in Tolman's view, as leading to the formation of goals. Once the goal has been established, an individual will take action to achieve the goal and thereby reduce the tension, meeting the inner need. More recent theoretical work in the cognitive area expands on this basic model. Weiner (1972) has proposed a cognitive model that involves antecedent stimuli leading to mediating cognitive events and resulting in behavior.

Another cognitive theory that has gained numerous followers in recent years is known as the expectancy-valence theory of motivation. It has its roots in the previously mentioned work of Tolman and Lewin, but it has been more completely developed by Vroom (1964) and Atkinson and Feather (1966). Expectancy-valence theories assume that human beings consciously anticipate (expect) rewards or outcomes that are desirable (valued), and this anticipation of something valued results in behavior designed to attain the valued outcome.

A comprehensive cognitive model of the expectancy-valence theory developed by Deci (1975) is represented in Figure 1. Stimulus inputs can come from internal states, external stimuli, or memory.

Figure 1. The Cognitive Model.

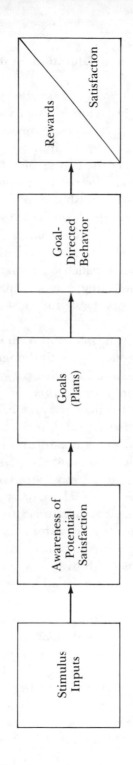

Source: Deci, 1975, p. 98.

Awareness that the organism can be satisfied provides the energy to set goals and engage in behavior. In other theories, this awareness has been referred to as affective states, drives, or intrinsic motivation. Next, goals or plans are set by the individual after evaluating the situation and determining the course of action that will lead to desired end states. This is followed by goal-directed behavior that Deci asserts will lead to accomplishment of the goals most valued by the organism. The result of this behavior is that the individual may experience some degree of satisfaction. If the reward-producing situation matches the original awareness, the awareness will be eliminated; if it does not match, the organism will reprocess through the cycle, establishing a new sequence of goal-directed behavior. Deci's model is probably the most comprehensive cognitive theory of motivation.

Another type of organismic approach is the *affective arousal theory*. As cognition is concerned with thought, affect is concerned with feelings. The affective arousal theorist would assert that affect is the basis of motivation in that it precedes, energizes, and directs behavior. Cues call up affect that motivates behavior in anticipation of reexperiencing an affective state previously experienced. If the past experience was positive, the organism is aroused to attend to the stimulus object (cue); the cue is avoided if past experience was negative. McClelland (1953), an affective arousal theorist, goes on to assert that motives can be acquired by associating a stimulus with an affective arousal and that all motives are learned. The strength of the motive is dependent upon the magnitude of the arousal. In other words, if one has a good or pleasurable experience, future cues associated with the experience will trigger behavior in anticipation of another pleasurable experience. In addition to McClelland, major theorists of affective arousal are Hebb (1967) and Young (1961).

A third organismic approach to human behavior consists of the *humanistic theories*. As noted in Chapter Two, humanistic theories focus on the importance and value of individual difference and how these differences affect day-to-day life. Humanistic theories are based on the assumption that man has a free will. As such, humanistic theorists assert that people are free agents who define their existence through making choices. These choices reflect the individuals' views of self in terms of the environment in which they find themselves. Action to define one's existence is present in the situation an individual is facing. Another situation would bring to the foreground other aspects of an individual's needs and goals. Various individuals will respond quite differently to the same situation because each perceives the situation uniquely and will rely on individual inner orientation in order to maximize the goal satisfactions. This means that that all individuals go through the same inner processes; however, based on their past accumulated experiences, they will respond differently.

Humanistic theories, for the most part, have not been based on empirical research; however, more recent writings by deCharms (1968) report the use of experimental methodology. Two of the more well-known humanistic theorists are Maslow (1954) and Rogers (1961).

Combination Approach. Some of the more recent motivational theorists suggest a combination of the mechanistic and organismic approaches. An early work advocating this approach is *Toward a General Theory of Action,* edited by Parsons and Shils (1951). This eclectic mix of external and internal forces appears to provide the practitioner, in this case the provider of CE, a much more comprehensive and usable body of knowledge on which to base educational activity. Other authors have also attempted to synthesize the literature identifying common factors in human behavior. Cofer and Appley (1964) place the more commonly accepted factors affecting motivation into the following categories: (1) biological—emotion, force, drive, instinct, and need; (2) mental—urge, wish, feeling, impulse, want, striving, desire, and demand; and (3) goal object—purpose, interest, intention, attitude, aspiration, plan, motive, incentive, goal, and value.

These three terms have in common the fact that they are used to represent states or conditions of the organism that affect the vigor, persistence, or direction of behavior. These common factors provide the avenue for describing motivational research and theory applicable to education. For instance, variations of these factors are probably involved in the decisions physicians make to learn new surgical procedures. Physicians may have the inner desire or need to function at the highest level of the state of the art. Equally plausible, however, is that mastering the procedure will enable physicians to increase their earnings.

The literature on motivation provides ample indication of the types of factors or forces that influence behavior. The following section discusses the application of this information to the practice of continuing education for the health professions.

Models of Application

While there are two major opposing points of view regarding human behavior—internal versus external control—it is not imperative to choose between the two when applying this research to continuing education. What does appear to be necessary, however, is to arrive at a definition of motivation that provides sufficient latitude to accommodate what is known and has been theorized about why people behave the way they do. An eclectic definition, not specific to any theory, says that *motivation represents the combination of forces, both intrinsic and extrinsic, that initiates and propels behavior and determines its intensity.* Of necessity, this definition is broad and all-inclusive; however, it is intended to focus on those forces that initiate and sustain behavior (in this case, involvement in learning) and to analyze which of those forces can be altered by the provider of continuing education. To examine these forces, recent attempts to convert the basic research already discussed into what might be termed "models of application" will be reviewed.

Boshier Model. Boshier (1973) developed a model focused on participation, nonparticipation, and dropping out by adult learners. The essence of his model is that congruence between the learners' self-concepts and key aspects of the educational environment are the determining factors of participation in continuing education. The Boshier model is based on an *affective arousal* theory wherein past experience causes the individual to attend to the stimulus or avoid it.

For instance, for a significant number of students, dental school may not be a positive experience that enhances their self-concept. If Boshier is correct, it is possible that holding continuing education courses in a dental school environment sets the stage for this incongruence to come into focus, thereby affecting participation in formalized continuing education. For those professionals experiencing such an incongruence between institution and self, the innovative provider of CE may offer CE services through another facility or at the professionals' own offices. The types of services should not resemble activities that typically occur in the professional school setting. Rather, it should focus more on self-directed, self-managed activities.

Dubin and Cohen Model. This is a systems model focusing on motivation to update knowledge and skills (Dubin and Cohen, 1970). The systems approach means that the model views the process as a whole rather than a collection of discrete components. Because it views the entire process and all the associated factors, it is an eclectic model. The model takes into account extrinsic factors that come to bear on the individual, as well as the individual's background and training. This model assumes that the professional works for an organization or an institution. Since the systems approach views the entire process as interaction, it examines and weighs all potential factors that may produce a given output. These collective factors constitute the input to the system.

In this *motivation to update* system, the input factors comprise the individual, including basic psychological factors and nonwork environment; formal education; on-the-job supervisory relationships; and management policies. These factors all feed into decisions to engage in updating practices, such as organizational training, professional organizational meetings, seminars, television and reading, self-study and formal study, and on-the-job learning. Once these updating practices have occurred, two specific feedback loops may affect future updating practices: group interaction and self-achievement. A simplified diagram of this model is presented in Figure 2.

Based on this model, Dubin and Cohen have a hypothesis that argues that "motivation to update can be simulated as a feedback control system by utilizing a mathematical model which incorporates the motivational and personality variables, the educational environment, and organizational factors" (1970, p. 366). They include the mathematical equations necessary to enable the user to determine which factor or factors are most important to the updating process in a given situation. A distinct advantage of this model is that it is all-inclusive. The updating practices can include activities

Figure 2. The Motivation to Update Model.

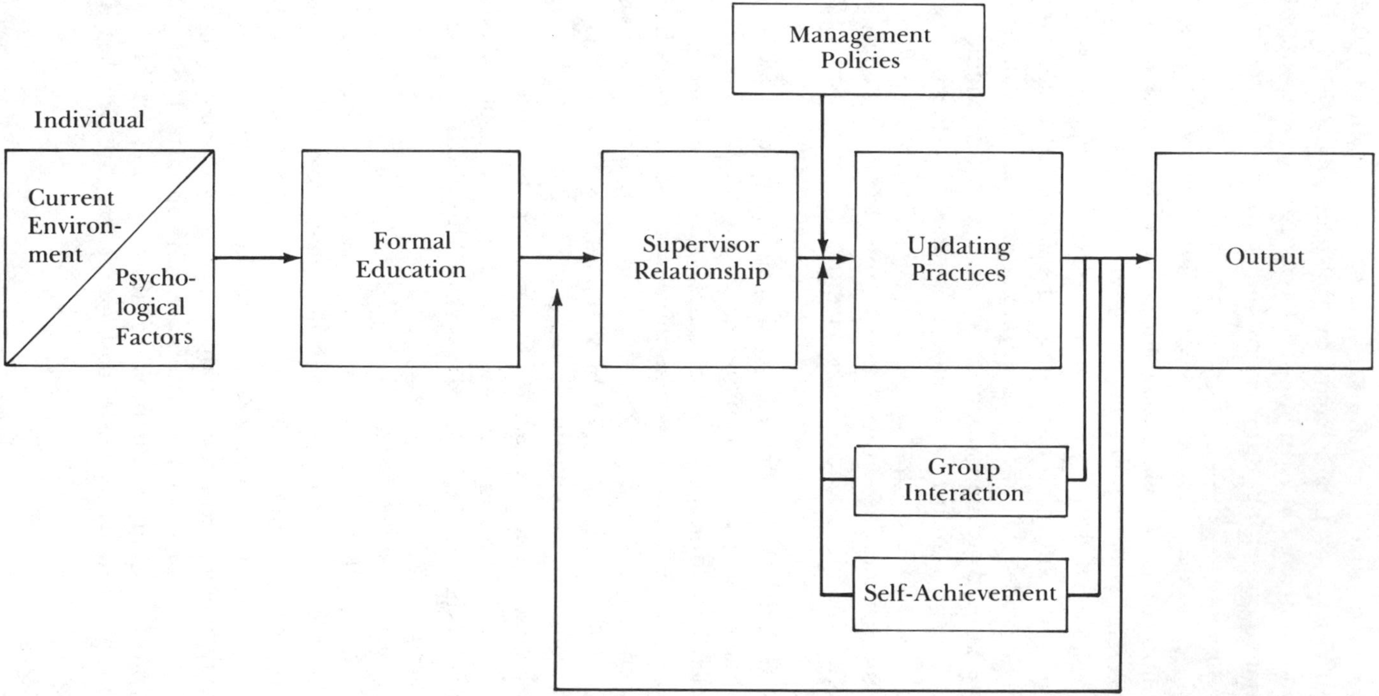

Individual

Current Environ-ment

Psycho-logical Factors

Formal Education

Supervisor Relationship

Management Policies

Updating Practices

Group Interaction

Self-Achievement

Output

Source: Dubin and Cohen, 1970, p. 366.

ranging from the most traditional to the most innovative, enabling the user to make programmatic changes as necessary to meet the CE needs of all constituents.

Cross Model. A third model is the so-called *chain-of-response* (COR) model (Cross, 1981). This is another eclectic model that draws from the various theories of motivation. According to Cross, the COR model "assumes that participation in a learning activity, whether in organized classes or self-directed, is not a single act but the result of a chain of responses, each based on an evaluation of the position of the individual in his or her environment" (p. 125). The concept of behavior as a sequence of discrete events suggests that understanding the factors of change within the sequence is more important than knowing the cause of the discrete behaviors. An additional concept of importance is that while the sequence flows toward involvement, the various forces affecting involvement may flow both ways. This is most easily understood by viewing a diagram of the model in Figure 3.

According to the COR model, participation in continuing education involves a sequence of linkages. Self-evaluation (A) represents a first linkage that, depending on accumulated experiences, influences the individual's attitudes toward education (B). The individual's attitudes may be influenced by "significant others." People who are likely to involve themselves in continuing education as a function of A and B can be thought of as intrinsically motivated. The third link (C) embraces the expectancy-valence approach to explain behavior. Goals are set that the individual feels can be met and are of value. The expected degree to which the highly valued goals can be met through CE determines the strength of the stimulus to participate. A fourth link (D) is related to events in the life of an individual that require change and readjustment. These are both the long-term transitions associated with aging, for example, and the more sudden, dramatic events such as the death of a spouse or loss of a job. These transitions influence the decisions individuals make regarding involvement in continuing education.

The next link in the COR model is that of barriers and opportunities (E). If an individual has a desire to participate in continuing education, the final decision to follow through may be determined by perceived or real barriers to participation or con-

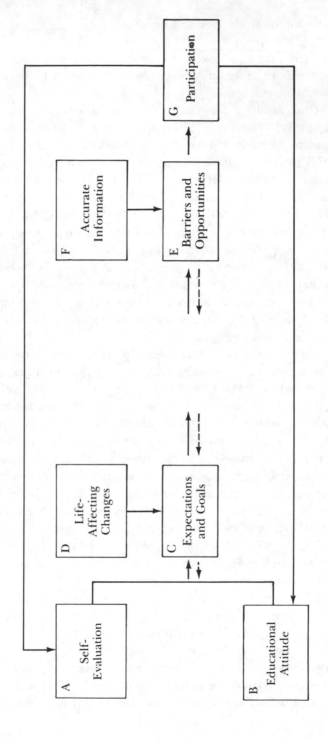

Figure 3. The Chain-of-Response Model.

Source: Cross, 1981, p. 124.

versely by special arrangements facilitating participation. If continuing education activities fail to match certain needs of the learner—for example, time, place, and format of the activity—all but the most determined learners will be deterred. This implies that removal of barriers is most likely to enhance participation.

Accurate information (F), relates closely to barriers and opportunities; lack of opportunities may represent a barrier to participation. Accurate information about educational offerings allows potential participants to match their needs to existing opportunities. Cross states that "without accurate information, point E in the model is weak because opportunities are not discovered and barriers loom large" (p. 127).

Point G in the model is involvement in continuing education. This involvement will impact upon the individual at points A and B. If the model holds, successful continuing education will stimulate additional participation in CE to meet new needs as the individual changes and grows.

The COR model is an excellent application model for CE for health professionals because at each step it offers the provider of CE opportunities to make conscious management decisions that can enhance the level and frequency of involvement with the learners. The involvement with learners may be providing an activity that meets specific needs or helping set up a management information system in a community hospital to help identify continuing education needs. As another example, refer to step F, that of providing accurate information. Most CE providers can improve the comprehensiveness of information they make available to potential learners. This may address the specificity of what learners can expect from an offered learning activity or it may include information about various opportunities to engage in nontraditional learning activities.

Mager-Pipe Model. Another approach to "motivating" behavior, referred to as *applied behavior analysis,* has in recent years gained increasing favor in the field of business management. Unlike the other application models presented, applied behavior analysis adheres rigidly to one theory of behavior, namely, behaviorism. Supporters of this approach adhere to the law of parsimony, which intimates that the simplest, most direct explanation for a phenomenon is the best explanation. Applying this law to human behavior, attention is paid only to those phenomena that are observable, and no effort is spent trying to analyze unseen "causes" of behavior. The approach is pragmatic, and its supporters contend that there is no value in asserting the presence of internal factors, even if they exist.

The management community is attracted to this approach because it focuses on tangible, bottom-line outcomes, such as productivity and sales. A case can be made that providers of continuing education in many settings are faced with similar situations. If this is so, it is indeed important to be able to assess the impact of various factors affecting involvement in continuing education by some measure of change. Operationally, a desired outcome of manipulating selected variables may be increased rates of participation in CE or use of self-assessment instruments by health professionals. Either change is easily measurable prior to and after the planned intervention.

Mager and Pipe (1970) describe a model, depicted in Figure 4, designed to analyze why desired outcomes are not being reached. As an example, the following discussion of the use of self-assessment by health professionals will demonstrate the model's relevance for CE. The first issue is performance discrepancy between what is and what should be—in this case, the frequency of using self-assessment instruments. If a deficiency is established, the importance of this deficiency must be assessed, a relatively easy matter. Once an important performance deficiency has been identified, it must be determined whether there is a lack of skills on the part of the health professionals or whether circumstances either punish the desired performance or reward nonperformance.

In general, continuing education experts agree that use of self-assessment instruments is desirable and that nonuse does not imply the lack of any specific skill. Thus, the cause for nonuse must either be lack of rewards, presence of punishment for performance, or rewards for nonperformance. The busy health professional may consider time spent on self-assessment as punishment when translated into loss of income or loss of time for patient care. The CE provider can remedy this either (1) by providing time in an employer-employee situation or making arrangements for the least time-consuming type of self-assessment activities or (2) by providing credit for relicensure or recertification.

Figure 4. The Applied Behavior Analysis Model.

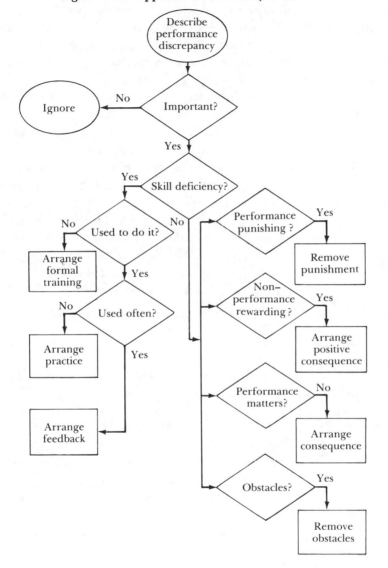

To make use of this model, the provider of continuing educa
tion must carefully specify the desired outcomes and determine if
there are discrepancies between what is and what should be. The
provider must also determine the values of the target audience in
terms of what will be reinforcing or rewarding to prospective continuing education participants. To take the necessary corrective
steps will require close collaboration between the CE provider, the
health professionals, and potential employers or regulators.

Implications of the Models. The provider of traditional or
nontraditional CE has multiple opportunities to apply motivation
research to the conduct of CE. All the application models discussed
emphasize the importance of attending to what the learner values. In
the day-to-day practice of CE, this requires identifying what learners
value as part of the needs assessment process and, in turn, designing
ways of providing what learners value. For example, providing CE
in the manner, time, and place most desired by the learner is a strong
initial positive step. How often is CE provided that more closely
matches the manner, time, and place most preferred by faculty rather
than by the learner?

Summary and Conclusion

Why adult human beings engage in learning or participate in
continuing education is an often-asked question. A frequent response to this question is that they were "motivated" to participate.
The term *motivation,* therefore, is used as if it were a cause of behavior rather than a description of the various forces that initiate and
propel behavior. Since the term *motivation* is used differently by
different people, its use as a meaningful communication aid is
seriously weakened. This situation is exacerbated by the fact that
neither lay use nor the professional use of the term is consistent.
Researchers tend to define motivation in a way that helps explain
the theory of behavior they espouse. Laymen tend to use the term as
a catchall that helps explain phenomena that otherwise are simply
too difficult to describe.

Motivation is a difficult word to define, because it is a theoretical construct and is neither observable nor empirical and cannot be
measured. Instead, behavior is observed, and the inference is made

that the individual is motivated. In the case of continuing education, individuals who assess their own educational needs and participate in educational activities to meet those needs would no doubt be labeled as motivated.

There are multiple theories of human behavior. These theories can be classified into two major approaches: the mechanistic approach and the organismic approach. In the mechanistic approach, the most popular theory—behaviorism—states that behavior occurs because it is reinforced by something in the environment. The most popular theory in the organismic approach is cognitive theory, which holds that human beings knowingly engage in behaviors to attain or accomplish things that they value. The primary distinguishing factor that separates these theories is locus of control. In cognitive theory the individual controls and thereby makes knowing choices, whereas in behavioristic theory the individual responds to reinforcement contingencies in the environment.

This dichotomy of viewing behavior that is "motivated" by either internal forces or external forces has a long history and appears to be rooted in the basic assumptions made about human nature. The dichotomy has spawned the associated terminology, intrinsic and extrinsic, as descriptors of motivation. Intrinsic motivation comes from within the individual and is comprised of urges, wishes, feelings, emotions, desires, and drives. Extrinsic motivation comes from outside the individual and is manifest in those environmental factors that precipitate behavior. The combination of intrinsic and extrinsic provides an eclectic mix that is manifest in the goal object. The goal object is found in the environment and is therefore extrinsic. However, the goal object has become such by virtue of the value placed on it from within the individual and is therefore intrinsic. This interplay of intrinsic and extrinsic factors is the basis of much contemporary research in motivation.

The systematic application of motivation theory and research to continuing education is a relatively new phenomenon. Most models of application are eclectic in nature. They view behavior as being initiated and propelled by a variety of forces, both within and outside the individual. However, a model of application gaining in acceptance, particularly in the management community, is known as applied behavioral analysis and is best represented by Mager and

Pipe (1970). It deals only with factors in the environment that are identified as being reinforcing to a given individual.

In applying the motivation research to continuing education, it is clear that the continuing educator does not have unlimited opportunity to affect the forces that initiate or propel behavior. For instance, change in the values or belief systems of an adult professional are highly unlikely. Therefore, resources expended to attempt these changes will most likely be wasted. On the other hand, identifying the values held by the individual and structuring continuing education activities congruent with these values is much more likely to end in success. In closing, it is fair to say that most providers of CE are but scratching the surface when it comes to using or applying what is currently known about motivating the adult professional learner.

References

Atkinson, J. W., and Feather, N. T. (Eds.). *Theory of Achievement Motivation.* New York: Wiley, 1966.

Bolles, R. C. *Theory of Motivation.* New York: Harper & Row, 1967.

Boshier, R. "Educational Participation and Dropout: A Theoretical Model." *Adult Education,* 1973, *23* (4), 255–282.

Brown, J. S. *The Motivation of Behavior.* New York: McGraw-Hill, 1961.

Cofer, C. N., and Appley, M. H. *Motivation: Theory and Research.* New York: Wiley, 1964.

Cross, K. P. *Adults as Learners.* San Francisco: Jossey-Bass, 1981.

Darwin, C. *The Origin of Species by Means of Natural Selection.* Oxford, England: Oxford University Press, 1951. (Originally published 1859.)

deCharms, R. *Personal Causation: The Internal Affective Determinants of Behavior.* New York: Academic Press, 1968.

Deci, E. L. *Intrinsic Motivation.* New York: Plenum Press, 1975.

Dubin, S. S., and Cohen, D. M. "Motivation to Update from a Systems Approach." *Engineering Education,* 1970, *60* (5), 366–368.

Hebb, D. O. *The Organization of Behavior.* New York: Wiley, 1967.

Hull, C. L. *Principles of Behavior.* New York: Appleton-Century-Crofts, 1943.

Lewin, K. *Principles of Topological Psychology*. New York: Mc-Graw-Hill, 1936.

McClelland, D. C., and others. *The Achievement Motive*. New York: Appleton-Century-Crofts, 1953.

McDougall, W. *An Introduction to Social Psychology*. London: Methuen, 1960. (Originally published 1914.)

Mager, R. F., and Pipe, P. *Analyzing Performance Problems or You Really Oughta Wanna*. Belmont, Calif.: Fearon Pitman, 1970.

Maslow, A. H. *Motivation and Personality*. New York: Harper & Row, 1954.

Miller, N. E. "Liberalization of Basic S-R Concepts: Extensions to Conflict Behavior, Motivation, and Social Learning." In S. Koch (Ed.), *Psychology: A Study of a Science*. Vol. 2. New York: McGraw-Hill, 1959.

Miller, N. E., and Dollard, J. *Social Learning and Imitation*. New Haven, Conn.: Yale University Press, 1941.

Parsons, T., and Shils, E. A. *Toward a General Theory of Action*. Cambridge, Mass.: Harvard University Press, 1951.

Rogers, C. R. *On Becoming a Person*. Boston: Houghton-Mifflin, 1961.

Skinner, B. F. *Science and Human Behavior*. New York: Free Press, 1953.

Tolman, E. C. *Purposive Behavior in Animals and Men*. New York: Appleton-Century-Crofts, 1932.

Vroom, V. H. *Work and Motivation*. New York: Wiley, 1964.

Weiner, B. *Theories of Motivation: From Mechanism to Cognition*. Chicago: Markham, 1972.

Woodworth, R. S. *Dynamic Psychology*. New York: Columbia University Press, 1918.

Young, P. T. *Motivation and Emotion*. New York: Wiley, 1961.

4

How Family Physicians
Use Information Sources:
Implications
for New Approaches

Robert P. Means

This chapter describes a study of the information-seeking behaviors of a group of family physicians in the state of Michigan, conducted in the late 1970s. Although this group is not representative of all health professionals in all states, it does offer insights as to the types of information sources that health professionals tend to use. An in-depth description of the manner in which health professionals use these information sources to seek answers to their practice-related problems is included. This chapter can assist the reader in understanding why continuing education (CE) provider units should develop their capacity to assist individual health professionals as they seek information to solve problems. Chapter Eleven, "Facilitating Self-Directed Learning," should be referred to for the more specific approaches to addressing the implications from this study.—Editors

The medical profession has long faced the problem of keeping abreast of new advances emanating from research and development in the natural, physical, social, and behavioral sciences. Today's health care professionals are confronted with the realities of dramatic social and technological changes. There exists a major discrepancy between what is known and what is used in medical science. The problem is compounded by the vast array of medical journals, pharmaceutical promotional literature, and educational opportunities from which practitioners must select the medical information that is most relevant to their particular needs and professional development interests.

For the family physician, the problem is further complicated. The family physician must maintain competence in a larger cross section of medical subspecialties than other types of medical practitioners. Heavy patient loads allow limited time to engage in continuing medical education (CME). Solo practice settings create some degree of professional isolation that limits interaction with colleagues and access to community hospitals or academic medical centers where desired CME activities are provided. The necessity for family practitioners to maintain competence through systematic acquisition of new knowledge and skills (information seeking) as part of a lifelong learning process has never been greater.

While it is well documented that practicing physicians rely heavily on the literature in their information-seeking efforts (Strasser, 1978; Stinson and Mueller, 1980), a recent study indicates that clinical faculty and medical students in their clinical years have limited skills at accessing library resources for resolving patient management–related problems (DaRosa and others, 1983). Yet to date, CME providers have done little to facilitate self-directed learning behaviors.

In general, CME is episodic and tends to be traditional in its use of instructional processes (Nakamoto and Verner, 1970; World Health Organization Expert Committee, 1973; Miller, 1975). A major focus of CME should be practice-based problems, gleaned from day-to-day real life encounters that involve the highest incidence of morbidity and mortality. Observers of medical education have repeatedly noted the need for CME providers to develop a variety of instructional methods and techniques that are compatible with individual physician's learning styles (McLaughlin and Penchansky, 1965; Miller, 1967; World Health Organization Expert Committee, 1973). Consequently, the CME planner must come to understand better those personal and situational characteristics of the physician that affect learning, as well as the various patterns of information seeking that the physician finds most functional in producing the desired outcome of increased competence in delivering patient care.

Study of Family Physicians

This chapter will examine the information-seeking behavior of a group of family physicians in Michigan in order to gain insight into the extent and sequence in which various sources of information are used for learning. The results of this study (Means, 1979), completed in 1978, will be examined in order to provide suggestions to CE provider units for facilitating the natural learning that goes on among a specific group of physicians. It is reasonable to assume that many of these suggestions will also apply to facilitating the learning of other physician groups and other health professionals.

The study was carried out in two phases. *Phase I* consisted of a mailed questionnaire designed to collect baseline data from a random sample of Michigan's population of practicing family physicians. Specifically, the focus was on those learning efforts aimed at resolving problems encountered in practice. *Phase II* of the study was designed to allow for a more in-depth examination of family physician's information seeking—why, how, with what difficulties and with what success physicians resolve practice problems using various sources of information. Phone interviews ranging from twenty minutes to one and one-half hours in length were conducted with 41 of the 172 family physicians who had completed Phase I of the study and volunteered for the interview. The criterion for problem selection was the physician's identification of two problems encountered during the previous twelve months. These encounters were to represent "critical incidents" in practice that prompted entering into a "learning effort" to gain and retain some new knowledge, clinical skills, or understanding. These were not to include problems resolvable by patient referral or by a quick reference to a medical text but rather problems that required resolution through more lengthy, deliberate, and systematic learning efforts in which a variety of sources of information might be used.

Sources of Information

The Michigan study determined which sources of information were most frequently used by family physicians to resolve problems encountered in their day-to-day practice.

Print Material. Family physicians reported using professional journals and medical texts for clinical problem solving more than any other source of information. The reasons for the extensive use of these print materials were their availability and close proximity to practice; their accessibility, that is, their ability to provide information quickly; and their reliability. This finding is substantiated by studies that showed that physicians use first and most frequently print material, principally medical journals, to seek information on new advances in medical science and technology (Murray-Lyon, 1977; Strasser, 1978; Clintworth and others, 1979; Manning and Denson, 1979).

Respondents reported skimming and scanning; they read only a limited number of articles in their entirety. They preferred to read at home, at work between patients, or over the lunch hour. The family physician's familiarity and confidence with print material greatly influenced persistent use. They primarily used textbooks to review basic science and clinical aspects of a problem, which, in turn, provided them direction for further information seeking. If time had permitted, physicians indicated, they would have doubled the amount of time devoted to reading. The physicians reported using digests, abstracted materials, and pharmaceutical promotional literature because of their compatibility with time constraints imposed as a result of heavy patient loads.

Family physicians identified several obstacles to using print sources. These included lack of relevance—material is often out-of-date by the time it is printed, or it is designed for the researcher rather than the clinician—and lack of time—family physicians find it difficult to locate clinically relevant information in the limited amount of free time they have, without the aid of abstracted or indexed materials.

Direct Contacts with Colleagues. Contacts with colleagues ranked as the second most frequent source of information. Formal patient referrals and informal conversations in practice settings, such as discussion over lunch, during staff meetings, and during phone conversations represent forms of colleague contact most frequently mentioned and preferred. In a given month, family physicians reported spending an average of close to eighteen hours using this source. Generally, conversations and interactions with colleagues provide the immediate feedback, clarification, and confirmation necessary when the clinical problem addressed is critical. The physicians were likely to seek the consultation and encouragement of three to four close colleagues, usually practice partners.

Obstacles to the use of interpersonal contacts as part of the information-seeking process included too much time between the initiation of a consultation and the receipt of a response and the assumption by consultants that the family physician understands more about a problem than is actually the case. The latter may lead a consultant to convey information that may be inappropriate. Family physicians placed great value on the opportunity to interact with colleagues. However, many felt opportunities for such interactions were not available in most continuing education settings, contrary to what institutional or organizational providers of CME often think to be the case.

Formal Educational Activities. The traditional continuing education activity using predominantly the lecture has been the mainstay of continuing medical education for physicians. Family physicians indicated that CME sponsored by a medical school, specialty society, or hospital staff was an important part of their information-seeking process for resolving clinical problems. However, the family physician has suffered from what has traditionally been a maldistribution of CE activities. This is partly the result of CME's primary focus on the educational needs of the specialist.

Family physicians are discriminating in their use of CE activities. They are more likely to attend an activity that addresses aspects of a current clinical problem. Topics of general clinical interest are less likely to be selected. For example, family physicians will prefer a discussion of the treatment of otitis media in children over a general presentation of advances in ear, nose, and throat medicine or in the treatment of childhood diseases. These physicians utilize postgraduate courses or CME as opportunities to review with colleagues and experts the latest advances in medical science. Attendance at these courses typically occurs last in a sequence of sources of information used. Further, they are used only when time is not a critical factor in resolving a problem.

The most prevalent obstacles to family physicians' participation in formal CME include heavy patient loads and an inability to find replacement coverage. The result has been an increased use of CME opportunities in the local practice community. These included staff meetings at the local hospital with formal lecture presentations, hospital staff–sponsored activities, such as grand rounds and clinical pathology conferences, and correspondence or home study options. Several physicians interviewed mentioned activities that included a combination of correspondence and residential study as part of a plan for continuous learning. The periodic monographs, self-assessment tests, and options to attend related postgraduate courses provided them with intermittent opportunities to continue formal learning at their own pace.

Nonprint Material. Nonprint sources of information such as audiotapes, computer-assisted instruction, and telephone dial access systems were mentioned infrequently as a source of information used to resolve clinical problems. An average of four hours per month was spent using nonprint sources.

The interviewed physicians preferred to use nonprint materials, such as audiotapes that come with indexed and supplemental reading materials, in combination with print materials. They were favorably disposed to correspondence courses that included a monograph or manual, combined with tape cassettes. In addition, 20 percent of the family physicians interviewed mentioned the desirability of a dial access system or a combination of a dial access and live consultation telephone network with a major medical center or medical school. The physicians reported that nonprint sources of information are more difficult to use because of the prohibitive cost of hardware and software systems, the difficulty of availability or access, and the lack of knowledge about what is actually available or how to use it.

The Act of Information Seeking

Family physicians engaged in clinical problem solving often confront conditions that they are unable to diagnose or treat unless they acquire new knowledge, skills, or understanding. The specific clinical problem may be acute or chronic and recurrent. In any case, the physician may be faced with a decision whether to refer the problem or acquire the necessary competence to resolve the problem. Family physicians who decided to resolve the problem themselves typically described multiple reasons for engaging in information seeking.

Motives. A major motive was *cognitive dissonance*—the felt need for knowledge about a presenting problem because of some anxiety based on a current deficiency in understanding. This represented the physician's need to understand a presenting problem in order to make an appropriate diagnosis and develop a treatment plan for the patient.

A second motive was the family physician's *curiosity* about the answer to a problem—knowledge for knowledge's sake. There was the desire to prove to themselves that they could develop a strategy that would lead to resolution of an issue, even if it did not relate to a current practice problem. In a number of cases, family physicians reported making these problems the subjects of mini-clinical research studies in which they systematically sought to use a variety of sources of information to formulate a solution.

A third but minor motive was receiving *credit* for the activity. In approximately half the reported cases of information seeking, physicians indicated that they used sources of information that fulfilled various credit requirements for state relicensure, specialty board certification, or membership in a professional association. This was generally, but not exclusively, the case for individuals who, in their efforts to resolve a clinical problem, used formal educational activities as one of several sources of information.

Sequences and Combination of Sources Used. Once motivated, family physicians' information-seeking behaviors aimed at resolving clinical problems did not represent a random choice of sources of information but rather a sequential process that was predicted on their previous use of sources. Sources of information served as stimuli to the physician's self-initiated learning, representing a series of consecutive transitions from awareness of the problem, to actively searching for a solution, to decision making, and finally, to problem resolution.

In the majority (73 percent) of the interviews, print materials, in particular medical texts, were mentioned as initial sources of information used as part of the information-seeking process. The next most frequent sources were professional journals or communications with colleagues or a combination of the two. In those cases where family physicians used formal educational activities, they usually came last in a sequence.

In many ways, this sequence of steps in the physician's information-seeking process resembles behaviors evident in the clinical reasoning process, namely, information gathering and interpretation, hypothesis generation, problem-oriented search strategy, problem formulation, and diagnostic or therapeutic decisions (Barrows and Tamblyn, 1980). With respect to the dissemination and utilization of knowledge, Havelock and others (1969) described this sequence as the problem-solver approach. This represents a psychological process whereby an individual senses a need, diagnoses and formulates a problem statement, identifies relevant resources, defines solutions to the problem, and tests those solutions. Feedback indicates the degree of need reduction.

Rogers and Shoemaker (1971) offer a further explanation in terms of a communication model. This study of family physicians' use of sources of information closely parallels those stages in the innovation–decision-making process. These include stages of knowledge, persuasion, decision, and confirmation. Family physicians' statements regarding why they selected sources and used them in the order they did are consistent with stages in the innovation–decision-making process. Print material was used at the awareness or knowledge stage to review background material concerning the basic and clinical science aspects of a problem. Interpersonal contact with colleagues was used at the analysis, hypothesis, and persuasion state in which physicians tested their diagnosis or treatment regimes by comparing them with peer judgments or some standard of quality practice. Formal educational activities were used at the decision-making and confirmation stage to provide the most current information on a topic, as well as a final opportunity to compare a decision with that supported by peers.

Although this sequence represents the major pattern of information seeking that emerged from interviews with family physicians, it was by no means the only pattern. The innovation-decision-making process itself is not always linear, proceeding from awareness of need to hypothesis testing and decision making. In this study there were a number of cases where information seeking was initiated, application in practice occurred, and additional information seeking was required before reaching a final resolution.

Another important observation derived from the interviews dealt with the combinations of sources used as part of every information-seeking process described. For example, a formal educational activity did not in itself result in the resolution of a particular clinical problem. Rather, it was a combination of reading material, attendance at a continuing education activity, and communications with colleagues that was most beneficial at different stages of the problem-solving process. Similar observations were made by Beal and Rogers (1960) and Coleman, Katz, and Menzel (1966). Their studies found that a combination of various sources of information at the persuasion and adoption stages is more likely to lead to the use of new innovations than when a single source is used.

The nature of the clinical problem and the urgency of the need for resolution were major determinants in the sequence, type, and number of sources used, as well as the time spent in the information-seeking process. In those cases where the problem was recurrent over an extended period of time, print material, consultation with colleagues, and attendance at continuing medical education courses was the sequence and combination of sources of information used. Physicians interviewed reported that 18 hours was the average time spent in using sources of information to resolve any one problem. However, some information-seeking efforts took as long as 130 hours.

For those problems that needed immediate resolution, print sources were used. Additional importance was placed on consultation with a well-known expert (not necessarily a close colleague or associate). These information-seeking efforts were much briefer and required as little as one or two hours during which sources of information were actively used. Many of these information-seeking efforts did not meet the minimum criteria of seven hours of time per learning project set by Tough (1971) and used in other research investigations of individual adult learning (McCatty, 1973; Fair, 1973). Instead, these efforts closely resembled those described by Collican (1974) as "quick learning," which occurs in less than seven hours but, if the stimulus is strong enough, can contribute to continuous learning. Many of these shorter efforts represented attempts by family physicians to relearn or refamiliarize themselves with basic concepts to allow for rapid assimilation and integration of new information.

As revealed by this study, sequence and content of information sought by physicians suggested a logical pattern of progression. The physicians seemed to proceed from the acquisition of new knowledge (cognition) to the more complex tasks of skill development, attitudinal change, and problem solving. Family physicians indicated that they went beyond information acquisition by reading or attending formal postgraduate courses. Their study pattern included personal contact with peers, which helped to modify or confirm appropriate attitudes essential for problem resolution. If formal educational activities were part of their learning plan, activities were chosen that offered more than simple information transfer from the academic medical centers. They gave preference to activities that offered opportunities for testing and simulating components of clinical performance.

In some instances, there emerged a sense of progression, continuity, and persistence in individual information-seeking efforts. Later in the study, when family physicians were queried further on this point, they indicated that some of the more valuable learning efforts were those that included components of self-assessment, followed by correspondence study, and, in some cases, by in-residence study in which they were able to increase medical competence and improve performance at their own pace. In reacting to correspondence formats, they developed a particular affinity for periodic learning modules that included self-assessment tests, monographs, or audiotapes that offered them an opportunity for continuous learning.

Criteria for Selection of Sources of Information

While physicians continue to spend a substantial amount of time in formal CME activities each year, almost thirteen days according to a recent study (American Medical Association, 1981), it is also apparent that considerable time is spent in the act of information seeking through informal and self-directed approaches. In information seeking related to clinical problem solving, family physicians initiated the majority of their own learning. In these self-directed efforts, a number of conditions influenced the family physicians' criteria for selection, organization, and use of various sources of information. These conditions or criteria for selecting information sources have implications for improving the quality of CME designed by the individual physician learner and CME provider (see Chapter Eleven).

Clinical Relevance. Sources of information are selected based on the extent to which they contribute to resolving a current clinical problem. Source selection was based on the potential application to the practice setting. For instance, family physicians reported that their decisions to attend a particular CE activity were based on the anticipated benefits they would receive regarding a specific practice problem.

Familiarity with Source. Sources of information with which family physicians have the greatest familiarity are likely to be those utilized most frequently. Family physicians' greatest obstacle to using new or different sources beyond the same medical texts, journals, and CE courses, was their lack of familiarity with what else was available and for what purposes it could be used, where it was located, and what skills were required for its proper use.

Availability and Accessibility. Sources of information used are those that (1) are in close proximity to the family physician's practice setting, such as print material available in the physician's office and personal library or formal CME in local community hospitals, and (2) require the shortest time to access, such as indexed medical texts or consultation with practice partners. Availability and accessibility are important to the practitioner because the closer in time the actual learning is to the need to apply the learning, the greater the chances are that the individual will maintain interest in learning and that learning will contribute to actual improvement in practice behavior.

Stage of Information Seeking. Sources of information are selected to closely parallel each stage in the physician's information-seeking process. For example, at the initial awareness stage, journal articles or medical texts tend to be selected at the point where a practitioner needs to develop a new skill. At the stage where a final decision has to be made to proceed with a therapeutic plan, consultation with colleagues is frequently used.

Active Involvement in Learning. Sources of information are used that are likely to actively involve the practitioner. The physician is not only interested in increased knowledge (basic transfer of new medical information) but also improved skills and changed attitudes. This requires the physicians to seek information that involves greater participatory or inquiry-oriented learning techniques. While listening and observing are important methods of gaining information, discussion and practice, which require the learner to take action, are more challenging and more apt to maintain interest and persistence in learning.

Progression in Learning. Preferred sources of information give learners the flexibility to move from understanding the fundamental aspects of the basic science to the more complex clinical implications. This transition should be feasible at the learner's own pace. Use of sources in this manner takes into account the differences in individuals' ability to process information.

Continuity in Learning. Sources of information are used that provide physicians with a sequence of experiences that are continuous and allow for the integration of information from a variety of sources. Sources are used that reinforce previous learning experiences, build on existing experiences, and integrate new information as part of a continuous process to link the medical practitioner with a resource system.

Conclusions

In recent years CME has received considerable criticism because of its tendency to emphasize the use of classroom instruction techniques and group learning to the exclusion of other more self-directed modes of learning. Houle (1980) notes the persistent failure of the professions to respond in meaningful ways to the needs of the professional and comments, "Each response to the need for assuring quality has had its unique influence, but the general effect of all of them has been to increase the provision of organized instructional activities. . . . In fact, many people are growing irritated by what seems to them to be a mindless proliferation of courses and conferences, each of which may be valuable but which are not collectively undergirded by any unifying conception of how education can be used in a mature, complex, and continuing way to achieve excellence of service throughout the life span" (p. x).

Studies in the past decade have shown that individuals' efforts to remain professionally competent reflect a preponderance of self-directed, inquiry-oriented approaches to learning (Tough, 1971). In order to improve the quality of continuing medical education, it is essential that CME providers give increasing attention to ways in which they can understand and facilitate better individual practitioners' independent and self-directed modes of learning.

References

American Medical Association. "Survey of Current Status of Continuing Medical Education." Report on the Council on Medical Education. *Continuing Medical Education Newsletter,* 1981, *10* (1), 2–3.

Barrows, H. S., and Tamblyn, R. M. *Problem-Based Learning: An Approach to Medical Education.* New York: Springer, 1980.

Beal, G. M., and Rogers, E. M. *The Adoption of Two Farm Practices in a Central Iowa Community.* Ames, Iowa: Agricultural Experimental Station, 1960.

Clintworth, W. A., and others. "Continuing Education and Library Services for Physicians in Office Practice." *Bulletin of the Medical Library Association*, 1979, *67* (4), 353–358.

Coleman, J. C., Katz, E., and Menzel, H. *Doctors and New Drugs*. Indianapolis, Ind.: Bobbs-Merrill, 1966.

Collican, P. M. *Self-Planned Learning: Implications for the Future of Adult Education*. Syracuse, N.Y.: Educational Policy Research Center, Syracuse University Research Corporation, 1974.

DaRosa, D. A., and others. "A Study of the Information-Seeking Skills of Medical Students and Physician Faculty." *Journal of Medical Education*, 1983, *58* (1), 45–50.

Fair, J. W., *Teachers as Learners: The Learning Projects of Beginning Elementary School Teachers*. Unpublished doctoral dissertation, University of Toronto, 1973.

Havelock, R. G., and others. *Planning for Innovation*. Ann Arbor: Center for Research on Utilization of Scientific Knowledge, Institute for Social Research, University of Michigan, 1969.

Houle, C. O. *Continuing Learning in the Professions*. San Francisco: Jossey-Bass, 1980.

McCatty, C. A. M. *Patterns of Learning Projects Among Professional Men*. Unpublished doctoral dissertation, University of Toronto, 1973.

McLaughlin, C. P., and Penchansky, R. "Diffusion of Innovation in Medicine: A Problem of Continuing Medical Education." *Journal of Medical Education*, 1965, *40* (5), 437–447.

Manning, P. R., and Denson, T. A. "How Cardiologists Learn About Echocardiography." *Annals of Internal Medicine*, 1979, *91* (3), 469–471.

Means, R. P. *Information-Seeking Behaviors of Michigan Family Physicians*. Unpublished dissertation: University of Illinois at Urbana-Champaign, 1979.

Miller, G. E. "Continuing Education for What?" *Journal of Medical Education*, 1967, *42* (4), 320–326.

Miller, G. E. "Why Continuing Medical Education?" *Bulletin of the New York Academy of Medicine*, 1975, *51* (6), 701–706.

Murray-Lyon, N. "Communication in Medicine: A Study of How Family Doctors Obtain Information on Recent Advances in the

Treatment of Rheumatic Diseases." *Medical Education*, 1977, *11* (2), 95–102.

Nakamoto, J., and Verner, C. *Continuing Education in the Health Professions: A Review of the Literature Pertinent to North America*. Washington, D.C.: ERIC, 1970.

Rogers, E. M., and Shoemaker, F. F. *Communication of Innovations*. New York: Free Press, 1971.

Stinson, E. R., and Mueller, D. A. "Survey of Health Professionals' Information Habits and Needs." *Journal of the American Medical Association*, 1980, *243* (2), 140–143.

Strasser, T. C. "The Information Needs of Practicing Physicians in Northeastern New York State." *Bulletin of the Medical Library Association*, 1978, *66* (2), 200–209.

Tough, A. *The Adult's Learning Projects*. Toronto, Canada: Ontario Institute for Studies in Education, 1971.

World Health Organization Expert Committee. "Continuing Education for Physicians." *World Health Organization Technical Report Series* no. 534, Geneva, Switzerland: World Health Organization, 1973.

5

Evolving Approaches to Continuing Medical Education: Efforts to Enhance the Impact on Patient Care

Donald E. Moore, Jr.

This chapter represents a historical analysis of continuing medical education from the early 1900s to the present. The reader is made aware of the many changes in medical education over the years that have had direct effect on continuing medical education. The different roles that continuing education (CE) has played within the health care setting are described in detail. The trend toward more practice-linked continuing medical education sets the stage for the discussion of the projected role of the CE provider unit that follows in Chapter Six. The editors felt that this historical perspective on CME, although not necessarily generalizable to the other health professions, does serve as valuable background for many of the concepts presented in this book.—Editors

The term *chaotic* probably best describes the present state of continuing medical education (CME). However, the annual increment in terms of numbers of courses offered and the number of physicians participating in them has been remarkably consistent. A comparison of the figures published for 1970 and 1980 by the American Medical Association (AMA) in the annual special issue on medical education of its journal shows the magnitude of the increment (American Medical Association, Division of Medical Education, 1972; Johnson and Gannon, 1981). Over this ten-year period, the number of course offerings reported (this by no means approaches all the courses actually offered) has increased over ninefold, and the number of physicians enrolling in these courses has increased nearly eightfold. During this same period, the total number of licensed physicians has increased less than twofold. These figures clearly indicate a greater involvement of physicians in formal, recorded, and documented CE activities. In 1977 an estimate by Miller suggested that CME at that time represented an annual investment of two billion dollars or 1.5 percent of the national health expenditures.

Presumably, the implementation of mandatory continuing education requirements has been a significant factor contributing to increased enrollment in CE. Twenty-five states now require physicians (and some other health professionals as well) to attend a designated number of hours of approved continuing education activities as a condition for relicensure (Johnson and Gannon, 1982). Similar requirements exist for membership in several specialty and state medical societies. In addition, the specialty boards have developed a schedule for implementing voluntary recertification, for which participation in CME represents one of various requirements. Finally, many hospitals now mandate evidence of participation in CME for continuation of hospital privileges. The net result has been an increase in interest, activity, and investment in CME across the country.

Many suggestions have been proposed to improve CME. They include applying adult learning principles and adult education procedures for planning and conducting continuing education for physicians; integrating CME with such quality assurance procedures as medical audit to increase relevance of programming; and locating CME in patient care settings, such as the community hospital and the office-based practice.

A review of the literature reveals some successful applications of these proposed suggestions but also indicates that there are still major problems with CME. Looking at the evolution of CME helps one understand why these suggestions were developed and what might be done to improve the quality of CME. Though the focus of the chapter is on continuing medical education, much can be learned about the present state of continuing education in general.

Medical Education

Medical educators and medical school administrators like to view medical education as a continuous process that begins with premedical education and ends with retirement or death. They define three phases of medical education, namely, premedical and medical education in the university (six to eight years); residency training in a teaching hospital (varies from three to seven years, depending on the requirements of the specialty board); and continuing education (thirty to forty years).

Currently, student physicians at the premedical, medical school, or residency level operate in an educational atmosphere and are kept informed of significant new developments by their peers, journals, the medical faculty, and the medical library. Through a delineation of specialties and subspecialties, the structure of residency training has changed so each physician need not attempt to absorb all scientific information available. Increased participation of physicians in CME activities demonstrates that there is also heightened awareness of the role that CME can play in responding to the accelerating rate of social and technological change. The growth and development of CME in the last two decades is the story of the adjustments that have been made in medical education in response to the rapid increase of biomedical knowledge.

Until early this century, medical education was available predominantly at proprietary schools that offered apprenticeship-type training. Entry requirements into these schools were nonexistent. There were no standards for curricula or for student and faculty selection; the program consisted predominantly of lectures with no laboratory and clinical teaching. Education beyond graduation was rare. The publication of the Flexner Report (Flexner, 1910) resulted in closure of many substandard schools and in restructuring the remaining schools and their programs. Major points of the Flexner Report were that (1) medical education must provide a scientific basis for medical practice, and thus there was a need for basic science faculty in the medical school; (2) the student must receive a supervised clinical experience in a teaching hospital; and (3) the medical school should be based in a fully accredited university.

The Flexner Report, together with a movement toward introduction of state licensure laws (Starr, 1982), initiated changes in both medical education and medical practice, the consequences of which are still felt today. Medical schools as diploma mills gave way to educational institutions responsible for the generation and dissemination of biomedical information, ultimately providing an expanding scientific base to medical education and patient care. Graduate medical education gradually expanded and in 1919 became formalized by the publication of guidelines by the American Medical Association, Council on Medical Education and Hospitals (1959). The subsequent development of residency training is further evidence that the profession of medicine perceived formal education as an appropriate response to an ever-expanding body of biomedical information, so that today nearly all graduates of U.S. medical schools enter residency training (Mayer, 1973).

Early CME Efforts

During the development of undergraduate and graduate medical education as formal responses to the "biomedical information explosion," formal continuing education was assuming an increasingly important role. Early efforts in CME were attempts at reparative education for the graduates of pre-Flexner medical schools. The primary goal of CME at that time was to correct deficiencies of physicians to make them more competent practitioners. Polyclinic hospitals and proprietary graduate-postgraduate schools were the primary institutions offering reparative CME programs (Shepherd,

1960), or as Flexner called them, "undergraduate repair shops" (Flexner, 1910, p. 174).

As early as 1906, however, the AMA initiated activities that contributed to the development of CME activities at the county level. The focus was on the local medical society as organizer and provider of CME, with no role identified for medical schools. These AMA-initiated programs were largely reviews of undergraduate medical education. This attempt failed, primarily due to the inadequacies of local practicing physicians as instructors and the absence of facilities for the programs. In 1911, after publication of the Flexner Report, the AMA reactivated these general review courses that, along with the proprietary and hospital programs, were the dominant forms of CME until around 1920 (Shepherd, 1960).

Although these programs remained the major CME opportunities in the early 1920s, there were signs of growing involvement by medical societies and medical schools. The role of the medical society in CME was fostered by a statement by the AMA Council on Medical Education in 1923. In this statement (see Shepherd, 1960), the council suggested increasing opportunities for county, state, and local medical societies to organize and operate diagnostic classes once or twice a year, as well as extension courses of lectures and clinics in cooperation with universities. This position of the AMA accounted for the increasing activity of medical societies during the 1920s and their assumption of leadership in CME during the late 1930s.

One of the first examples of university involvement in CME was the program developed by the University of North Carolina Extension and the state Department of Health. During 1916–1919 and in 1921, two instructors traveling on circuits at opposite ends of the state offered classes to practitioners on public health topics, similar to the agricultural county agent approach. The program was discontinued briefly because of financial difficulties but was resumed when the University of North Carolina agreed to assume operating expenses of the program (Shepherd, 1960).

Postgraduate Medical Education. The most significant example of university involvement in CME during this perioid was the creation in 1927 of the Department of Postgraduate Medicine at the University of Michigan Medical School in Ann Arbor. The department was to assume responsibility for educational activities beyond the M.D. degree, an increasing concern of medical educators of that time. This developed at a time when the distinction between graduate medical education (GME) and CME was not yet clearly drawn.

Many hospitals began to offer internships, following the publication of the Flexner Report. By 1919 the first general standards for GME were established and published by the Council on Medical Education of the AMA (American Medical Association, Council on Medical Education and Hospitals, 1959). Initial programming of GME by medical schools reflected an approach that combined CME with GME. In the early 1930s, for example, regional programs developed by the University of Michigan, Albany Medical College, and Tufts Medical School were designed primarily for the education of interns, with continuing education of hospital staff as a spin-off (Richards, 1978).

Specialty training and practice became well established, and specialty board certification was increasingly recognized by physicians as a valuable professional and economic asset during the thirties. As the internship developed and additional graduate education was recognized as necessary, the concept of a continuum of medical education began to emerge, to include three separate and essentially independent entities. Undergraduate medical education was generally viewed as the primary educational concern of the medical school and its faculty. The traditional rotating internship was isolated as a hospital staff activity and had little or no educational integration, either with undergraduate programs or the subsequent residency years. In some instances, however, straight internships in medicine, surgery, and pediatrics were part of some residency programs. Graduate medical education within an institution or a hospital traditionally has been the responsibility of individual department and program directors. Only recently has the academic medical center begun to assume some authority over graduate medical education comparable to that found in undergraduate medical education (Kinney, 1972).

The concept of continuing medical education as a separate entity of medical education did not emerge until after the development of residency specialty programs and their subsequent recognition by specialty board certification. Specialty training and CME were considered together, and the differences in objectives and educational values of meetings and formal courses of various kinds were not recognized (Shepherd, 1960).

In 1938 the AMA Council on Medical Education initiated the first national survey of CME programs. The report of that survey indicated that state medical societies had assumed leadership in CME, a major transition from commercial postgraduate school sponsorship common in the early days of CME. With the increasing activities of medical schools, a bipolar CME system was developing. Local CME activities were being coordinated by medical societies, while formal postgraduate programs were being coordinated by medical schools (Council on Medical Education and Hospitals, 1939).

At the same time, the focus of CME was beginning to change from reparative education to keeping up-to-date, a change that was made necessary by the advances in graduate training, specialization, and research. The flow of new knowledge was relatively slow-paced until the 1930s, and CME had the comfortable role of reinforcing, updating, and expanding the practitioner's knowledge base. The resultant CME programs were comparatively simple, not because they were not effectively planned and implemented but because the task was limited (Meyer, 1973). Educational methods used in the activities of CME were rarely different from medical school lectures and amphitheater demonstrations to which physicians had become accustomed.

After World War II, the increasing demand for postgraduate courses among physicians led to a steady rise in postgraduate offerings, with peaks in 1948 and 1952 (Vollan, 1955). A subtle shift in sponsorship patterns occurred after World War II, when medical schools gradually assumed a leadership role in CME. This was due in part to the fact that the AMA and its constituent state societies focused their activities on socioeconomic and political matters and in part due to the fact that medical schools were equipped to handle the influx of physicians who returned from World War II wanting refresher courses or specialty training. To assist medical schools in this postwar effort, the W. K. Kellogg Foundation supported the CME activities of eighteen medical schools in 1947–1948 (Shepherd, 1960). Commenting at a conference that reviewed the results of that funding, A. C. Furstenberg, Dean of the University of Michigan Medical School, stated, "acceptance of responsibility by the medical school for GME and CME is an outstanding feature of recent medical education. . . . Many of us will agree that the schools are not well organized to accept the responsibility, and the medical educators still do not have the best methods of providing graduate and postgraduate medical education" (Kellogg Foundation, 1947, p. 3).

In 1951–1952 Norwood surveyed the eighteen Kellogg Foundation–supported programs. He determined that nearly every school had a formally appointed postgraduate committee or its equivalent with a director or an assistant dean or chairman of the committee as the responsible official. Norwood concluded that these people were most effective when they were directly responsible to the dean, although the author recognized that there was no single pattern of administration that was universally applicable. Norwood further noted that a cooperative relationship existed between medical schools and medical societies, despite occasional difficulties that emerged as a result of the lack of coordination and the duplication of effort in program planning (Norwood, 1952).

Recognition of Problems in CME. From September 1949 through May 1951, Deitrick and Berson (1953) surveyed medical schools and medical education in the United States for the American Medical Association and the Association of American Medical Colleges. A sample of forty-one schools was visited. Although the authors were interested primarily in undergraduate medical education and, to a certain extent, graduate medical education, some of their attention was devoted to the postgraduate medical education or continuing medical education activities of these medical schools. The authors stated that the development of internship and residency training replaced the need for traditional postgraduate medical education, which had been considered as specialty training for M.D.s. They did indicate, however, that some physicians still enrolled in postgraduate courses to meet basic science and other requirements of specialty boards.

Deitrick and Berson identified three forms of formal postgraduate medical education prevalent around 1950: courses of free-standing postgraduate medical schools, medical school programs with an assistant dean or director, and entrepreneurial activities of medical school departments and individual physicians.

According to the authors, these institutions produced two major types of postgraduate medical education, in-residence courses and extension programs. In-residence courses consisted of refresher courses and longer courses. Refresher courses were conducted by clinical departments and were three days to two weeks in duration. Longer courses were generally two to nine months long and were preparation for specialty board examinations. Extension programs were offered in areas easily accessible to the practicing physician and usually at the request of local medical societies. Their findings replicate those of the AMA study during 1938–1940.

Another study, conducted by Vollan (1955) for the AMA, reviewed postgraduate medical education in the United States. The study identified a gradually increasing demand for postgraduate courses among physicians and a steady rise in offerings. It also identified two basic types of course offerings, the refresher course and the special course. The refresher course was designed to review basic medical knowledge and acquaint the physician with recent developments in a particular area. In 1952–1953, even though refresher courses represented only 5 percent of the offerings, they accounted for 20 percent of the attendance. According to Vollan, the difference reflected greater physician demand for refresher courses at that time, an important shift in emphasis. Special courses were designed to expand the physicians' understanding of one narrow field or aspect of their own area of practice. Some of the special courses were graduate medical education cram courses for residents. Others were long-term programs accepted by boards as equivalent to residency training or represented training in specialties that did not yet enjoy board status. A large number of general practitioners used special courses to acquire competence in various specialties.

The persistence of special courses, identified by both Vollan and Deitrick and Berson, indicates that there was still no clear distinction between CME and GME in the minds of practitioners and some medical school directors of postgraduate education. In addition, despite what Deitrick and Berson said about residency training substituting for postgraduate medical education, the lack of suitable resident training opportunities was a serious problem. With federal support of hospital building programs beginning in the late 1940s, however, the number of available residency positions increased, while the use of formal postgraduate education courses for graduate medical education began to diminish.

Vollan stated that 75 percent of all postgraduate hours were didactic instruction. He further stated that he thought didactic courses were more valuable for practicing physicians because they permitted them to readily relate new factual knowledge to their own practice needs. He did admit, however, that didactic presentations did not allow physicians to develop clinical judgment or improve technical skills. Small group discussion was the educational method ranked highest by physicians in his study.

Vollan reported that the vast majority of all postgraduate hours was offered by medical school faculty, even though sponsors included medical societies, government health agencies, hospitals, and public organizations, in addition to medical schools. Medical school programs represented 33 percent of the attendance in 1952–1953. According to Vollan, schools in public universities were more active than those in private universities. Independent postgraduate schools offered over half the hours, but the majority of their programs were not well attended. By this time, general medical societies had slipped from their previous position of leadership in CME.

Vollan's findings showed that only a few institutions had a full-time director to administer their postgraduate programs. Most commonly, the director was also responsible for graduate medical education, which may have contributed to the confusion that persisted between GME and CME.

The studies conducted by Deitrick and Berson and Vollan were critical of CME as it was practiced during the early 1950s. They reported lack of organization, absence of administrative mechanisms, confusion between graduate medical education and CME, minimal direction, and no evidence of educational planning. At the same time, some medical schools recognized the importance of CME and expanded their efforts. Increasing concern was expressed by a number of leaders in medicine, and a number of solutions were proposed to improve CME.

Improving CME: A Focus on the Practice Setting

Organized medicine and medical education responded quickly to the reports describing problems in CME and proposed various remedies and solutions. Some of them proved to be successful, and others were either ineffective or not feasible. These efforts fell roughly into three categories: administrative intervention, such as the Physicians Recognition Award coupled to accreditation; technological solutions, such as the "university without walls" for physicians; and educational solutions.

Physicians Recognition Award. By 1957 the AMA Council on Medical Education had published solutions and recommendations prepared by its Advisory Committee on Postgraduate Medical Education under the title *A Guide Regarding Objectives and Basic Principles of Postgraduate Medical Education.* Following publication of these guidelines, the Journal of the American Medical Association used these guidelines for selecting and publicizing programs. These criteria included recommendations made by Vollan to remedy the observed deficiencies.

In an effort to assure the quality of continuing education for physicians, the AMA established an accreditation program for CME that would provide the basis for rewarding physicians for voluntary participation in accredited CME. The program, implemented in 1968, called for questionnaire and on-site survey of CME providers, using a 1967 revision of the guide. The implementation of the program aggregated ten years of work after the publication of the Vollan Report (Ruhe, 1968).

Through the AMA program called the *Physician Recognition Award* (PRA), established in December 1968 and still functioning, physicians can participate in a variety of CME programs offered by sponsoring organizations and institutions accredited by the ACCME and be awarded credits, based on the category to which the program belongs. Physicians are given awards when they have earned at least 150 credit hours, in accordance with the schedule and categories shown in Table 1.

Several years later, Ruhe (1975) suggested that the link between the Physicians Recognition Award and the quality of care was at best indirect, since there were many steps between registration

Table 1. Schedule and Categories for
Physician Recognition Award Program.

Category		Credit Hour Limit
1. CME activities so designated by an accredited sponsor (60 credit hour minimum)		No limit
2. CME activities that do not meet specific criteria for category 1.		45 hours maximum
3. Medical teaching		45 hours maximum
4. Articles, publications, books, and exhibits		40 hours maximum
5. Non-supervised Individual CME		45 hours maximum
(a) Self-instruction	22 hours	
(b) Consultation	22 hours	
(c) Patient care review	22 hours	
(d) Self-assessment	22 hours	
6. Other meritorious learning experience		45 hours maximum

Source: American Medical Association, 1983, p. 3.

for educational programs and improved performance in caring for patients. He also acknowledged critics of the program and their contention that PRA was essentially a "brownie point" system. In response to their criticisms, Ruhe indicated that PRA was never meant to do more than identify participation in CME, that the standards could and would be expanded to encourage more relevant programming, and that in any case, the PRA served predominantly as an incentive for physicians to participate in CME.

Educational Technology. Initial proposals to remedy the problems of CME identified in the reports published in the 1950s focused on the application of educational technology to CME. One of the first technological solutions was a proposal for a "National Academy of CME" (Darley and Cain, 1961). This proposal had two major components. First, a national faculty would be appointed with responsibility to develop a comprehensive curriculum based on review and application of the constantly changing pool of biomedical information. Second, using the latest communications technology, this curriculum would be transmitted to practitioners to make participation as convenient as possible.

In response to the proposal, the AMA appointed a commission to outline the dimensions of the academy. The report of the commission's efforts (Dryer, 1962) describes a "university without walls" for physicians. The report advocated a distribution system (television and videotape) that would serve the physician learner anywhere, at any time, and at reasonable cost; a clinically oriented curriculum developed by a national coordinating organization and made available through the distribution system; and a self-evaluation program based on the best techniques available.

The thrust of the Dryer plan was improved communications from medical researchers and faculty to practitioners to provide physicians with access to a resource system of biomedical information. The use of television, according to Dryer, would facilitate the distribution of this information, codified into a core curriculum by a national faculty. By using self-evaluation instruments that would be provided, practitioners could test their learning after viewing a television program. Dryer claimed that the university without walls would close the gap between knowledge and application because it would correct the maldistribution of opportunities for physicians to participate in formal CME courses.

Several of the "innovative" approaches, such as the Darley and Cain and the Dryer proposals that had been developed to use educational and communications technology in CME, were critically reviewed by Miller (1963). He stated that the major goal in all the systems studied was dissemination of information, and he did not think that increased amounts of information was what physicians primarily needed. A major problem, according to Miller, was the approach of traditional CME, which neither involved the physician learner in planning or participatory learning activities nor provided educational experiences that were relevant to practice. Miller was one of the first in the medical profession to recognize the applicability of adult learning principles and adult education procedures to CME.

The purpose of CME, Miller contended, was to improve the quality of patient care. CME had failed to achieve this purpose because conventional approaches to program design, emphasizing subject instruction, had not been effective in changing physician behavior. He recommended instead a new model based on the way adults learn. He explained that there is ample evidence demonstrating that adult learning is made most effective by involving learners in identifying problems and seeking ways to solve them rather than through systematic subject instruction. Adults, Miller stated, learn what they want to learn.

Bi-Cycle Model. The approach described by Miller reached its fullest form in the bi-cycle model that was developed by Brown and Uhl (1970). Arguing that the central challenge of continuing medical education was to relate learning directly to patient care, Brown and Uhl enlarged upon the model described by Miller to develop the bi-cycle model. The approach consists of two cycles (see Figure 1). The outer cycle, patient care evaluation, is connected to the inner cycle, educational development, to relate learning directly to patient care. Both cycles start with the patient and the interaction with the physician learner.

According to the authors, continuing education programs developed in this way would be more relevant to physician practitioner needs than to the interests and assumptions of the education program planner or the instructional staff. The concept is quite different from the traditional approach to continuing medical education.

Patient Care Evaluation and CME. Linking CME to patient care evaluation programs was proposed as an approach that would make CME more relevant and would increase learner involvement in planning and conducting CME. A number of projects followed on the heels of Miller's remarks that suggested an integration of patient care evaluation and educational development activities. Some earlier studies, described in the following, examined the link between CME and patient care.

One of the first attempts to determine the impact of CME on patient care was a study done by Youmans (1935) that included a follow-up evaluation on the implementation of postgraduate courses from 1929–1934. The evaluation procedure consisted of unannounced visits to thirty of the general practitioners who attended the course and a comparison of their practice with an ideal, high standard of practice determined by Youmans and his associates. After comparing scores that practitioners received in the spot check with scores that they had received in an informal precourse

Figure 1. The Bi-Cycle: Relationship of Patient Care Evaluation and Education Cycles.

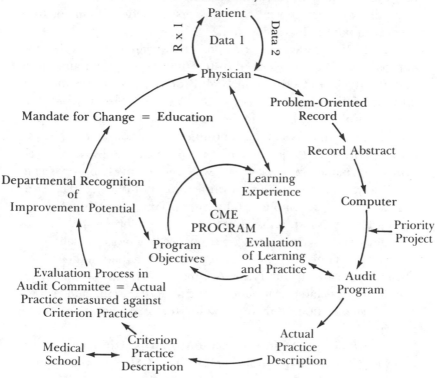

Source: C. R. Brown and H.S.M. Uhl, "Mandatory Continuing Education: Sense or Nonsense." *Journal of the American Medical Association,* 1970, *213* (10), 1663. Copyright 1983, American Medical Association.

test, Youmans reported a moderate improvement in practice behavior.

While Youmans's study suggested a positive impact of CME on the practice behaviors of physicians, Peterson's study (Peterson and others, 1956), conducted in North Carolina, indirectly questioned his conclusions. Peterson concluded that physicians who averaged fifty hours of postgraduate study per year provided a somewhat better quality care to their patients. Some of the highest-rated physicians, however, had taken little CME, and some of the poorest-rated physicians were frequent participants. Peterson concluded that CME had a "nebulous influence" on physician performance and suggested a reappraisal of the methods of CME (Peterson and others,

1956). In another study, similar to Peterson's, Clute (1963) indicated that there was no correlation observed between the quality of the work of Canadian general practitioners and the amount of time devoted to postgraduate education.

The first evidence of a comprehensive patient care evaluation approach in CME is described in the final report of an ambitious undertaking by the AMA in the Utah Project between 1963 and 1966 (Storey, Williamson, and Castle, 1968; Castle and Storey, 1968). The purpose of the project was to develop a continuing education process directly responsive to the continuing education needs of physician practitioners. Project activities were aimed at improving physician performance in a systematic way and at involving physician practitioners in the program. An integration of practice and learning would be accomplished by identifying educational needs through analysis of practice situations and developing specific educational activities directed toward those needs. The steps included in this proposed approach were (1) organization of national faculties, (2) development of criteria for optimal patient management, (3) review of physician performance using a set of criteria, and (4) provision of educational "therapy" with the assistance of a faculty expert.

In order to obtain information from practitioners, a form entitled "Physician Inventory of His Own CME" was developed. This form was designed to collect baseline information on the professional environment and felt needs for CME. It included professional characteristics of the physicians, circumstances under which they practice, opportunities currently available to them in CME, their own perception of their educational needs, and patient problems encountered in practice.

The procedures were pilot-tested in Utah during 1967–1968. A regional resource system was developed to include the medical school, the medical society, and hospitals. The operational unit consisted of the individual physicians and their advisor, members of the national faculty.

The authors contend that this approach differed from traditional CME by making the faculty and the organization responsible for responding to specific practice problems encountered by physicians and by generating educational activities aimed at these problems. Unfortunately, no final conclusions about the effectiveness of this process were reached by the authors because the study did not proceed far enough in acquiring evaluation data.

A similar project was initiated on a smaller scale, in Rockford, Illinois, by Williamson, Alexander, and Miller (1967, 1968). Addressing the fifth element of the Physician Inventory of His Own CME from the Utah study, dealing with patient problems encountered in practice, Williamson and his colleagues conducted a pilot study in which a community hospital and a university medical center explored the feasibility of improving the quality of care by integrating programs of continuing education and patient care research. Specifically, the pilot study was designed to measure physician responses to abnormal and unexpected results of routine admission tests (needs assessment); determine what, if anything, these physicians needed to learn to improve their responses (objectives); provide the required education (instruction); and reassess the responses to these screening tests (evaluation).

The success of this model depended on the willingness of hospital staff to participate in the project, the capability to obtain and review patient charts, the accessibility of staff, and a permission to intervene in the patient care process in the hospital. It also demonstrated clearly the necessity of a linkage between a medical school office of CME and hospitals.

Many of the patient care evaluation procedures that had been proposed to link CE for physicians with their practice-based problems were approaches for hospital settings. The Individual Physician Profile (IPP), developed at the University of Wisconsin, related CME directly to an individual physician's practice (Sivertson and others, 1973; Sivertson and McDonald, 1977). The IPP consisted of three components—practice profile, examination, and educational consultation and design of a CME program. The profile was obtained from information for a specified time period provided by the physician via tape recorder. The information included patient demographic data, presenting symptoms, significant findings, major diagnosis, test orders, and disposition. Diagnoses were coded according to *The International Classification of Diseases*, or ICD (1978), and practice profiles were developed for each physician based on the number of diagnoses in each category. Examination questions, filed on a computer according to ICD codes, were then administered to physicians based on their practice profiles. When test results were available, a consultant met with the physician to study the results, the practice profile, and whatever additional information was necessary. An appropriate educational program was then designed. The IPP approach required computer resources because of the large number of test items and the great amount of information needed. The authors indicated that it had been difficult to assess the success or failure of the approach, but they suggested that there was little doubt that the method did relate to individual practices.

Community Hospital and CME. Escovitz (1973) reported that a significant trend in CME has been the shift of responsibility for CME to the community hospital. The AMA has supported this trend in its accreditation program by encouraging state medical societies to accredit programs offered at hospitals for their staff.

Freymann (1965), Rosinski (1968), and Gaintner (1975) identified several reasons for the community hospital to serve as the focus for CME activities. First, continuing education should relate to the outcomes of medical care. This could best be accomplished at the physicians' work place in the context of their patients and practice. Second, the community hospital and the ambulatory care system reflect a realistic distribution of patients. Third, there are many competent physicians and specialists already in the community who could serve as instructional staff. And fourth, the decision-making structure in community hospitals is sufficiently flexible to allow innovation and change.

Eisele (1967) suggested that patient care audit in the community hospital would improve CME. Findings of the medical audit committee could be used to define areas of greater need, and CME programs developed in this fashion would use the physician's own patients and experience. All members of the staff would be involved, increasing the motivation for the formal as well as informal CME. Sandlow, Bashook, and Maxwell (1981) later reported that the medical audit process itself was a powerful learning experience.

Randle (1966) envisioned a dual role for the community hospital in CME. First, the medical staff of a community hospital could establish standards of practice in the community. When properly organized and operated, the medical staff would possess the necessary authority to supervise the work of the individual physicians and would have the power to withhold hospital privileges from those demonstrating poor performance. Second, activities establishing standards of care for the community could be directly related to continuing education. In order to accomplish this, Randle stated that the community hospital would have to (1) implement sound medical audit procedures; (2) develop learner-based teaching conferences; (3) maintain liaison with medical schools; (4) establish a comprehensive consultation network; and (5) under the supervision of a trained medical librarian, provide medical library services that include learning resources such as audiovisual materials. The 1970 standards of the Joint Commission on Accreditation of Hospitals underscored these recommendations by including continuing education in standards that would be used to review community hospitals for accreditation.

The federally funded Regional Medical Program (RMP) was viewed by some as an appropriate mechanism to prepare the community hospital for cooperation with a national program similar to that described in the Dryer Report (Dimond, 1968). In Dimond's proposal, the RMP would link community hospitals with such national resources as the National Library of Medicine, the National Medical Audiovisual Center, and a national graduate medical education center for national continuing education programs. Roles were described for (1) community hospitals, to collect and provide information about practitioner needs; (2) professional societies, to develop performance standards; and (3) medical schools, to provide educational resources.

A study by the Association for Hospital Medical Education (1975), designed to examine the role of community hospitals in the continuing education of health professionals, described the development of consortia among community hospitals in some areas for continuing medical education. A total of 127 consortia were identified, most forming after 1970. In the majority of instances, CME was a purpose of the consortium from the onset. Many consortia had graduate medical education and noneducational functions as well. Most programs offered by consortia were of the traditional CME format, though some effort was made in some consortia to use Professional Standards Review Organization (PSRO) and other audit findings as data for needs assessment. In addition to community hospitals, a variety of organizations participated in consortia, including nursing homes, community colleges, libraries, and professional associations, with some consortia having linkages with medical schools.

Stearns and others (1974) proposed an approach to assist community hospitals to develop CME programs. A method of educational consultation was developed in which brief, periodic inputs by medical center–based physicians trained in relevant principles of continuing medical education were used to establish working relationships with local hospital representatives, review ongoing activities, identify educational needs and local resources for program development, provide access to extra hospital resources, and recommend appropriate changes for restructuring existing programs or initiating new ones.

The authors also reported a study that examined the effectiveness of this approach as implemented in forty hospitals in New England. The CME activities at the experimental group of hospitals were compared with those at a control group of forty hospitals in the same area. The results of the study showed that the use of consultants facilitated the development of hospital-based CME programs. No attempt was made to assess the impact of consultation on the quality of CME or patient care. According to the authors, the implication of the study was that many medical school–based physician educators, with only a minimum of additional training and guidance, could bridge the gap between medical schools and community hospitals to facilitate the development of hospital–based CME programs.

Professional Standards Review Organization. To implement the patient care evaluation approaches to CME, access to information about physician performance in the practice setting is necessary. Access depends on the willingness of physicians and hospital administration to participate, the capability to obtain and review patient charts, the accessibility of staff, and permission to intervene in the patient care process at the hospital or in the physician's office.

Initially, it was thought that PSRO could be a source of standardized information about physician performance in a given region. PSROs were established by Congress in response to concerns about the cost and quality of medical care provided under the Social Security Act. The PSRO system included 203 regional organizations of physicians with responsibilities to conduct peer review of health care in a given geographical area. The mission of the PSROs was to review the medical necessity, quality, and appropriateness of services for which payment may be made under the Medicare, Medicaid, and Maternal and Child Health Programs (Goran and others, 1975; Jessee and Goran, 1976). Components of the PSRO review system included utilization review, medical care evaluation studies (audit), and profile analysis. The role of the PSRO with respect to CME was to provide information regarding existing knowledge and performance deficiencies that educators could then address by developing CME programming.

Some proponents of the PSRO system saw a central role in the process for academic medical centers to help these groups develop criteria, set standards, and provide educational activities to remedy deficiencies. One of the major thrusts of the PSRO program was to stimulate the development of CME to address problems discovered through review. In this way, PSRO would serve to make continuing education programs of academic medical centers more relevant by identifying practice-based problems (Jessee and Goran, 1976). Many hospitals and individual physicians, however, were uneasy about releasing information describing performance, and many hospitals lacked the staff for such activities.

The success of the PSRO in its initial years was spotty. In fact, there was not one fully operational PSRO even four and one-half years after the legislation was signed (Sanazaro, 1977). Consequently, the full potential of PSRO as a valuable information source about practice-related problems has not been realized. If PSRO had functioned effectively, it could have provided the necessary linkage and been a single contact point for a wealth of information about physician behavior.

Even when access to information is obtained, there have been problems associated with the data available. Review of medical records is central to the patient care evaluation approach to CME, but most charts do not provide adequate information. Linn, Stephenson, and Smith (1977) reported that poor record keeping prevented the accumulation of representative data for evaluation of care provided. Gonnella and others (1970) expressed concern about the limitations of equating actual clinical performance with that inferred from chart analysis.

A critical flaw in the PSRO model has been the training of those individuals involved in it. The PSRO process requires that those involved bring to their tasks refined skills as well as perceptiveness regarding both the factual measures of the quality of patient care and the more subtle patient behavior and health systems variables. Moreover, in separate literature reviews, both Donabedian (1966) and Barro (1973) criticized the rigor and precision of methods and procedures for quality assurance. Work continues to refine current approaches, and the necessity for CME providers to understand the process and the information it provides remains important.

Effectiveness of Quality Assurance–Based CME. Sanazaro (1977) reported some instances of significant improvement after an audit cycle including CME but suggested that there were many more examples where there was no impact. Donabedian (1969) and Barro (1973) reported in literature reviews that they could not find clear evidence that audit and CME were effective in assuring quality of care in the studies they reviewed. Sanazaro (1976) also concurred, adding that there was a lack of hard data to demonstrate that the combination of audit and CME had changed physician behavior substantially. Success in quality assurance activities, according to Donabedian (1969), can be attributed to two factors. First, physicians are aware that their activities have been made visible to their colleagues and others and that professional and administrative supervision is in force. Second, educational activities are associated with the analysis and review of medical care patterns and specific instances of patient management. Sanazaro (1977) concluded that it was easier to discern a correlation between the changing quality of care and administrative conditions, such as top management support and encouragement, than between the change and CME activities. However, more recently the same author outlined in precise terms various groups of factors reported to improve physicians' performance or to enhance the effectiveness of CE in changing physicians' behavior (Sanazaro, 1983).

Conclusion

This brief historical review of CME raises the question as to why the many efforts made over the years to enhance the effectiveness of CME have not yielded better results. The answer eludes most workers in the field, except for the recognition that there probably are limits to the human capability of voluntary change and that we have not yet found the best approach. Possibly the new information management technology that is being introduced at all levels of education will indicate new options for providing continuing education for individuals and groups.

The sentiment of many involved in continuing medical education is summarized by George Miller (1975, p. 701). In the paper entitled "Why Continuing Medical Education?" he stated:

I present this paper with mixed feelings. I am not optimistic about the usefulness of gatherings which merely place before an audience a group of speakers, particularly a group whose views are generally predictable from what they have already said and written about continuing education. Some of us have been saying essentially the same things for at least a decade; I sometimes wonder whether anyone listens. For, despite a seemingly endless round of conferences, symposia, round table discussions, and panel debates over the last twenty years, continuing medical education in 1974 is not greatly different than what it was in 1964, or in 1954, for that matter. There is simply a greater quantity of the same familiar things.

Despite the initial pessimism, the essence of his talk was a reaffirmation of the principles that had characterized the suggestions for improving CME and toward which this book is aimed: maximum involvement of the health professionals in their continuing education by relating it to their work experience and providing more interactive educational methods.

References

American Medical Association. *The Physician's Recognition Award Information Booklet.* Chicago: American Medical Association, 1983.

American Medical Association, Council on Medical Education and Hospitals. *A History of the Council on Medical Education and Hospitals of the American Medical Association, 1904–1959.* Chicago: American Medical Association, 1959.

American Medical Association, Division of Medical Education. "Medical Education in the United States, 1971–1972." *Journal of the American Medical Association,* 1972. *222* (8), 961–1048.

Association for Hospital Medical Education. *Role of Community Hospitals in Continuing Education of Health Professionals: Final Report to the National Library of Medicine.* Arlington, Va.: Association for Hospital Medical Education, 1975.

Barro, A. R. "Survey and Evaluation of Approaches to Physician Performance Measurement." *Journal of Medical Education,* 1973, *48* (11, Supplement), 1048–1093.

Brown, C. R., Jr., and Uhl, H. S. M. "Mandatory Continuing Medical Education: Sense or Nonsense?" *Journal of the American Medical Association,* 1970, *213* (10), 1660–1668.

Castle, C. H., and Storey, P. B. "Physicians' Needs and Interests in Continuing Medical Education." *Journal of the American Medical Association,* 1968, *206* (3), 611–614.

Clute, K. F. *The General Practitioner: A Study of Medical Education and Practice in Ontario and Nova Scotia.* Toronto, Canada: University of Toronto Press, 1963.

Council on Medical Education and Hospitals. "Medical Education in the United States and Canada." *Journal of the American Medical Association,* 1939, *113,* 757–792.

Darley, W., and Cain, A. S. "A Proposal for a National Academy of Continuing Medical Education." *Journal of Medical Education,* 1961, *36* (1), 33–37.

Deitrick, J. E., and Berson, R. C. *Medical Schools in the United States at Mid-Century.* New York: McGraw-Hill, 1953.

Dimond, E. G. "National Resources for Continuing Medical Education." *Journal of the American Medical Association,* 1968, *206* (3), 617–620.

Donabedian, A. "Evaluating the Quality of Medical Care." *Milbank Memorial Fund Quarterly,* 1966, *44* (3), Part 2, 166–206.

Donabedian, A. *A Guide to Medical Care Administration,* Vol. 2, *Medical Care Appraisal—Quality and Utilization.* New York: American Public Health Association, 1969.

Dryer, B. V. "Lifetime Learning for Physicians: Principles, Practices, Proposals." *Journal of the American Medical Association,* 1962, *180,* 676–679.

Eisele, C. W. "The Medical Audit Is Postgraduate Education." In C. W. Eisele (Ed.), *The Medical Staff in the Modern Hospital.* New York: McGraw-Hill, 1967.

Escovitz, G. H. "The Continuing Education of Physicians: Its Relationship to Quality of Care Evaluation." *Medical Clinics of North America,* 1973, *57* (4), 1135–1147.

Flexner, A. *Medical Education in the United States and Canada.* Bulletin no. 4. Boston, Mass.: D. B. Updike, Merrymount Press, 1910.

Freymann, J. G. "Wither the Director of Medical Education?" *New England Journal of Medicine,* 1965, *273* (23), 1253–1257.

Gaintner, J. R. "Continuing Medical Education in the Community Hospital." *Bulletin of the New York Academy of Medicine,* 1975, *51* (6), 739–744.

Gonnella, J. S., Goran, M. J., Williamson, J. D., and Cotsonas, N. J., Jr. "The Evaluation of Patient Care: An Approach." *Journal of the American Medical Association,* 1970, *214* (11), 2040–2043.

Goran, M. J., and others. "The PSRO Hospital Review System." *Medical Care,* 1975, *13* (4, Supplement), 1–33.

The International Classification of Diseases: Clinical Modification: ICD-9-CM. 9th Revision. Ann Arbor, Mich.: Commission on Professional and Hospital Activities, 1978.

Jessee, W. F., and Goran, M. J. "The Role of the Academic Medical Center in the PSRO Program." *Journal of Medical Education,* 1976, *51* (5), 365–369.

Johnson, M. E., and Gannon, M. I. "Continuing Medical Education." *Journal of the American Medical Association,* 1981, *246* (25), 2945–2947.

Johnson, M. E., and Gannon, M. I. "Continuing Medical Education." *Journal of the American Medical Association,* 1982, *248* (24), 3285–3287.

Kellogg Foundation. *International Professional, Educational, and Educational, and Special Programs, Cumulative to September 1, 1947.* Battle Creek, Mich.: W. K. Kellogg Foundation, 1947.

Kinney, T. D. "Implications of Academic Medical Centers Taking Responsibility for Graduate Medical Education." *Journal of Medical Education,* 1972, *47* (2), 77–84.

Linn, B. S., Stephenson, S. E., Jr., and Smith, J. "Evaluation of Burn Care in Florida." *New England Journal of Medicine,* 1977, *296* (6), 311–315.

Mayer, W. D. *Evaluation in the Continuum of Medical Education.* Philadelphia: National Board of Medical Examiners, 1973.

Meyer, T. C. "Toward a Continuum in Medical Education." *Journal of Medical Education,* 1973, *48* (12, Part 2), 67–73.

Miller, G. E. "Medical Care: Its Social and Organizational Aspects: The Continuing Education of Physicians." *New England Journal of Medicine,* 1963, *269* (6), 295–299.

Miller, G. E. "Continuing Education for What?" *Journal of Medical Education,* 1967, *42* (4), 320–326.

Miller, G. E. "Why Continuing Medical Education?" *Bulletin of the New York Academy of Medicine,* 1975, *51* (6), 701–706.

Miller, L. A. "The Current Investment in Continuing Medical Education." In R. H. Egdahl and P. M. Gertman (Eds.), *Quality Health Care: The Role of Continuing Medical Education.* Germantown, Md.: Aspen Systems, 1977.

Norwood, W. F. *An Evaluation of Programs of Postdoctoral Medical Education in Eighteen Medical Schools.* Battle Creek, Mich.: W. K. Kellogg Foundation, 1952.

Peterson, O. L., Andrews, L. P., Spain, R. S., and Greenberg, B. G. "An Analytical Study of North Carolina General Practice, 1953–1954." *Journal of Medical Education,* 1956, *31* (12, Part 2), 1–165.

Randle, R. E. "The Community Hospital and Continuing Medical Education." *Northwest Medicine,* 1966, *65* (11), 933–934.

Richards, R. K. *Continuing Medical Education: Perspectives, Problems, Prognosis.* New Haven, Conn.: Yale University Press, 1978.

Rosinski, E. F. "The Community Hospital as a Center for Training and Education." *Journal of the American Medical Association,* 1968, *206* (9), 1955–1957.

Ruhe, C. H. W. "Problems in Accreditation of Continuing Education Programs." *Journal of Medical Education,* 1968, *43* (7), 815–822.

Ruhe, C. H. W. "Governmental and Societal Pressures for Programs of Continuing Medical Education." *Bulletin of the New York Academy of Medicine,* 1975, *51* (6), 707–718.

Sanazaro, P. J. "Medical Audit, Continuing Medical Education, and Quality Assurance." *Western Journal of Medicine,* 1976, *125* (3), 241–252.

Sanazaro, P. J. "The PSRO Program: Start of a New Chapter?" *New England Journal of Medicine,* 1977, *296* (16), 936–938.

Sanazaro, P. J. "Determining Physician's Performance: Continuing Medical Education and Other Interacting Variables." *Evaluation and the Health Professions,* 1983, *6* (2), 197–210.

Sandlow, L. J., Bashook, P. G., and Maxwell, J. A. "Medical Care Evaluation: An Experience in Continuing Medical Education." *Journal of Medical Education,* 1981, *56* (7), 580–586.

Shepherd, G. R. "History of Continuation Medical Education in the United States Since 1930." *Journal of Medical Education,* 1960, *35* (8), 740–758.

Sivertson, S. E., and McDonald, E. "Medical Practice Related to Continuing Education by Practice Profiling." In R. H. Egdahl and P. M. Gertman (Eds.), *Quality Health Care: The Role of Continuing Medical Education.* Germantown, Md.: Aspen Systems, 1977.

Sivertson, S. E., Meyer, T. C., Hanson, R., and Schoenenberger, A. "Individual Physician Profile: Continuing Education Related to Medical Practice." *Journal of Medical Education,* 1973, *48* (11), 1006–1012.

Starr, P. *The Social Transformation of American Medicine.* New York: Basic Books, 1982.

Stearns, N. S., Getchell, M. E., Gold, R. A., and McCombs, R. P. "Impact of Program Development Consultation on Continuing Medical Education in Hospitals." *Journal of Medical Education,* 1974, *49* (12), 1158–1165.

Storey, P. B., Williamson, J. W., and Castle, S. H. *Continuing Medical Education: A New Emphasis.* Chicago: American Medical Association, 1968.

Vollan, D. D. *Postgraduate Medical Education in the United States: A Report of the Survey of Postgraduate Medical Education Carried Out by the Council on Medical Education and Hospitals of the American Medical Association, 1952–1955.* Chicago: American Medical Association, 1955.

Williamson, J. W., Alexander, M., and Miller, G. E. "Priorities in Patient-Care Research and Continuing Medical Education." *Journal of the American Medical Association,* 1968, *204* (4), 303–308.

Williamson, J. W., Alexander, M., and Miller, G. E. "Continuing Education and Patient Care Research." *Journal of the American Medical Association,* 1967, *201* (12), 938–942.

Youmans, J. B. "Experience with a Postgraduate Course for Practitioners: Evaluation of Results." *Journal of the Association of American Medical Colleges,* 1935, *10*, 154–173.

6

Interaction of Continuing Education Clients and Providers: Increasing the Impact of Education

Joseph S. Green
Linda K. Gunzburger
Emanuel Suter

This chapter describes the health care professional as a client of the continuing education (CE) provider unit. Health professionals are categorized along several dimensions that have relevance to understanding the role CE provider units do and could play. CE organizations are also described in terms of their functions in providing continuing professional education. CE settings, the traditional CE provider unit role, and new roles are discussed in detail. Finally, from the descriptions of the type of health care professionals served

*by the CE provider unit, several implications are drawn, based on
the philosophy expressed in the quality elements in Chapter One.*
                                                              —Editors

What are the roles the health professional and the CE provider unit should play to make CE more relevant? CE provider units'
goals are to have impact upon health care processes by facilitating
the learning of health professionals. This learning ideally leads to
enhancement of the health professionals' competence (knowledge,
skills, attitudes, and judgment), a significant factor in determining
how health professionals perform in interactions with patients. For
anyone involved in providing CE activities, products, or services, it
is important to understand the realities that affect the professionals'
ability to learn, to change, and to provide patient care. The health
professionals are those served by the individual and group educational projects of the CE provider unit. Who are these health professional learners? Of what significance is it that they are defined as
health professionals? What are the implications for the CE provider
unit?

Health Care Professionals: Clients of the CE Provider Unit

The clientele served by the CE provider unit may include any
or all of those with direct or indirect responsibility for patient care
in the various settings. This includes professionals who (1) provide
direct patient service independently, such as physicians, dentists,
and clinical psychologists; (2) usually provide services under direction of a physician, such as nurses, therapists, social workers, dieti-
cians, pharmacists, and many others; and (3) render mostly indirect
services, such as technologists and medical record librarians.
Whether a given CE provider unit serves one particular group or
many, it should know as much as possible about its clients. Familiarity with the dimensions on which one could describe health care
professionals can have implications for facilitating their learning
and can offer insight for CE providers.

Professionalism. A precise definition of the health professional is difficult, mainly because "today's health field is both complex and changing. Where 100 years ago less than a handful of

health professions existed, today's health environment includes more than 200 different occupations" (Nassif, 1980, p. 18). Each of these occupations claims professional status based on a standard definition of professionals—individuals who, through advanced study, have mastered a discipline. Professionals have been described as intellectual, learned yet practical, technically taught, organized, and altruistic (Flexner, 1915). They have also been defined as individuals who practice a full-time vocation (which is the major source of income) and have made a commitment to a particular calling. Another definition views professionals as individuals who follow a vocation with an identifiable body of knowledge applied to the affairs of others or in the practice of an art or science founded upon the application of that knowledge. Professionals can be considered as those who maintain a current knowledge of the chosen field and integrate it with previous learning in the performance of professional activities (Schein, 1972).

Another approach is to consider membership in a professional group as a condition of being recognized as a professional (Hepner and Hepner, 1973). The individual derives professional status from the organization and, in reverse, the organization's standing depends on the status of its membership. As Cogan (1953) summarizes, a "profession is a vocation whose practice is founded upon an understanding of the theoretical structure of some department of learning or science, and upon the resulting abilities accompanying such understanding" (p. 48). In many instances, the goal of professional organizations is self-policing through establishing performance standards, offering self-assessment programs, and providing appropriate educational experiences for their membership (McGuire, 1977). The ethos established by a professional organization may also influence the degree of initiative and sense of responsibility with which the individual approaches continuing education.

Houle (1980b) offers a definition in light of some of the attributes of a profession. According to his definition, the members of a profession should individually or collectively strive toward:

- mastering the rudiments of knowledge and theory that have been derived for theoretical and descriptive rather than practical reasons

- using these bodies of knowledge to deal with a category of specific problems and concerns that arise in the vital practical affairs of mankind
- transmitting this body of knowledge and technique to all recognized practitioners, both before they enter service and throughout their careers
- testing the capacity of individual practitioners to perform their duties at an acceptable level of accomplishment and to license those who are qualified
- maintaining associations that will advance and protect the interests of practitioners and maintain their standards of performance
- securing legal recognition of the special rights and privileges of the vocation
- establishing a tradition of ethical practice, sometimes reinforced by a formal code or by legislation
- establishing formal and informal relationships between the profession's practitioners and those of allied occupations

Autonomy. Another dimension on which to characterize health professionals is their relative degree of autonomy, which often relates to decision-making authority and power within the health care setting. Understanding these nuances should assist in providing CE that is more responsive to these realities. "Among the professions, medicine is both the paradigmatic and the exceptional case: paradigmatic in the sense that other professions emulate its example; exceptional in that none have been able to achieve its singular degree of economic power and cultural authority" (Starr, 1982, p. 28–29). Depending upon the type of tasks performed and the specific health care setting, a given type of professional will exhibit various degrees of autonomy. The extent of autonomy is determined not only by belonging to a profession but also by the hierarchical organization of health or medical care. In general, the highest level of clinical autonomy in the health care setting is accorded to those professionals with the most arduous or advanced educational requirements for licensure or certification, such as medicine, dentistry, and nursing. Others such as hospital directors and chiefs of staffs and services are at the highest levels of the organization and have a degree of autonomy that is dictated by their position as well as their professional standing. Their autonomy is based on the fact that they are involved in the most complex and consequential level of judgment. Their decisions may have considerable impact, affecting potentially large numbers of people in a decisive fashion.

At the other end of the continuum, other health professionals have little autonomy or decision-making authority. Their freedom of judgment frequently is limited by organizational rules or algorithms set by more autonomous professionals or by the organization itself. Organizational rules dominate their professional as well as their continuing education behaviors. These professionals are accountable to an organizational superior who is usually their employer.

Educational Requirements. The educational requirements for recognition as a member of a profession will profoundly affect the professional's later approaches to continuing education. The nature of the terminal degree will determine the level of sophistication and depth of knowledge acquired, and the inclusion of graduate education will be an indicator of the extent of specialization and expertise. Usually, formal graduate education or advanced educational experiences will raise the level of autonomy of the professional, often resulting in greater motivation. Requirements for professional education may also differ in the emphasis on conceptual versus technical skills. This will influence the type and methodology of continuing education needed.

Regulatory Requirements. Most health professions are governed by statutory or voluntary professional regulations that may include requirements for continuing education, either for licensure, certification, or acquiring and maintaining professional privileges. Mandatory continuing education has an impact on motivation of the professional and may influence the conduct of CE activities. The demand for CE opportunities is greatly influenced by compulsory CE requirements.

Nature of Patient Care Tasks. The nature of the day-to-day activities undertaken by various health professionals offers another contrasting view. Some health professionals are involved in very technical skills that require a great deal of manual dexterity. Others are involved in very complex decision making, applying theoretical concepts to practical problems. Still others need to be more sensitive to the subtleties of human emotion. And finally, some are involved in motivating their colleagues or handling administrative details.

Openness to Change. While the previous categorizations have considered primarily differences among professions, Houle (1980b) suggests that individuals within professions vary in relation to their willingness to adapt to changes in their work environment. Houle, whose work has been adapted from earlier works on the diffusion of innovation by Havelock and others (1969), describes five categories of professionals on this dimension.

The *innovators* are those who strive for the highest level of performance and who seek and carry out continuing education activities on their own. They search for new approaches to their tasks and may be in conflict with the established order. They are leaders of their profession, on whom others depend for new information and for stimulation. Often they are involved informally and formally in education of either colleagues or students and on their own may carry out scientific investigations. It is obvious that these individuals are found at all levels of professional standing. While their impact may be greatest in the autonomous professions, in the lower echelons they may have significant influence on work morale and efficiency.

The *pacesetters* seem to be less anxious to be the first but have considerable influence on their own professional group as role models. Their predominant posture is toward independence in regard to professional behavior and continuing education. Their influence is particularly strong on the middle majority who exhibit considerable dependency in their professional behavior. The pacesetters' attitudes toward innovative, quality performance and continuing education are strongly molded by their immediate work environment.

The *middle majority* makes up the largest percentage of practicing professionals. Innovations are much more gradually incorporated into their practice behaviors. Since this group is so large, the openness to change varies tremendously between those who are near the pacesetters and those who are near the laggards. There often tends to be a rather large gap between the realities and perceptions of vast numbers of the middle majority and the innovators.

Of concern to the profession and the public are the *laggards.* They usually perform at the lowest permissible level and require surveillance on a continuing basis. They need a structured environment to function at their optimal level. Regulations are most likely to be necessary because of their tendency to transgress their professional code of behavior.

The last category, the *facilitators,* have removed themselves from the direct practice of the profession and have become full-time teachers, investigators, administrators, or any combination. They usually work in educational and research institutions, professional organizations, or as administrators in a health organization.

Characteristics of the Work Setting. Another dimension on which to compare various clients of the CE provider unit is the setting within which they work. The work setting can greatly influence the motivation for and attitudes toward continuing education for any level of professionals. The provision of continuing education in a health care organization, hospital, or HMO, with clearly defined continuing education requirements for all health professionals, must be approached differently by the CE planner than in a setting that has no such official policy regarding CE. Likewise, the health professionals working in such an organization are differently motivated toward CE, depending on the extent of CE demands made by the organization in which they work.

With legal and regulatory provisions, the work setting establishes the policies and procedures that determine the extent of autonomy for each professional group in the organization. This may also influence the attitudes and approaches toward CE. Autonomous professionals may be more likely to seek opportunities for self-directed learning that can be promoted and assisted by the CE provider unit.

An analysis of the work setting of the potential participants provides an insight into the extent and way the professionals relate to patients, including the extent of their contact with patients, the level of critical decision making, and the potential consequences of the decisions made by these professionals. The learner who works directly with patients will be stimulated by learning about patients or by directly seeing the impact of new approaches on patients. The nature of the interaction with patients in the learning situation should be representative of that which the professional encounters in the work setting.

Finally, the work environment determines the mode by which the health professional is compensated, either by wages or fee for service, and who pays for the CE costs. On the surface, these variables may seem irrelevant to an educational planner, but in reality they may significantly strengthen or weaken motivation and thus influence the response of the potential participant to the CE effort.

CE Provider Unit: Serving the Client

Continuing education is in the process of change. Because of the rapid proliferation of CE provider units in almost all the health professions and health care organizations, there has been little organized growth (Moore, 1982). Most CE provider units now must generate enough income to cover their expenses; state support for CE is dwindling. There are calls for accountability and for CE to have a greater impact on health care delivery.

Continuing Professional Education. Health professionals have an obligation to maintain and, in fact, expand their competencies by learning about the latest developments of diagnostic techniques and treatment modalities. Continuing education, therefore, should be at the heart of the professionals' approach to their daily work. Professionals should be aware of this responsibility and of the need to maintain competence in practice, maintain an awareness of the theories and techniques of innovative practice, be aware of the new developments in the basic disciplines, examine ethical principles that are presented by new situations and influence practice, know how to provide leadership for the profession itself, and escape the boredom that comes from long, continued, and monotonous work (Houle, 1980a).

Houle (1980b) concluded that continuing professional education is distinct from other forms of adult education. Continuing professional education should be viewed as a means to help professionals be better problem solvers by providing them with new information and showing them how the information relates to their experience in the patient care situation (Gunzburger, 1983).

CE Settings. CE is available to health professionals in a multiplicity of settings, ranging from one's personal library to a hospital or a national association meeting. The definition of CE offered in Chapter One implies that CE can occur at any place at which health professionals spend their time. This includes home, office, professional school, professional and specialty society, primary work place (such as hospital or HMO), CE center, and other locations. For each locale, the activity best suited may be different and the relative contribution of the CE provider unit to the learning experiences will differ.

The *work place* probably represents the most influential and flexible setting for continuing education. CE in this setting may vary from checking a precise prescription dosage or brushing up on a specific technique (be it for the operating room, the laboratory, or the bedside) to more careful study of difficult patient care problems or calling a colleague for consultation. These activities all have in common that they seek answers to an immediate problem and thus are directly applicable to patient care. In addition, health care professionals at their work place may embark on CE directed at long-range goals. For instance, in an emergency room, a review of hospital admissions may reveal a high frequency of a particular condition. The health professionals involved may then decide to obtain greater competence in this area, although there may be no immediate cause for concern. Also in the practice setting, the health care organization may develop CE activities that are aimed at preparing staff for new patient care services hitherto not offered, such as introducing new technologies, or activities may be aimed at correcting identified patient care deficiencies. In all instances, the objectives are to optimize patient care, whether it requires institutional or personal effort.

In the work setting, the initiative for CE can be taken by the individual health professional, the health care team within the health care organization, the organization, or any combination in a cooperative fashion. While the approaches may differ, the expected outcomes usually remain the same. Although the general principles of quality CE should be applicable to all health professionals, the specific activities may differ, not only in content but also in process. For instance, in the hospital setting, the approach to continuing education of nurses may differ from that of physicians or housekeeping personnel.

Another important setting for CE is the *professional school* that assumes the initiative for offering CE activities, products, and services. CE activities represent, in many respects, a common format—a course given by a school on its premises or nearby or, in some instances, at a remote place. The planning, in general, is done by the CE provider unit, with relatively little contribution by the prospective participants. If involvement of the participants is solicited, it is usually done in collective rather than personal terms, that is, surveys, questionnaires, or other methods. The objective is usually not immediate problem solving but rather the general transmission of knowledge and skills considered relevant to patient care. Overall, the activity is designed for groups rather than the individual professional. The participant chooses an activity that is already planned, on the basis of announcements of that activity. However, many professional schools are turning to a more personalized or individual approach to CE.

One of the major goals of *professional societies* is the maintenance and enhancement of professional competencies of their membership. As mentioned earlier, the approaches taken by these organizations include setting standards for professional performance, developing self-assessment programs, participating in certification programs, and offering CE activities, products, and services. As in professional schools, the tradition has been toward group-oriented activities. However, the trend toward individualization is now growing.

Regionalization is considered a mechanism that may facilitate and render more cost-effective the dissemination of educational services throughout an area. Regional or national education centers serve this purpose in both the federal and private sectors. The Regional Medical Education Centers (RMECs) of the Veterans Administration (VA) provide a sophisticated structure for offering continuing education services to the health professions and technical professions employed in the VA health care system. The RMECs are staffed and funded to assume responsibility for total CE program development. RMECs respond to needs perceived by the top management of the VA health care system, as well as by constituent hospitals and professionals. Area Health Education Centers (AHECs) represent regional education consortia usually under the leadership of a medical school. Their goal is the advancement of patient care through offering CE opportunities using local and institutional resources. Both RMECs and AHECs serve multiprofessional audiences.

Other settings where CE is offered include voluntary organizations such as the Red Cross, the American Heart Association, the Arthritis Foundation; colleges, long involved in providing update courses to many of the associated health professions; and, entrepreneurs who may be affiliated with pharmaceutical houses, publishing companies, or organizations that develop and sell technologically sophisticated equipment to the health care industry.

Traditional Role. What has been, and still remains, typical for CE provider units is the offering of educational activities made up primarily of lectures, with minimal opportunities for discussion. Needs assessment activities include surveying a few individuals as to their desires and having selected faculty members determine the content of the talks. "What those people need is" remains a commonly heard phrase from planning committees. The underlying assumption, of course, is that what those people need is what the selected expert had to offer. Evaluation consists of a "happiness index" to determine how well participants liked the faculty, the hotel, and the coffee. The two most important factors for the success of a CE activity are where it was held and what "big names" were chosen as speakers. Oftentimes a hospital, the university medical school, and a local specialty society will be offering a similar activity during the same month. Little collaboration and much fragmentation of purposes still characterize the CE scene in any geographic area.

Of course, these are all only examples of suboptimal arrangements, not a description of the rule. However, a most serious consequence of this kind of system is the reliance on a limited "type" of continuing education, domination by the subject experts, and instruction that rarely involves the learner in the process. "Widespread dissatisfaction with a purely content-centered approach to continuing professional education arose in the 1960s because of the all-too-apparent fact that it was not working satisfactorily" (Houle, 1980b, p. 225). In this seminal work on *Continuing Learn-*

ing in the Professions, Houle notes that "the broadest outcome has been the widespread realization that the maintenance of learner attention and involvement requires the use of varied educational techniques. The same effect has also been reinforced by the growing realization that the achievement of an objective calls for the use of the methods suited to its accomplishment" (p. 224).

New Role. "There must be movement away from the content model, which encourages dependence upon teachers, to a process model, which demands a significant measure of self-reliance—a shift away from preoccupation with courses and methods toward an augmented concern for educational diagnosis and individualized therapy" (Miller, 1967, p. 324). As can be noted, this call for change occurred in 1967. While there has been some change, the pace must be quickened. What is needed is a new philosophical orientation toward the purpose of CE. CE provider units need to begin viewing themselves as agents for change, not merely passive providers of formal instruction. As presented in Chapter One, this new model focuses primarily on learning rather than teaching and, more importantly, on the application to the practice setting of what is learned in CE. Learning can be defined as changes in behavior, and education as changes in behavior that are planned and organized (Fleisher, 1973). This begins to expand the role possibilities of the CE provider unit. Potential new approaches can be summarized in two new aspects of the CE provider unit roles—facilitating individual learning and supporting organizational development of health care institutions. In both cases, CE provider organizations need to see the ultimate value in using new approaches. They need to learn the methods necessary to accomplish new goals and develop ways to fund the effort. Other chapters throughout this book will address the "how to's" of some of these issues in more detail.

In *facilitating individual learning,* the CE provider unit should be determining ways it can help physicians and other health professionals to organize their practice in such a way as to learn from it (Manning, 1983) and particularly to learn from their patients (Osler, [1906], 1953). This would involve teaching health professionals how to profile and categorize their patients and practice problems. Using one's practice and patients as a basis of continual learning is the essence of professionalism and of assuming responsibility for learning. This encourages the individual health professional to become the driving force within the CE arena. The provider unit can then more easily facilitate learning activities that are responsive to the "real needs" (see Chapter Eight) of their clients. Additionally, CE provider units should be making available multiple formats for their group learning activities—conferences, workshops, individualized readings, problem identification sessions, and others described in detail in Chapter Nine. Teaching the skills necessary to become a more effective self-directed learner should be a primary focus in working with individual health professionals. Using the new information management technology to facilitate interactive learning and linking the learner to national data bases are examples of new opportunities for self-directed learners. These are discussed in depth in Chapter Eleven.

Facilitating the organizational development of health care institutions is a second new dimension of the CE role. This may require some new thinking on the part of CE provider units located within hospitals and other health care institutions. Rather than being a fragmented series of seemingly unrelated activities, education and staff development should be an integral part of the strategic planning (see Chapter Twelve) of the hospital administrators and staff. CE should not be viewed as merely an expense item but rather as an investment in the organizational development of the health care institution. Education is only one of the tools available to management as it determines its present and future course. All CE within the organization should be administered centrally in order to share expenses and to allow staff to learn from each other. For example, the quality assurance and utilization review activities and the operations of the medical library should be integrated with the educational operations. Educators should be part of the hospital committees involved in problem identification. When problems are uncovered that have causes that lend themselves to educational interventions, CE projects would become an automatic outcome (see Chapters Seven and Eight). As hospital top management begins to translate long-range goals into yearly operational plans and resource allocations, educational staff should be involved in order to represent the capabilities of the CE provider unit. CE staff can also serve to facilitate interdisciplinary communication that may be hindering hospital operations. CE providers in regional education centers can assist hospital CE staff in their developmental role within the health care institution (Green, 1981). Finally, CE provider units should work together in a coordinated way, each taking advantage of their obvious strengths and mitigating any weaknesses, as they attempt to meet the needs of health professional learners and the organizations within which they work. Maximizing the possible educational approaches to meet the needs of both is the task. "The number of possibilities and ideas is not only growing but accelerating in its growth. Therefore, anyone who becomes dominated by some preexisting notion of how education should be planned is locked away not only from all present alternatives but also from those which are certain to arise in the future" (Houle, 1980b, p. 236).

Additional Implications. In reviewing the description of the client, other implications for the CE provider unit are apparent. Whenever possible, those involved in facilitating learning of health professionals should use peer review, patient care audit, or performance standards data as a starting point for identifying practice-related needs and concerns. The design of educational activities should always take into consideration the sensory demands of the relevant tasks performed in the practice setting by the learner. As an example, it is usually preferable to use hands-on approaches for teaching psychomotor skills.

CE provider units should be aware of who the innovators are in various health content areas. These individuals can be extremely useful when the goal of a CE project is to bring about certain behavior changes in health practitioners. Both the innovators and the pacesetters can have a major influence over the middle majority. It should also be kept in mind that most CE activity audience members would fall into this large category of middle majority and will not, therefore, be as open to change and innovation. This group needs to see the results of improved patient care in order to consider changing long-held beliefs or behaviors.

Bringing about change within a health care organization such as a hospital also requires some different educational "approaches." Decision makers (hospital leadership or department chairmen) need to be involved early in the planning of any CE activity aimed at behavior or procedural changes required of those with whom they work. Without the support of decision makers, these changes become very difficult to implement.

Providing CE opportunities for different groups of health professionals involves being sensitive to the differences among the various clients. Some health professionals work multiple shifts, requiring either different educational formats or a series of educational activities provided at different times. Some health professionals can be expected to select their own CE and attend on their own time, while for others with less autonomy, CE must be available at the work setting and must be designed with the needs of the individual and the organization in mind. Reading levels of different groups may vary drastically and should be taken into consideration when developing any educational materials. Time of the day or day of the week may be critical in the planning of educational or in-service training activities. When educational sessions are multidisciplinary, the perceptions of status discrepancies should be taken into consideration. It is not usually productive to make the pre- or posttest scores known by name or profession when certain individuals or groups will obviously score lower. Anonymous scores allow for needed feedback without sacrificing personal or professional pride.

Conclusion

This chapter has described the client and the CE provider unit and has drawn implications for a new role that should facilitate improving the impact of CE on the health care setting. Understanding the characteristics of health professionals as learners should assist those in CE provider units to be more responsive to their clients' needs. Based on an analysis of the described characteristics of health professionals, this chapter proposes a new or modified role for the CE provider unit. Moving from an organization providing workshops and conferences for large numbers of learners, CE provider units are urged to become more helpful to the health organizations within which they exist and to facilitate the self-directed learning efforts of individual professionals by providing assistance in learning how to learn from one's practice, linking learners into relevant data bases through existing modern information technologies, involving learners in the entire systematic educational devel-

opment process, and using CE as a more effective vehicle for the
organizational development of health care institutions.

References

Cogan, M. L. "Toward a Definition of Profession." *Harvard Educational Review,* 1953, *23* (1), 33–50.

Fleisher, D. S. "Priorities and Data Bases: Their Relationship to Continuing Education." In Project Continuing Education for Health Manpower, *Fostering the Growing Need to Learn: Monographs and Bibliography on Continuing Education and Health Manpower.* Rockville, Md.: Health Resources Administration, Public Health Service, U.S. Department of Health, Education, and Welfare, 1973.

Flexner, A. "Is Social Work a Profession?" Address before the National Conference of Charities and Corrections, Baltimore, Md., May 17, 1915. *Studies in Social Work,* no. 4. New York: New York School of Philanthropy, 1915.

Green, J. S. "Regionalizing Continuing Medical Education: Building Multi-Institutional Support." In J. C. Votruba (Ed.), *New Directions for Continuing Education: Strengthening Internal Support for Continuing Education,* no. 9. San Francisco, Jossey-Bass, 1981.

Gunzburger, L. K. "Can Lifelong Learners Be Identified During the Selection Process for Professional Schools?" *Mobius,* 1983, *3* (3), 45–52.

Havelock, R. G., and others. *Planning for Innovation.* Ann Arbor: Center for Research on Utilization of Scientific Knowledge, Institute for Social Research, University of Michigan, 1969.

Hepner, J. O., and Hepner, D. M. *The Health Strategy Game: A Challenge for Reorganization and Management.* St. Louis, Mo.: Mosby, 1973.

Houle, C. O. "Continuing Education of Physicians: Conclusions and Recommendations." *Journal of Medical Education,* 1980a, *55* (2), 149–157.

Houle, C. O. *Continuing Learning in the Professions.* San Francisco: Jossey-Bass, 1980b.

McGuire, C. "Peer Assessment in the Medical Profession," University of Illinois at the Medical Center, Chicago. Presentation at the third annual conference on the Professions sponsored by the Board of the Department of Education, New York City, 1977.

Manning, P. R. "Continuing Medical Education: The Next Step." *Journal of the American Medical Association,* 1983, *249* (8), 1042–1045.

Miller, G. E. "Continuing Education for What?" *Journal of Medical Education,* 1967, *42* (4), 320–326.

Moore, D. E., Jr. "The Organization and Administration of Continuing Education in Academic Medical Centers." Unpublished doctoral dissertation, University of Illinois at Urbana-Champaign, 1982.

Nassif, J. Z. *Handbook of Health Careers.* New York: Human Sciences Press, 1980.

Osler, W. *Aequanimitas.* 3rd ed. New York: Blakiston, 1953. (Originally published 1906.)

Schein, E. H. *Professional Education: Some New Directions.* Sponsored by the Carnegie Commission on Higher Education. New York: McGraw-Hill, 1972.

Starr, P. *The Social Transformation of American Medicine.* New York: Basic Books, 1982.

7

Planning
and Developing Programs
Systematically

Patrick L. Walsh

*Systematic program development encompasses all the components
necessary to provide quality continuing education activities, products, and services. These components actually incorporate several
development processes that include the identification and analysis
of educational needs, the design and implementation of educational
activities, and the evaluation of those activities and their possible
impact on the health care setting. This chapter provides the reader
with some theoretical and practical aspects of program development
and serves as an overview for Chapters Eight through Eleven, which
describe in detail the individual components of educational development. The chapter assimilates various models of program development and suggests a proposed approach that emphasizes impact
on the health care setting. At the end of the chapter, an example
illustrates the application of the suggested approach to systematic
program development in continuing education (CE).—Editors*

There are compelling reasons for health care professionals to continue their education: the knowledge explosion alters existing theory and provides new diagnostic and therapeutic tools; society is ever-changing and becoming increasingly complex; professionals are required to improve the quality of services rendered to meet increased demands for accountability; some individuals change roles within a profession (for instance, from direct care provider to administrator) or even change professions; and some health professions require documentation of participation in continuing education for relicensure or recertification to practice (*Compendium on Continuing Education Accreditation in the Health Professions,* 1977; Katz, 1979).

Learning occurs continuously throughout life. For health professionals much learning occurs incidental to performing their daily activities, for example, during medical audits or drug utilization review studies. Many learning projects are conducted entirely by the learners themselves (Tough, 1978). However, most health care professionals realize they must continue to learn in an organized fashion and seek activities that assist them to do so. Individuals who are engaged in offering continuing education for health care professionals are concerned with learning activities that are deliberate, systematic, and sustained (Szczypkowski, 1980). Deliberate learning activities are those that are engaged in for the main purpose of increasing proficiencies, with an application in mind; systematic learning activities reflect attention to needs, resources, objectives, activities, and evaluation; and sustained learning activities include a series of learning episodes. A systematic approach to educational development is a means of providing these types of learning activities in order to obtain desired outcomes and thus have an impact on health care professional performance.

Why a Systematic Approach?

A systematic approach to educational development is justified by the results that can be expected from its implementation. To inquire into the worth or value of an educational project is both reasonable and important. These inquiries become increasingly important as the economic philosophy moves from the view of "add

on" to one of "redistribute finite resources." There are finite resources available to provide the many activities, products, or services
that might be supported. If a new or different project is desired,
funding for that project might be obtained at the expense or exclusion of some other project or projects. Hospital administrators,
therefore, may want evidence that the continuing education activities that they finance actually have an effect on the competence and
performance of the health care professional and, ultimately, on the
quality of patient care.

In addition to the competition for resources, there is the more
general issue of accountability. Accountability is basically an obligation to reveal, explain, and justify what one does or how one
discharges one's responsibilities (Smith and Hague, 1971). Accountability, however, means something more than mere responsibility.
While the latter implies a commitment by an individual or group to
perform ethically or fairly, accountability is an implicit or explicit
contract between an individual or group who provides services and
another group whose expectations must be satisfied by the provider
(Samph and Templeton, 1979).

Continuing educators in the health care professions are
accountable to many, such as the learners and administrators, for
many things, such as instruction, income, and public relations.
Unfortunately, there has been a significant lack of data to document
the effectiveness of continuing education in the health professions
(Lloyd and Abrahamson, 1979). While there may be many explanations for this dearth of evidence, data indicate that the program
development processes used to design CE activities are a critical
variable in CE effectiveness (Stein, 1981). Therefore, CE provider
units are accountable to the health professionals they serve to use
those procedures that have the greatest chance of bringing about the
desired learning outcomes.

Most health care professionals are familiar with the medical
model for patient care, which includes diagnosis, treatment planning, treatment implementation, and follow-up. Planning for continuing education follows a similar logical pattern. It begins with
an identification of needs (diagnosis), followed by setting objectives
(treatment planning), selecting educational activities (treatment
implementation), and evaluation (follow-up). The most essential

step for appropriate medical care is diagnosis. Without an accurate diagnosis, any intended effects of treatment occur only by happenstance. Such is also the case in educational planning. Without an accurate identification of needs, any desirable outcomes will occur only serendipitously. Ultimately, a congruence must be established among needs, objectives, activities, implementation, and evaluation. Without such a match, the effectiveness of continuing education activities is purely a matter of chance. As diagnosis (needs identification) is a necessary but not sufficient step in effective health care, needs identification is an absolute necessity for effective continuing education.

The staff directly involved in designing educational activities will have a greater chance of realizing their goal of assisting learners to learn if they understand this rationale for a systematic process. As Stein (1981) pointed out in his article summarizing eight studies that reported impact on physician performance and patient care outcomes, the reason for the effects was that each CE project had been organized around sound educational principles.

The results of accountability and competition for resources, therefore, demand a close look at the methods used to plan and evaluate continuing education. A program development approach that focuses on the impact of continuing education activities could respond to the demands of each of these accountability factors. Impact is the effect of the educational activity and may include a range of consequences. Impact may be reflected by changed health professional performance, elimination of a problem, or improved patient health status. If continuing educators can generate data concerning the impact of their activities on health care professional competence and patient health status, they will be in a better position to compete for limited resources. If accountability is the obligation to disclose those acts for which an individual, group, or institution is responsible, then an approach that documents processes and outcomes can also satisfy that demand. Finally, if such an approach enables program developers to set goals and measure the success of their efforts, their continued motivation and growth as educators will be maintained.

It is the thesis of this chapter that the program development processes used to build continuing education projects are a critical variable in the resultant program's ability to foster impact. Therefore, a discussion of the theoretical evolution of program development follows.

Evolution of Program Development

Program development is the organized and systematic means by which educational experiences are shaped by continuing educators into structured sequences of events within given time frames (McKinley and Smith, 1965). A variety of educators, both in and out of the health professions, has proposed program development models. The unique contributions of a sample of important approaches are described here.

The classic program development model described by Tyler (1950) begins with a definition of purposes determined by considering studies of the learners, contemporary life, and the suggestions of subject matter specialists. Data derived from these studies are screened by the educational and social philosophy of the program developer and by the findings from studies of the psychology of learning in order to define specific objectives that will guide instruction. These objectives are stated in a fashion that makes them useful in selecting learning experiences and guiding teaching. Experiences then are chosen according to certain principles to conform to various categories of goals and are organized to produce desired results. The process of evaluation is designed to measure the degree to which identified objectives are achieved. The information produced through evaluation is used in future planning.

George Miller (1963, 1967) was one of the first health professionals to recognize the applicability of adult learning principles and adult education procedures to continuing education in the health professions. In Miller's (1967) opinion, CE had failed to improve the quality of patient care because conventional approaches to program design had not contributed to a change in the behavior of health care professionals. This failure, in turn, was attributed to the use of a content model, which emphasizes systematic subject instruction. He maintained that traditional CE for health professionals was not grounded in the practice problems of the learners who attended the activity and did not include enough participative methods to allow health care providers to develop the problem-solving skills they needed to perform effectively.

The process model proposed by Miller includes identifying problems and concerns faced by the potential learners in their professional activities, setting priorities of the problems according to their frequency and severity, writing educational objectives, developing an inventory of resources available to meet the objectives, using more interactive techniques for learning, and evaluating the results.

Brown and Uhl (1970) described a refinement of the Miller model (see Figure 1 in Chapter Five). Arguing that the central challenge of continuing medical education (CME) was to relate learning directly to patient care, Brown and Uhl developed the bi-cycle model in which an outer cycle (patient care evaluation) is connected to an inner cycle (educational development) to relate learning directly to patient care. Both cycles start with the patients and their interaction with the physician learner. In educational projects based on the bi-cycle approach, needs of the learners are identified by audit and possibly examinations; learners are actively involved in setting criteria for and reviewing their own performance; educational experiences are relevant to the practice of the learners; educational experiences include not only information transfer but also problem-solving activities; and learners receive immediate feedback.

Knowles (1970) drew a distinction between androgogy, the art and science of helping adults learn, and pedagogy, the art and science of teaching children. He described a number of phases in the process of program development to be followed when the principles of androgogy are considered. In 1980 Knowles revised the concept of androgogy to relate the principles to education for all ages. The unique aspects of Knowles's formulation include establishing a climate conducive to learning, creating an organizational structure for participative planning, and rediagnosing the need for learning based on the results of the evaluation.

Knox (1973) described a general approach that emphasizes lifelong self-directed learning. The approach places the main responsibility for continuing education on the individual professional. Unique features of Knox's framework are not only the focus on the health care professional as a self-directed learner but also the effort to recognize the importance of the work setting as it relates to continuing education, including the criterion of patient care and the facilitators and barriers of continuing education.

Charters and Blakely (1973), in discussing their model of continuing education for the health care field, made an important suggestion. They state that it is not enough to identify needs; high-priority needs must be identified and then analyzed to define whether or not the need represents a learning problem. Not all needs or problems are educational in nature. Oftentimes, needs present themselves as problems, but once analyzed, they may be found to be the consequence of noneducational factors. The discrimination of educational from noneducational causes allows program developers to invest resources where there is a likelihood of making an impact.

The concepts of Charters and Blakely reflect the fact that ideal program development has evolved from a subject-centered approach to a problem-centered approach. It is also evident that some elements of the different approaches are compatible and therefore can be incorporated into a combined approach.

Weaknesses in Current CE Planning Efforts

Studies (Pennington and Green, 1976; Stein, 1976; Richardson, 1981) have documented that CE activities are not planned according to adult learning principles or the previously described adult education program development procedures. Most current continuing education efforts in the health professions have several elements in common. They are based on a survey of participants' interests, focused on topics of interest identified by survey, oriented to specific disciplines, didactic in presentation, and provide but a single educational intervention to meet the need. This approach relies on several assumptions: health care problems with educational solutions will surface as topics in surveys; continuing education activities planned to respond to interest surveys will have an impact on the health professionals' competence and performance or on patients' health status; significant problems related to patient care are specific to single medical or health disciplines; didactic presentations will foster changes in professional performance or patient health status; and once participants have engaged in a single continuing education activity, they no longer have the need that originally stimulated their participation in the activity.

These assumptions appear to be invalid for several reasons. Often, topics evidenced in surveys are only a symptom of a problem, while the target for educational programming must be the causes of the problem, not the nominal problem; and frequently, topics produced by surveys do not even have an educational cause. If continuing education activities are to have an impact upon health professionals' competence and performance or on patient health status, the nature of the problems related to each of these outcomes must be considered. Topics from surveys rarely relate specifically to any of these impact dimensions.

The focus of continuing education should, whenever possible, be on practice-related problems and concerns and include all the disciplines involved. Planning for continuing education, therefore, begins with identification of practice-related problems or concerns that are further analyzed for their causes. Those disciplines associated with each cause that has an educational basis can be included in appropriate educational activities. If a problem indicates a need to develop teamwork on the part of a variety of disciplines, a multidisciplinary approach with the objective of building a functional team might be developed.

Reliance on didactic presentations limits the range of outcomes that may result from educational activities. Health professionals' lack of manipulative skills and the presence of negative attitudes, which are frequently component educational causes of practice-related problems, are not easily corrected by a didactic approach. Further, the opportunity to apply new information and receive feedback are severely limited by an exclusively didactic approach.

Health care problems represent complex educational challenges. It is misguided to believe that a single intervention could be an effective or, at times, even a desirable way to address these problems. The lasting effects of distributed practice as compared to massed practice is a well-known phenomenon in learning (Arney, Little, and Philip, 1979). Furthermore, as discussed previously, a patient care problem may involve many causes with educational bases, each of which must be addressed by learning activities in an integrated fashion in order to achieve the desired results.

Proposed Approach to Program Development

As a result of analyzing the weaknesses in current CE planning efforts and synthesizing what is known about how educational projects should be planned, a list of suggested program development processes is presented. The proposed approach is designed to increase the probability that continuing education activities will have an impact on professional competence and performance. This approach is premised on a set of assumptions: salient problems in medical care are detected through the use of multiple sources of data, with an emphasis on health care practice data; problems are identified that focus on practice-related concerns; not all practice-related problems have an educational cause; once practice-related problems with educational causes are determined, relevant target audiences (disciplines) may be identified; practice-related problems are complex and may require an integrated series of educational activities for a variety of disciplines in order to have an impact; the choice of educational format is best served by considering the nature of the objectives, as well as the learning style preferences of the participants and the available resources; educational activities that provide an opportunity for participants to apply new information and receive feedback will facilitate learning; and needs should not be assumed to be eliminated after educational activities are implemented—formal assessment of participant achievement of objectives and subsequent impact must be conducted as evidence for making that judgment.

The following paragraphs detail the tasks that should be addressed by the program planner in collaboration with the learners in order to develop high-quality CE activities, products, or services.

Identify problems that focus on health care. Data must be collected that allow planners to make informed decisions about the practice-related areas most in need of educational resources for a given period of time. One cannot respond to all needs in a limited period of time. A concerted effort in a few areas will have a higher probability of producing impact than will a diffuse approach in which many get little.

A variety of types of data is already available that can provide a planner with information to select practice-related programming areas: admissions and discharge records, patient care audit results, utilization review studies, morbidity and mortality rates, tissue committee reports, recidivism rates, critical incident reports, surveys of hospital staff, patient satisfaction surveys, and frequency of diagnoses (Green and Walsh, 1979).

When collecting needs assessment information, there are two principles to keep in mind: the faculty and participants involved in CE projects should have input in determining the focus of the assessment (Cole and Glass, 1977); when possible, data from different sources (for example, patient care audit, staff survey, and patient survey) should be combined to increase the validity and reliability of conclusions drawn from them (Webb, 1970). After the areas for possible programming are identified, the planner may want to make an initial attempt to set priorities among the areas. Because of fixed resources, all problem areas usually cannot be addressed during a single limited time period. Criteria, such as most frequent diagnoses, potential for loss of life, number of staff involved, number of patients affected, and materials available, should be established for setting priorities (Williamson, Alexander, and Miller, 1968; Green and Walsh, 1977). The introduction of new techniques and the professionals' desire to expand knowledge and expertise in specific practice-related areas also need to be addressed. Again, those involved in the CE program should be included in developing the criteria and establishing priorities. (See Chapter Eight for more detailed discussion of needs assessment.)

Analyze needs or problems to determine if there is a potential educational solution. Several steps may be necessary to complete this critical process. (1) Existing data are reviewed and additional data are collected that will help to further specify problems in the selected problem area. (2) Specific indicators of the problem are identified, which may be used later as indices of change. This allows planners to gather baseline data by which to judge the impact of educational activities after interventions have been implemented. (3) Causes are hypothesized for the top-priority problem. Most frequently, the problem is a symptom of an underlying cause or causes (Atwood, 1973). The causes that create the problem must be identified. (4) The causes are sorted according to whether they are amenable to educational intervention. Much time and effort are expended in developing educational interventions to eliminate problems that have no educational cause or basis. It is important, therefore, to differentiate between those problems that can be affected educationally and those related to the "system." Educational problems have a basis in lack of knowledge, psychomotor skill, or appropriate attitude to perform as expected. All other causes are systems problems and are as varied as lack of equipment to perform, lack of time to perform, lack of reinforcement for performing, lack of punishment for not performing, and undesirable consequences of performing as desired. One method of differentiating the causes is to attempt to state the educational strategy that might be used to affect each of the causes identified. (5) Priorities are set for education-based causes on the basis of those that have the most potential for impact on the problem. Each cause does not contribute equally to the problem. Therefore, it is important to identify those causes that have most impact on the problem.

Identify potential facilitators of and barriers to the learning process. Both professional performance and educational activity occur within societal and professional contexts that influence the performance of the individual practitioner. The program developer should be aware of the major influences in the professional setting in order to identify whether potential activities might increase professional competence, performance, or patient health status.

One type of contextual factor is the set of positive influences and resources that facilitate participation in continuing education. Facilitating influences include the high value the health professions place on lifelong learning; the encouragement and help available from project sponsors such as universities, professional associations, and community hospitals; the educational materials available; hospital quality assurance programs; requirements for relicensure; and the growing public concern about quality control in the health care field. A second type of influence is the barriers to continuing education participation. Examples include widespread professional insulation from normative standards, insistent demands for patient care, an overwhelming amount of new information and developments, and the increasing costs of many of the methods of continuing education.

A third contextual factor to be considered is whether the participant will have the opportunity to apply the newly acquired skills, be they cognitive, psychomotor, or attitudinal. If the equipment, patients, and organization necessary to apply the skills are not present, the skills will not be used and will soon decay. While these considerations may seem self-evident, they are all too often overlooked.

Select educational needs based on a priority system. The resultant causes are identified and the top-priority causes of a problem that have a realistic probability of change are selected. This priority system may also be based on feasibility and cost factors.

State educational goals and objectives for the selected needs. Once priorities have been set, it is possible to state educational goals and objectives related to each cause. Objectives should be stated so they relate to the causes, are understandable, are assessable, and focus on the learner (see Chapter Nine).

Select or design a learning experience to meet the goals and objectives. For any instructional objective or goal, there are a variety of alternative approaches. It is pointless to make decisions about content, methods, media, techniques, and devices without full consideration of the prospective participants, objectives, situation, and setting, in light of their systemic relationships in the flow from planning through implementation. Program developers at times reflexively select a particular approach, such as a workshop or a videotape. The key to effective programming is to be problem-oriented rather than method-bound in selecting a methodological approach. Method-bound programmers have a favorite method and spend all their time applying it. At times the method fits; however, more frequently it does not. Problem-oriented programmers start with the premise that the choice of methodology should follow, not precede, the delineation of the characteristics of the instructional task and be considered in conjunction with the characteristics of the prospective participants.

A review of resources available to implement the instructional intervention should be conducted. While the array of alternatives may be limited only by the characteristics of the task and of prospective participants, the reality is that not all appropriate options may be within the resource capabilities of the CE provider unit because human, material, and monetary restrictions set limits on the choice of an approach.

It may be possible to identify a variety of approaches that will reach the objectives effectively. However, programmers should be concerned about selecting the approach that will accomplish the objective in the most inexpensive way, not only for the CE provider unit but also for the prospective participants. The best-planned activity will have no impact if prospective learners cannot participate because of cost.

Inability of CE to result in impact on health professionals' behavior and on patient care may be attributed to a failure to use participative methods stimulating health care providers to develop the problem-solving skills needed for effective performance (Miller, 1967). Therefore, program developers must make every effort to provide learners with enough participative opportunity to develop the skills desired. Chapter Nine contains a detailed discussion of developing continuing education activities.

Implement the learning experience. It is important to implement the educational plan as developed for two reasons: first, after having invested effort and time in systematically planning the activity, the implementation provides feedback regarding the success of planning. Second, if for some reason the subsequent evaluation does not demonstrate achievement of objectives, the designer will be able to analyze the project to determine if there was a flaw in design or in implementation.

Evaluate the extent to which learners achieved objectives. Competence is a necessary but not sufficient condition for successfully eliminating causes and, thus, problems. That is, if professionals do not have the knowledge, skills, and attitudes necessary to perform, they will never be able to perform appropriately in practice. If planners intend to foster impact through individuals' participation in their CE activities, it is imperative that the competencies occasioned by participation be determined. Further, accountability in programming may be judged by results of measuring participant achievement of objectives.

If it is concluded that participants did not accomplish activity objectives, there is reason to believe that the project was either not effectively designed or not implemented as designed. A careful review of the planning process and the implementation should be carried out. The specific methods that may be used to evaluate participant achievement of objectives are described in Chapter Ten.

Determine the extent to which the original problem has been reduced. A problem is identified by monitoring a variety of indicators. Then causes of the problem are hypothesized to be educational in nature. After the activity is completed, the planner should return to those indicators to determine whether the original hypothesis about educational causes was correct and whether the indicators have been affected as intended. The test is to review the indicators to determine if the problem has been reduced to an acceptable level or eliminated. While achievement of educational objectives is important, the critical test of the success of a project is its final outcome or impact.

It would be unrealistic to expect a dramatic change in indicators after a single educational intervention. However, after a series of activities aimed at the causes of the problem have been implemented over a period of time, some changes in the indicators would be expected. If such changes are not found, it may be suspected that the hypotheses concerning the nature of the causes are incorrect.

Identify any additional tasks necessary to meet the need based on evaluation data. If data fail to demonstrate participant achievement of objectives, corrective action must be taken by the programmer. That is, the programmer must identify what caused the activity to fail, such as content, faculty, or planning. If appropriate, the programmer should offer a subsequent activity to bring about the desired accomplishments.

If data demonstrate achievement but fail to evidence any desirable impact, the programmer has another analysis task ahead. The failure to demonstrate impact may be a function of faulty needs identification. The causes hypothesized for the problem may have been inaccurate. Alternatively, the number of activities designed to address the causes may have been insufficient to occasion desired impact. It would be the responsibility of the programmer to trace back through the process steps to determine the most probable cause of failure. When the cause of the failure has been identified, new program design should begin.

Example

In order to highlight the critical aspects of program development, an example from a CE provider unit is presented. This example starts with a regionwide survey of hospitals, aimed at identifying broad problem areas related to patient care. The survey revealed a number of indicators from several hospitals that uncovered such health problems as emphysema and chronic obstructive pulmonary disease (COPD), diabetes, benign hypertension, alcohol addiction, and others. Because of the prevalence of patients with alcohol addiction within these hospitals and the lack of data on the impact of treatment programs on addiction, this problem was high on the priority list.

The CE planners then initiated an in-depth analysis of the possible problems in the alcohol addiction treatment programs. Several factors emerged, such as a lack of continuity of care for alcoholics, lack of compliance by patients with treatment regimes, the burnout of counselors working with alcoholics, and the lack of knowledge on the part of counselors about the new developments in treating alcoholism.

For the purpose of this example, the first area that was studied in more depth was the staff burnout problem. After interviews with several treatment units and an analysis of existing data, a list of several indicators of staff burnout was generated. These indicators included:

- high turnover rate due to transfer or separation
- frequent use of annual and sick leave
- incident reports related to abuse or neglect of patients
- poor health behavior as manifested by heavy smoking, overeating, and drinking
- incident reports related to medication errors
- health problems such as ulcers, dermatitis, and gastritis
- observable behavior and personality changes, such as social withdrawal, loss of interest in nonwork activities
- domestic problems, particularly divorces and separations

These indicators not only helped focus the nature of the problem, but they would also be used to determine the nature of the impact any resultant educational activity might have.

In analyzing the causes of the burnout problem, several possible hypotheses were developed. The CE planners then identified possible educational strategies to solve each of the causes of the problem. In this way, noneducational or systems causes were sorted. Table 1 shows the hypothesized causes and the strategies for eliminating the causes of the problem. As can be seen from the table, causes d, h, i, and l all were possible causes where no educational activities could provide solutions. (These causes were then referred to hospital directors for possible solutions.) Of the nine remaining causes, a planning group made up of CE planners, experts, and alcoholism counselors determined which solutions would have the greatest chance of solving the problem. This is depicted in the table in the left-hand column entitled "Rank Order" (systems problems are not ranked).

The next step was to identify goals of an educational activity aimed at solving the high-priority causes. Some generalized goals related to nonsupport from alcoholics' families: for example, describe the holistic approach to treatment of alcoholism (for alcohol treatment teams); identify the role of the family in treatment of alcoholism (for family members); and describe logistical guidelines for including the family in treatment (for both treatment teams and families). These goals are stated at a fairly general level and may require one or more interventions to accomplish each one. Further, the specific learner objectives were formulated after an analysis of each of the goals.

The next steps included designing and implementing a series of educational activities to meet the objectives that were developed to address the causes of burnout. The evaluation then focused on the degree to which these objectives were met and what changes had occurred in the health care setting, using the initial list of indicators of staff burnout. The same process was used for each possible cause, with the educational activities usually focusing on the solution to several causes.

Summary

This chapter reviewed a number of factors—such as economic competition, accountability requirements, lack of data to demonstrate the effects of educational projects, and the lack of rigor in

Table 1. Causes of Alcohol Counselor Burnout and Educational Strategies to Address Them.

Rank Order		Cause		Educational Strategies
9	a.	Chronic nature of disease	a.	Teach counselors adaptive coping behaviors
2	b.	Inability to reach short-term goals	b.	Teach counselors to set realistic goals
4	c.	Low success rates	c.	Teach staff more successful treatment approaches
—	d.	High patient dropout rates	d.	System problem
5	e.	Counselor's position and authority on health care team	e.	Develop team building, communication group process, and assertiveness
8	f.	Public attitudes toward alcoholics and people who work with them	f.	Provide community education program to change attitudes
7	g.	Quasi-medical stigma attached to alcohol treatment workers by house staff	g.	Educate health care professionals in hospitals
—	h.	Rotation of shifts worked	h.	System problem
—	i.	Nonvoluntary nature of patient's status in treatment	i.	System problem
1	j.	Nonsupport from patient's family	j.	Increase family involvement and teach holistic approach
6	k.	Inability to identify burnout early	k.	Develop assessment tool for health care professional—both staff and management
—	l.	System-reinforced dependency of patients	l.	System problem
3	m.	Lack of strategies to evaluate treatment effects	m.	Teach staff evaluation methods

considering adult learning principles for designing instruction—that build an argument for a reexamination of the methods used in developing continuing education for the health professions. A short history of the evolution of program development described the shift from content-centered approaches to a problem-oriented approach. The unique features of each approach were then consolidated into a suggested plan for program development that has impact as its goal. Each step in the proposal was then described, and an example of the entire process provided.

How might this approach be implemented? Each part of the process should be considered in developing continuing education, whether the programmers are solo practitioners or have a staff of twenty to assist them. The depth in which the processes are covered is not as critical as the fact that each is considered. If a phase had to be chosen as the most critical, it would be that phase related to needs assessment and analysis. As discussed previously, without an appropriate diagnosis in medical care, any desirable outcomes of treatment are purely serendipitous. Such is also the case in continuing education program development; without a valid diagnosis and analysis of needs to identify the educational causes, any desired outcomes from activities would simply occur by happenstance.

References

Arney, W. R., Little, G. A., and Philip, A. G. S. "Effects of Multiple Continuing Education Programs in Perinatal Nursing." *Evaluation and the Health Professions,* 1979, *2,* 365–372.

Atwood, H. M. "Diagnostic Procedure in Adult Education." *Viewpoints,* 1973, *49,* 1–6.

Brown, C. R., Jr., and Uhl, H. S. M. "Mandatory Continuing Education: Sense or Nonsense?" *Journal of the American Medical Association,* 1970, *213* (10), 1660–1668.

Charters, A. N., and Blakely, R. J. "The Management of Continuing Learning: A Model of Continuing Education as a Problem-Solving Strategy for Health Manpower." In Project Continuing Education for Health Manpower, *Fostering the Growing Need to Learn: Monographs and Annotated Bibliography on Continuing Education and Health Manpower.* Rockville, Md.: Health Resources Administration, Public Health Service, U.S. Department of Health, Education, and Welfare, 1973.

Cole, J. W., Jr., and Glass, J. C., Jr. "The Effect of Adult Student Participation in Program Planning on Achievement, Retention, and Attitude." *Adult Education,* 1977, 27 (2), 75–88.

Compendium on Continuing Education Accreditation in the Health Professions. Arlington, Va.: Association for Academic Health Centers, 1977.

Green, J. S., and Walsh, P. L. "The Use of Medical Audit Data to

Determine Educational Needs in Continuing Medical Educa-
tion." Paper presented as part of symposium on Alternative
Methods of Needs Assessment in Continuing Medical Education.
Annual meeting of Association of American Medical Colleges,
Washington, D.C., 1977.

Green, J. S., and Walsh, P. L. "Impact Evaluation in Continuing
Medical Education—The Missing Link." In A. B. Knox (Ed.),
*New Directions for Continuing Education: Assessing the Impact
of Continuing Education,* no. 3. San Francisco: Jossey-Bass, 1979.

Katz, S. "The Debate Over Continuing Medical Education: Continuing Medical Education Is Still a Controversy Among Medical
Societies." *Medical Meetings,* 1979, *6,* 6–10.

Knowles, M. S. *The Modern Practice of Adult Education: Androgogy Versus Pedagogy.* New York: Association Press, 1970.

Knox, A. B. "Lifelong Self-Directed Education." In Project Contin-
uing Education for Health Manpower, *Fostering the Growing
Need to Learn: Monographs and Annotated Bibliography on
Continuing Education and Health Manpower.* Rockville, Md.:
Health Resources Administration, Public Health Service, U.S.
Department of Health, Education, and Welfare, 1973.

Lloyd, J. S., and Abrahamson, S. "Effectiveness of Continuing Medical Education: A Review of the Evidence." *Evaluation and the
Health Professions,* 1979, *2,* 251–280.

McKinley, J., and Smith, R. M. *Guide to Program Planning for
Adult Education.* New York: Seabury Press, 1965.

Miller, G. E. "Medical Care: Its Social and Organizational Aspects:
The Continuing Education of Physicians." *New England Journal of Medicine,* 1963, *269* (6), 295–299.

Miller, G. E. "Continuing Education for What?" *Journal of Medical
Education,* 1967, *42* (4), 320–326.

Pennington, F., and Green, J. "Comparative Analysis of Program
Development Processes in Six Professions." *Adult Education,*
1976, *27* (1), 13–23.

Richardson, G. E. "A Sexual Health Workshop for Health Care
Professionals." *Evaluation and the Health Professions,* 1981, *4,*
259–274.

Samph, T., and Templeton, B. (Eds.). *Evaluation in Medical Education: Past, Present, and Future.* Cambridge, Mass.: Ballinger,
1979.

Smith, B. L. R., and Hague, D. C. (Eds.). *The Dilemma of Accountability in Modern Government.* New York: St. Martin's Press, 1971.

Stein, D. S. "The Continuing Medical Education Short Course: A Comparison of Adult Education and Traditional Education Approaches to Program Planning." Unpublished doctoral dissertation, University of Michigan, 1976.

Stein, L. S. "The Effectiveness of Continuing Medical Education: Eight Research Reports." *Journal of Medical Education,* 1981, *56,* 103–110.

Szczypkowski, R. "Objectives and Activities." In A. B. Knox and others (Eds.), *Developing, Administering, and Evaluating Adult Education.* San Francisco: Jossey-Bass, 1980.

Tough, A. "Major Learning Efforts: Recent Research and Future Directions." *Adult Education,* 1978, *28* (4), 250–263.

Tyler, R. W. *Basic Principles of Curriculum and Instruction.* Chicago: University of Chicago Press, 1950.

Webb, E. "Unconventionality, Triangulation, and Inference." In N. K. Denzin (Ed.), *Sociological Methods.* Chicago: Aldine, 1970.

Williamson, J. W., Alexander, M., and Miller, G. E. "Priorities in Patient Care Research and Continuing Medical Education." *Journal of the American Medical Association,* 1968, *204,* 303–308.

8

Identifying
and Assessing Needs
to Relate
Continuing Education
to Patient Care

Harold G. Levine, Donald L. Cordes
Donald E. Moore, Jr., Floyd C. Pennington

Needs assessment as part of systematic educational development is
described in detail in this chapter. For anyone within a continuing
education (CE) provider unit with the responsibility of assessing the
needs of the target audience, this chapter provides an approach to
how this might be accomplished. The authors and editors realize
that CE provider units vary tremendously in the resources they have
available for this activity. The approach described here can be
adapted to the capabilities of the CE provider unit, using methods of
information collection that are most feasible. The major part of the
chapter explains how to develop a needs assessment plan that speci-

fies the purpose, the audience for the assessment results, issues to be dealt with in the needs assessment, resources available, information required, analysis procedures, and means of reporting findings that allow use of those data.—Editors

If a continuing education provider unit is to influence the provision of health care, it must develop systematic methods for gathering data about the role the organization can perform in improving the health care system—it must conduct effective assessment of the needs of the health professionals it serves. Needs assessment is as essential for designing educational activities (see Chapters Nine and Eleven) as it is for evaluating the effectiveness of learning activities offered (see Chapter Ten).

In an atmosphere of cost containment in health care, CE providers must maximize the use of scarce educational resources. Concurrent with this push for cost containment is an increasing concern that CE produce observable results. Needs assessment can be used by those responsible for CE to identify relevant problems and to focus on areas of maximum benefit to the organization and the individual health care professional. To be most effective, needs assessment should be conducted as a rational, planned process, so that the findings are readily usable in program development.

Definitions

Needs assessment is defined as a decision-making process that provides information about the necessity and feasibility of an educational intervention. In the broadest terms, a need is a discrepancy between an existing set of circumstances and some desired set of circumstances (Knox, 1965). Discrepancies can be described in terms of knowledge or attitude, performance, or system deficits. In the case of discrepancies in knowledge or attitude, it is assumed that a need is based on lack of knowledge or the need for a change in attitude on the part of the individual. The advantage of this definition is that need can be reduced or eliminated by using well-known methods of education that emphasize information transfer. In terms of knowledge deficits, its disadvantage, however, is that failure to perform optimally may be the consequence of not applying knowledge already possessed (Miller, 1967).

McKinley (1973) describes what is called "real needs" and suggests two subcategories of real needs—performance discrepancy and performance enrichment. Performance discrepancy, the gap between desired and actual performance, can be based upon normative, scientific, or comparative data. This definition encourages the development of criteria for effective performance, which in itself is a learning experience with potential for increasing the proficiency of those involved (Sandlow, Bashook, and Maxwell, 1981). The disadvantages of this approach are the cost of appraisals (Sivertson and others, 1973; Brown, 1977) and the current state of technology for effective measurement of performance within many settings in which health care occurs (Coordinating Council on Medical Education, 1979).

Performance enrichment is defined as identifying areas where health professionals desire to expand their competence. This usually requires a comparison of the status of a practitioner group and the most recent scientific and technological information. The approach resembles a performance deficit analysis in that it relies heavily on expert opinion about what would improve the functioning of the practitioner group or health care organization. An analysis of needs for performance enrichment differs from performance deficit analysis by focusing on improvement and growth rather than remediation.

When needs are defined as a systems deficit, it is assumed that the setting in which health care is delivered influences the quality of care as much as the health professionals' competence or proficiency. The advantage of this definition is its economy. Resources are committed only to critical problems in the system that have a significant effect on health care delivery. The disadvantage is that it offers little help to continuing educators unless education and assessments of quality of care are conducted together at the institution. Persons responsible for planning and conducting CE can do little to influence directly deficiencies in health care systems unless they have a link to the assessment and delivery of care. If quality assessment is used to identify needs, definitions of acceptable care should be based on valid standards of care, which are not always easy to obtain (Sanazaro, 1976).

Some experts use the term *real needs* to describe the discrepancies between optimal and actual care. Educational needs as defined by potential learners are called "felt needs" (Atwood and Ellis, 1971). Felt needs may be real needs. Practitioners often decide what they are going to learn based upon felt needs. One task of CE provider units is to assist health care professionals in identifying which of their needs can be solved through education. Health care professionals may articulate their felt needs into expressed needs or requests for action. Responding to expressed needs and ascertaining real needs that can be met through education is a continuing challenge. It is also a task of the CE provider unit to assist health care professionals in perceiving as *felt needs* those that have been identified as *real needs*. Unless the professional recognizes an identified discrepancy, it does little good to offer "solutions."

Levels of Needs Assessment

The desired final product of needs assessment is an ordered specification of educational needs in a form that can be readily used in developing educational projects. A complete and systematic needs assessment is one that is conducted at three different levels: the strategic level, the programmatic level, and the individual project level. The distinction between levels is based on the purpose of acquiring the information and the focus of the assessment. Because each level provides information for different purposes in the educational development process, all three levels are not necessarily assessed each time a needs assessment is conducted. A strategic level needs assessment may only be conducted once every three to five years, while a programmatic level needs assessment is usually carried out at least once a year, and, whenever possible, project level assessment is completed for each educational offering. The issues at each level must be defined and examined as thoroughly as possible. The results of assessment at each level help focus planning for the next level of assessment. Regardless of the size or type of CE provider unit, each of these levels of assessment should be undertaken in order to develop educational projects that are responsive to the needs of health professionals.

Strategic Level. Needs assessment at this level provides information for long-range planning for the CE provider unit. Assessment results identify general content areas and the professions that will be addressed by the CE provider unit during a specified period of time. Information gained from the strategic level needs assessment usually indicates the direction of programming for three to five years.

Data sought for strategic level needs assessment include current health care issues, new knowledge and technology affecting health care delivery, and social, cultural, and environmental issues. For example, identification of problems and concerns at this level may reflect the recent needs of Vietnam veterans, the higher median age of the population, or the prevalence of hypertension among various ethnic groups. A needs assessment at the strategic level should examine local community needs, institutional needs, and national health issues.

The results of an assessment at this level will aid administrators and CE planners in making decisions concerning long-term focus and the future direction of program development within their organization. Although a complete needs assessment at this level may only be conducted every few years, the long-term goals should be reviewed yearly to determine if any changes are necessary.

Some of the issues that should be examined for a strategic level needs assessment include:

- major health problems under the jurisdiction of the parent institution and the CE provider unit
- significant changes in health care delivery that warrant education of health care delivery personnel
- organizational or mission changes of the institution(s) served by the CE provider unit or those of the CE provider unit itself
- technological, scientific, and biomedical advances that require dissemination to health care providers through CE
- demographic patterns of those served by the health care facility and those served by the CE provider unit
- local environmental, social, or cultural factors that influence health care
- health manpower distribution

These issues establish the framework in which the CE provider unit functions with respect to its parent organization, the community it serves, and the changes and advances that affect the delivery of health care. From the results, decisions are made concerning the general subject areas the CE provider unit will address, where it will spend resources, and which general target audiences will be involved.

Programmatic Level. Needs assessment at the programmatic level provides information about specific concerns within the general areas identified at the strategic level. For example, if as a result of national or community demographic changes, concerns about health problems of the aged were identified at the strategic level as one content area to be addressed by the CE provider unit, assessment at the programmatic level would identify specific topics of focus for educational programs, such as nutritional assessment of the elderly.

Those responsible for developing programs are predominantly concerned with this level of needs assessment. Where a strategic level assessment establishes the general direction for the programmatic concerns of the organization, results of a programmatic needs assessment will help continuing education administrators, planning committees of CE provider units, and instructional designers make decisions that determine the specific topic areas of the continuing education activities.

Areas of emphasis established as a result of the strategic level assessment are examined in some detail during the programmatic assessment. Issues that should be reviewed at the programmatic level include:

- specific problems or concerns that exist relative to the content areas identified at the strategic level
- specific groups or individuals that are affected by the problem or concern
- factors (educational, managerial, or both) that contribute to the prevalence of the identified problems
- the expressed educational needs and interests of the health professionals as related to the content area

The outcome of a programmatic needs assessment is a list of program topics that will be offered by the continuing education provider unit. The topics are within the general areas previously established, relate to the causes of the problems or concerns, and address the needs and interests of those health providers most involved.

Project Level. Currently, many CE providers are conducting needs assessment at the programmatic level to determine which programs to develop. However, program planners often do not give adequate attention to on-the-job performance and the actual knowledge, skills, and attitudes of the learners. With a clear understanding of the actual performance of those involved in the delivery of health care, the educator will be able to focus the programs identified at the programmatic level so they are appropriate for the audience. For example, if the problem identified at the programmatic level is one of performance deficit, an assessment of the present level of the learners' performance can be used to focus an educational intervention on specific content at the appropriate level for the learners.

Although this may seem like an additional step to those units that are small and have limited budgets, it is a major factor in designing relevant educational projects. Too often project level needs assessment is not undertaken. Assumptions are made about the participants' knowledge, skills, and attitudes; as a result of incorrect assumptions, activities often miss their mark. The desired outcome is not obtained and valuable resources are depleted.

Projects that are based on professionals' practice situation and present levels of knowledge will be more interesting and beneficial to learners and will have a greater impact on learners' performance than projects that unnecessarily review information already known to learners or that present information at too complex levels. The assessment results can also be used to develop project objectives and to aid faculty in developing content that will best meet the needs of the identified audience.

Table 1 provides a brief description of the three levels of assessment and gives two examples of the results of the issues assessed at each level.

The description of the three levels of assessment represents the ideal plan for determining learner and institutional needs. The scope of the assessment at each level will depend on the continuing education responsibility and size of the CE provider unit. For

Table 1. Examples of Needs Assessment Outcomes.

Needs Assessment Level	Outcomes of Needs Assessment	
	Example 1	Example 2
Strategic Needs Assessment Long term planning to address major issues, such as new technology and mission changes	Health Care of the Aged Increasing age of patient population indicates this as a problem area to be addressed in the coming years.	Automatic Data Processing (ADP) An institutional shift to use of minicomputers for all record keeping will require staff training.
Programmatic Needs Assessment Specification of problems and concerns within content areas identified in strategic needs assessment, including decisions on education or management action	Nutrition of the Aged Providing for proper nutritional care of patients is indicated as a specific problem requiring programmatic effort.	Accessing Patient Information Health professionals' skills and understanding of minicomputers as applied to patient record keeping is assessed to develop program at appropriate level.
Project Needs Assessment Actual learner knowledge, skills, and attitudes related to specific programmatic area	A Nurse's Ability to Conduct a Dietary Assessment Individuals' performances are measured and compared to desired performance, to identify what learning is necessary.	Application of ADP to Patient Record Keeping Health professionals' specific needs are identified, such as learning how to use ADP for entering and obtaining information about patients.

example, needs assessment for a national association may require the collection of data on innovations in practice, statistics on national demographics, prevalence data, and political issues. A strategic level assessment at a small hospital would have a different focus. The data generated by the national association could provide an existing source of information for the hospital. Other strategic level information might include the opening of a new wing or the closing of an alcoholism clinic in the community, which could influence the educational needs of the health professionals served by the hospital CE provider unit.

Systematic needs assessment is also influenced by unanticipated programming needs. If there is a sudden outbreak of infection
after surgery in a community hospital, an immediate assessment
may be called for, to investigate the causes of the problem and to
suggest the corrective interventions needed. If new regulations or
procedures are issued by a national organization, local institution,
or by specialty boards, educational programs may be required, even
though they did not result from programmatic assessment and were
not included in earlier planning. In these cases, program and project
level assessments are still appropriate to determine the specific needs
of the audience.

Developing a Needs Assessment Plan

A plan for needs assessment may be viewed as as blueprint
that provides information about the intended needs assessment
activities. Since there are many ways to assess needs and many techniques that can be employed, a needs assessment plan will help the
educator identify specific decisions required and activities to be
accomplished. The specifics of a needs assessment plan will, of
course, differ from project to project, but the basic elements are the
same for all plans.

Purpose. The needs assessment plan begins with a statement
of purpose—the reason for conducting the assessment. The purpose
distinguishes the level of the needs assessment (strategic, programmatic, or project level), states the specific problem areas that will be
examined, and specifies who will be involved. The general issues
that relate to the appropriate level of assessment are the basis for
identifying the focus of the needs assessment. Based on these issues,
statements can be developed that reflect why the needs assessment is
being conducted and what outcome is expected. In some cases all the
problem areas are explored, and in other cases only selected issues
are examined.

Audience. The audience for needs assessment results must be
identified at the outset. Typical audiences include hospital educators, program planning committees, potential faculty, potential participants, program funders, organizational sponsors, professional
societies, and various levels of administration. The special interests
of these individuals and groups in the needs assessment activities, as
well as in the project that might follow, should be considered in the

formulation of a needs assessment plan. Because audiences have different requirements and preferences, individuals who conduct needs assessments should be aware of the information desired by these audiences so that the design and conduct of the assessment can reflect those interests. It is important to consider the legitimacy and urgency of each audience. Their support will be important to the success of the project.

Issues. Each needs assessment should focus on specified concerns to ensure that the results contribute to program planning. Issues may be general, focusing on major health problems, new technology requiring information dissemination, or needs of the community that the CE provider unit serves. They may also relate to the identification of specific problems or needs within a particular area, such as cardiology, thus defining project topics and the appropriate audience.

Issues are identified by talking with the audience, potential participants, and faculty experts in the subject area or by past experience. It is important that the educational planner and the primary users for needs assessment concur on issues and their priority established on the basis of importance and available resources.

Resources. It is also necessary in the planning stages to determine the resources that will be available for the needs assessment activity. The available resources will influence the scale of the effort, the types and amount of information that can be collected, and the methods used to collect the information. Planners should determine the type of expertise and number of staff available to work on needs assessment, the amount of money available, personnel time that can be used for the project, and the supplies and services available.

Types of Data. An important decision when planning a needs assessment project is selecting the data to be collected to address identified issues. Generally, there are four categories of data: individual performance, individual characteristics, the work setting, and health status indicators. The focus of the data search often will differ, depending on the level of the need assessment.

The major issues addressed at the strategic and programmatic levels are characterized by their generality. Assessments at these levels define the major issues by focusing on individual characteristics, the work setting, and health status indicators, rather than specific levels of individuals' performances. Project level assessment is centered primarily around performance data. An examination of the individual's characteristics, their work setting, and relevant health status indicators adds to the planner's understanding of individuals' performances.

Performance data consist of descriptions of identifiable current behavior of health professionals in the work setting, as well as specification of accepted standards of practice, if available. Data describing *individual characteristics* of the professional include age, sex, professional responsibilities, learning style preferences, and CE participation patterns. They help the planner get a picture of the audience that will be attending future projects and can sometimes help in identifying the causes of problems. Data about the *work setting* describe the environment in which the health professional works. Information about the scope of practice, patient mix, staffing, organization, and professional requirements, for example, provide a perspective of the organizational framework and the day-to-day job requirements of the professional. These data are often used to help determine if a problem is primarily educational or managerial. *Health status indicators,* usually referred to as epidemiological data, describe the incidence and patterns of particular diseases, morbidity and mortality, and the environmental, social, cultural, and economic influences among the population served by the institution and the CE provider unit.

Planners should exercise care when selecting types of data because the quality of data selected will ultimately have an impact on the outcome of the needs assessment. Some data are considered to be "hard" data because they are objective and quantifiable. Self-reported or subjective data are considered to be "soft." Planners should not rely exclusively on either subjective or objective data; a mix of both provides a better data base upon which to make decisions. Attempts should be made to determine the reliability and validity of either type of data; gathering either type systematically increases the validity of the data. Planners should also try to use as many types of data as possible to explore a given issue. Since all data and data-gathering techniques have potential sources of invalidity (Campbell and Stanley, 1963), it is helpful to triangulate (Webb,

1970) by looking at issues from all available perspectives in order to make the best possible judgments about the problem or its cause.

Sources of Data. Data collected in needs assessment should match the level of importance assigned to the problem and should be balanced by the availability of resources to collect, collate, analyze, and report the data. At least five sources of data can be used in assessing the educational needs of a group of health professionals. *Professional standards* for practice are used to detect possible discrepancies between ideal practice and the observed performance by practitioners. For example, based on accepted standards of performance and data about professionals' level of practice, Kattwinkel and others (1979) determined that the community hospitals in Virginia were not providing as high quality of care to infants and mothers at risk as the current state of medical knowledge allowed. The researchers then developed educational projects to address the identified deficiencies.

Health professionals' *perceptions* of needs arising from daily practice provide a relevant source of information. Professionals often encounter problems that are easily remedied by referring to an article in a recent journal or by turning quickly to standard references. Other situations require more extensive processes of information seeking and problem solving (see Chapter Four). These situations represent important sources of information for needs assessment of the individual practitioner, though it is difficult for CE providers to gather these data in a systematic fashion.

Normative sources of data are those from which needs can be inferred from the study of the comparative characteristics of similar individuals, groups, or communities. For example, significant differences in the infant mortality rate in two communities with very similar populations, health care facilities, and socioeconomic and racial distribution might reveal a discrepancy in practice that signals a need for specific education about treatment methods. Data from the numerous studies of the National Center for Health Statistics can be used to identify such needs.

Scientific research, new technology, and developments from new discoveries can be used to identify needs. For example, Mahan, Philips, and Costanzi (1978) identified relevant scientific research and provided South Texas physicians with information about cancer treatment, which altered the physicians' referral patterns. Scientific data differ from quality standards for identifying needs in that a scientifically based need is dictated by the research or technology itself, whereas quality standards are derived from the opinion of experts.

Patient opinions and attitudes can be an important source of needs assessment data regarding patient care outcomes. Patients can be an especially useful source of information regarding health professionals' needs for knowledge and skills in patient communication, patient education, and patient counseling.

Data-Gathering Techniques. Once a decision is reached as to what is to be assessed and specific questions to be asked have been formulated, the next task is to ascertain whether enough data already exists to permit a reasonable assessment or whether additional data must be gathered from the sources just described. In selecting a data-gathering technique, it is important to decide what questions to pursue, who can provide answers to the questions, where these respondents can be found, and when and how they will be most willing to provide the required information. Cost, time, and utility should be considered in selecting data-collection techniques. Some of the strengths and weaknesses of the techniques used to gather data are discussed briefly in the following paragraphs (see Knowles, 1970; Morris and Fitz-Gibbon, 1978; Levine, 1978, for more details on many of the procedures discussed).

Searches of documents, articles, and texts produce relevant information or can provide clues to problems; however, they do not always show causes of problems and at times do not reflect current situations. They can serve as a good beginning for focusing on particular needs that should be investigated more thoroughly.

Interviews will yield facts but also can be used to reveal feelings, perceptions of causes, and possible solutions for problems. Since some goals of instruction include changing attitudes, interviews can be used as measures of performance, with the gap between desired attitudes and actual attitudes as one direct indication of needs. Interviews also afford the maximum opportunity for free expression of opinion. Respondents are much more likely to elaborate on their comments during human interaction, and can be more strongly urged to respond. Since potential clients should be involved in identifying their needs, interviews can serve to stimulate positive attitudes toward the proposed projects. Interviewers, however, should be careful not to use the interview to interpret, sell, or educate. Among the limitations of interviews are that they are time-consuming and difficult to quantify; respondents may feel they are on the spot. Interview questions should be field-tested and revised before being used.

Questionnaires and surveys can reach many people, are relatively inexpensive, provide anonymity (which relieves respondents of fear of embarrassment and reprisals), permit time for reflection before answering, and are cost-effective. They can be given to large numbers of people simultaneously, are more easily standardized than interviews, and are relatively easy to analyze. Questionnaires, however, do not have the flexibility of interviews, in which an idea can be explored in depth. Therefore, causes of problems or possible solutions are less likely to emerge. Like interview questions, questionnaires should be validated and revised before use (Kempfer, 1955; Eastmond, 1969; McMahon, 1970).

Observations can provide firsthand information about activities and problems rather than relying on others' perceptions. Often observations are the only way of obtaining direct measures of performance. However, observations can be impractical and costly since they require qualified observers who are usually well paid. Observations may be biased by the attitudes, perceptions, and expectations of the observers. Furthermore, the presence of an observer can change the behavior of those being observed. Despite the drawbacks, however, observations can be useful as pilot studies. Observations can also be used to confirm hypotheses generated from data obtained by other techniques.

Inspection of medical records and other types of formal health care reports, such as mortality and morbidity charts, can provide clues to problems and can be used as direct measures to assess discrepancies. Most administrators and practitioners understand the data from records. Often, however, records are incomplete, and medical records may have only a vague relationship to what actually happened during the practitioner-patient interaction. Records are often extremely hard to retrieve and analyze, especially when the record was not designed for retrieval of the desired data.

Formal cognitive testing is useful to identify specific areas of knowledge deficiency. The results of tests are easy to compare and report and are obviously useful in evaluating the immediate outcome of CE programs. Tests also can be useful in selecting those that are most likely to profit from CE experiences. The fact that a group scores well on a test, however, does not guarantee performance, since possessing knowledge does not mean that health professionals will choose to apply that knowledge. Furthermore, knowledge is only a part of competence, which requires application of skills as well.

Clinical performance testing has been the focus of much developmental activity in the last few years. Such techniques as oral examinations, peer review, performance checklists, patient management problems, and other simulation exercises (Senior, 1976) require application of learning and have improved the ability of tests to relate to performance (Lloyd, 1982). Many problems still exist, however. Many practitioners are reluctant to take any type of test, even under anonymous conditions, because they are skeptical of the relationship between the types of abilities measured by tests and their own ability to deliver patient care.

Self-assessment and peer review as data collection methods give the professionals some perspective on their needs. Learners' individual activities are often compared to normative standards. Sivertson and McDonald (1977) conducted an individual appraisal by developing a profile assessment of a number of physicians using a pocket-sized tape recorder. After a practice profile was obtained, a test was developed based on the profile. The test results and the analysis of the profile were used to determine educational needs and make recommendations for meeting the needs. However, with a few exceptions, the process has not been able to document that either recommended education was completed or that behavior was changed as reflected in performance and outcome of patient care rendered. The disappointing results with initial attempts at individual appraisal systems do not mean that such approaches may not eventually be fruitful.

Group problem analysis is a method in which groups seek to identify needs and causes of problems. Sometimes planners utilize both formal and informal groups to assist them in the determination of educational needs. In some cases, a planner may periodically set up meetings of small discussion groups that focus on the expression of educational concerns.

In group problem analysis, various methods can be used to encourage health professionals to voice their opinions about educational needs. Eastmond (1969) described several ways in which this can be accomplished. The *speak-up procedure* is designed to encourage a wide range of health professionals to express their perceptions of educational needs with a minimum of structure that might limit such expressions. An organization of discussion groups is developed to provide a vehicle for input into educational planning. The *brainstorm technique* uses small discussion groups to generate ideas and opinions about educational needs. One ground rule is that all criticism or judgment of such ideas and opinions is withheld during the initial brainstorming session. After all the ideas are suggested, the group begins to discuss the relative merits of each. By process of elimination, members of the group arrive at a collective decision about the nature of educational needs. Research has suggested that such brainstorming groups in which the members are familiar with the general problem can make significant contributions to the assessment of needs.

Unmet needs conferences involve a considerable amount of representative participation and call for effective planning. Such a conference consists of a large meeting with numerous small group discussions held simultaneously. Discussion in each group is centered on a broad theme such as "educational needs of nurses." The participants are asked to write down their thoughts and ideas on the topic prior to any discussion. The unmet needs conference can reveal the nature and extent of the needs of individuals, departments, and hospitals. At the same time, they provide an opportunity for beginning cooperatively to address such problems. Encouraging groups of health professionals to share perceptions of educational needs creates more awareness of both the complexity of such needs and the necessity for a systematic and cooperative approach to meet them.

Nominal group process is specifically directed at problem identification rather than at problem solutions (Delbecq, Van de Ven, and Gustafson, 1975). Nominal group process is a structured group meeting that involves the silent generation of ideas in writing, round-robin recording of ideas, discussion of ideas for clarification and evaluation, individual voting, and mathematical computation to determine rank ordering. In this manner, nominal group process overcomes a number of critical problems typical of interacting groups. In particular, it facilitates the involvement of individuals who may be reluctant to participate in regularly conducted meetings.

In some cases, more *formal groups* are utilized by program planners to assist in the assessment of educational needs (Kempfer, 1955; Knox, 1969; Watson, 1972). Among these more formalized groups are two types, the advisory committee and the task force. Although advisory groups or committees may vary greatly in size and responsibility, they are basically of two kinds. Kempfer (1955) has referred to these as "special area committees"—those that address specific need areas and are considered most effective—and "general committees"—those that usually provide a rough estimation of needs.

Other techniques using groups include the *critical incident technique* in which respondents provide particular occurrences of effective or ineffective performance (Campbell and Markle, 1968). This technique is actually a special type of questionnaire that provides a basis for identifying problems in an empirical fashion, but it can be costly and complex. Kaufman (1972) and Eastmond (1969) describe the *Delphi technique,* in which expert respondents achieve a consensus on some issue or problem based upon a series of questionnaires. Although the Delphi technique is a precise method of determining priorities, it lacks the face-to-face interaction inherent in other group techniques.

Analysis. In analyzing needs there are four main questions that should guide the educator: (1) do any needs exist, (2) are those needs identified as educational needs, (3) what are the causes of the identified needs, and (4) what are the priorities among the identified needs? Analysis consists of judging and comparing one set of data with another that represents some standard to determine if there is any variance. In educational needs assessment in CE, the analysis would aim at comparing collected data describing current circumstances with some standard that describes a more desirable condition.

The next step is to determine which of the identified needs are educational needs and which would be more appropriately reduced by administrative or other noneducational means (Knowles, 1970; Zacharewicz and Coger, 1977). As mentioned earlier, educational needs can be defined in terms of deficiencies of knowledge, skills, and attitudes and can be addressed through educational means. Noneducational needs require administrative action, such as changes in staffing patterns, purchase of new equipment, or policy changes. Some needs contain elements of both, and careful attention should be paid to their interaction.

When assessments are conducted at both the strategic and programmatic levels, several areas may be identified for educational efforts; a decision must then be made as to which topics are more important. Factors to consider when making these decisions include severity of health-related problem, number of patients affected, number of health professionals and staff involved, potential for solving the problem through education, available resources, relationship to CE provider unit and institution goals, time investment required, availability of previously developed relevant educational projects, and capability and willingness of learners to make necessary changes.

These factors can be weighted and assigned as they apply to topics under consideration, or topics addressing the most factors can be established as most important. A priority list is then established, indicating those needs that should be addressed first and those that will be addressed if time and resources permit.

Reporting Findings. Whatever the size and scope of the needs assessment, some form of report should be compiled. The needs assessment then can be used for documentation of decisions for programming and later can be used in evaluation to determine if needs have been eliminated or reduced. The type of information included in the report and the way in which the results are presented will depend on the user of the needs assessment findings. Different users will be interested in specific information and may require different methods of presentation. The educational planner may only require sketchy notes that can be included in the documentation for program development while institutional administrators may require a formal report to justify fund allocations. Results might be reported to potential learners through publicity for educational activities.

The primary information that should be included in the documentation is a description of purpose and issues of needs assessment, a brief review of those professionals involved in the needs assessment, the information sought, the process used to collect the data, analysis procedures, and a summary of results.

Summary

Needs assessment is a critical part of a systematic approach to developing educational projects. More and more educational institutions are incorporating needs assessment into curriculum development procedures. The approach to needs assessment in continuing education for the health professions contained in this chapter describes a systematic process based on a carefully developed plan. This plan calls for describing the purpose of the needs assessment activity, the users of the findings, the issues that will be examined, and specification of the resources required. The plan also calls for the selection of types of data, sources of data, data-gathering techniques, and data-analysis methods. Finally, the plan includes a prescription for reporting findings.

There are many reasons for conducting needs assessment activities and many benefits that are derived from the process. The ultimate purpose is to obtain information—whether quantitative or qualitative—so that educators can determine better the nature, extent, and priority of educational needs to develop continuing education projects that address the needs of a constituency of learners and do so within a context of limited resources. The framework described in this chapter can be applied to both large and small CE provider units. Its scope will depend on the responsibilities and size of the unit. A properly conducted needs assessment can be the most powerful mechanism for linking CE to the health care setting.

References

Atwood, H. M., and Ellis, J. "The Concept of Need: An Analysis for Adult Education." *Adult Leadership*, 1971, *19* (1), 210–212, 244.

Brown, C. R., Jr. "The Continuing Education Component of the Bi-Cycle Approach to Quality Assurance." In R. H. Egdahl and P. M. Gertman (Eds.), *Quality Health Care: The Role of Continuing Medical Education*. Germantown, Md.: Aspen Systems, 1977.

Campbell, D. T., and Stanley, J. C. *Experimental and Quasiexperimental Designs for Research*. Chicago: Rand McNally, 1963.

Campbell, V. N., and Markle, D. G. *Identifying and Formulating Educational Problems—A Final Report to the Far West Laboratory for Educational Research and Development*. Palo Alto, Calif.: American Institutes for Research, 1968.

Coordinating Council on Medical Education.*The Continuing Competence of Physicians: A Report of the Coordinating Council on Medical Education*. Chicago: Coordinating Council on Medical Education, 1979.

Delbecq, A. L., Van de Ven, A. H., and Gustafson, D. H. *Group Techniques for Program Planning*. Glenview, Ill.: Scott, Foresman, 1975.

Eastmond, J. N. *Needs Assessment: Winnowing Expressed Concerns for Critical Needs in Education*. Washington, D.C.: Educational Resources Information Center, 1969.

Kattwinkel, J., and others. "Improved Perinatal Knowledge and Care in the Community Hospital Through a Program of Self-Instruction." *Pediatrics*, 1979, *64* (4), 451–458.

Kaufman, R. A. *Educational System Planning*. Englewood Cliffs, N.J.: Prentice-Hall, 1972.

Kempfer, H. *Adult Education*. New York: McGraw-Hill, 1955.

Knowles, M. S. *The Modern Practice of Adult Education: Androgogy Versus Pedagogy*. New York: Association Press, 1970.

Knox, A. B. "Clientele Analysis." *Review of Educational Research*, 1965, *35* (3), 231–239.

Knox, A. B. "Continuous Program Evaluation." In N. C. Shaw (Ed.), *Administration of Continuing Education*. Washington, D.C.: National Association for Public School Adult Education, 1969.

Levine, H. G. "Selecting Evaluation Instruments." In M. K. Morgan and D. M. Irby (Eds.), *Evaluating Clinical Competence in the Health Professions*. St. Louis, Mo.: Mosby, 1978.

Lloyd, J. S. (Ed.). *Evaluation of Noncognitive Skills and Clinical Performance.* Chicago: American Board of Medical Specialties, 1982.

McKinley, J. "Perspectives on Diagnostics in Adult Education." *Viewpoints,* 1973, *49,* 69–83.

McMahon, E. E. *Needs—of People and Their Communities—and the Adult Educator: A Review of the Literature of Need Determination.* Washington, D.C.: Adult Education Association of the U.S.A., 1970.

Mahan, J. M., Philips, B. U., and Costanzi, J. J. "Patient Referrals: A Behavioral Outcome of Continuing Medical Education." *Journal of Medical Education,* 1978, *53* (3), 210–211.

Miller, G. E. "Continuing Education for What?" *Journal of Medical Education,* 1967, *42* (4), 320–326.

Morris, L. L., and Fitz-Gibbon, C. T. *How to Measure Achievement.* Beverly Hills, Calif.: Sage, 1978.

Sanazaro, P. J. "Medical Audit, Continuing Medical Education, and Quality Assurance." *Western Journal of Medicine,* 1976, *125* (3), 241–252.

Sandlow, L. J., Bashook, P. G., and Maxwell, J. A. "Medical Care Evaluation: An Experience in Continuing Medical Education." *Journal of Medical Education,* 1981, *56* (7), 580–586.

Senior, J. R. *Toward the Measurement of Competence in Medicine: The Development and Validation of a Computer-Based System for Testing and Teaching Clinical Competence in Medicine.* Philadelphia: John R. Senior, 1976.

Sivertson, S. E., and McDonald, E. "Medical Practice Related to Continuing Education by Practice Profiling." In R. H. Egdahl and P. M. Gertman (Eds.), *Quality Health Care: The Role of Continuing Medical Education.* Germantown, Md.: Aspen Systems, 1977.

Sivertson, S. E., Meyer, T. C., Hansen, R., Schoenenberger, A. "Individual Physician Profile: Continuing Education Related to Medical Practice." *Journal of Medical Education,* 1973, *48* (11), 1006–1012.

Watson, C. D. *Educational Needs Assessment.* Little Rock: Arkansas Department of Education, 1972. (ERIC: ED 084 293)

Webb, E. "Unconventionality, Triangulation, and Inference." In N. K. Denzin (Ed.), *Sociological Methods*. Chicago: Aldine, 1970.

Zacharewicz, F. A., and Coger, R. "Educational Needs Assessment: A Systematic Approach." *Journal of Allied Health*, 1977, *6* (1), 54–60.

9

Designing Effective Educational Activities for Groups

Sarina J. Grosswald

*Once needs have been identified and priorities have been estab-
lished, educational activities must be designed to meet those needs.
This chapter, after a brief theoretical treatment of educational
design, presents the design process in depth. This process includes
setting goals, selecting subject matter experts, establishing objectives, selecting methods and media, and selecting delivery approaches. The final section includes a discussion and examples of
implementing educational activities for groups of learners. This
chapter ties together some familiar concepts about educational
design to present a logical and concise approach. Many of the
activities that are listed and described are also appropriate for individual health professionals or for continuing education (CE) provider units that are developing activities for groups and individuals.
This chapter can also serve as a useful complement to Chapter
Eleven.—Editors*

The primary goal of a continuing education experience is to have some impact on the professional, whether the purpose of the specific activity is to assist the professional in learning something new, to change present practice, or to verify that present practice is appropriate. Among the conditions that contribute to the ability of an educational activity to create an impact, two are predominant. First, the activity must be based on something the learner has the need and motivation to learn; second, the activity must be designed to present what the learner needs to know in a manner that will promote learning. The second condition is the subject of this chapter.

Designing educational activities is part of the broader process of program development. As described in Chapter Seven, there are many models of program development; nevertheless, the major components include identifying needs, analyzing and selecting educational needs based on priorities, developing educational objectives, designing activities, implementing activities, and evaluating the outcomes. Simply speaking, programs are developed to meet identified needs and are then evaluated as to how well they actually met the needs. This chapter will focus on a process that can be used by CE provider units to design educational experiences, primarily for groups rather than for individual learners. Though the approach is similar for both individuals and groups, Chapter Eleven will look more closely at the considerations for working with individual learners.

The success of an educational activity, from the standpoint of outcome, relies strongly on the needs assessment effort (see Chapter Eight). The more thoroughly the areas of educational need are examined, the greater the validity of the data available for designing the activity. The more that is known and the fewer assumptions that have to be made about learners' needs and interests, the closer the activity can be designed to meet those needs and result in the desired outcomes.

When decisions about the content and presentation of an educational experience are being made, an orderly process of design and development can enhance the activity's value to the learner. By using a systematic process, the planner can develop an activity that matches what the learner needs to know with the most effective means of learning that information.

As with program development, there are many models of educational design. This chapter provides a synthesis of the most important concepts, presenting those aspects that are most critical for planning a learning experience that will have an impact on professional knowledge and performance.

Theoretical Background

An organized process for the development of activities has emerged from educational research over the past fifty years and from experiences of how adults learn. One need not have extensive knowledge of educational theory and research to apply the principles of educational design. However, a brief explanation of the major concepts that have influenced educational design can help illustrate the essence of such a process.

As discussed in greater detail in Chapter Two, theoretical foundations of educational design lie in educational psychology. (For a review of the literature, see Lovell, 1980.) Early theories of learning were based on animal research and centered around the concepts of eliciting desired responses to specific situations (Thorndike, 1898; Guthrie, 1935; Skinner, 1938). These theories were widely accepted in their time, though they met with some criticism (Tolman, 1932) because they did not consider the internal motivations of the learners as influencing the response. Behavior modification, the system of rewards and punishments to mold responses, grew out of these theories.

In contrast to those emphasizing the conditioning of single responses were the Gestalt psychologists (Kohler, 1929; Koffka, 1928; Wertheimer, 1945), who were concerned with the learning situation as a whole. From the Gestalt perspective, the learner tries different responses; then the solution seems to come abruptly as a flash of insight. Gestalt psychologists emphasized the learner's perception of relationships and the sensible solution of problems rather than mechanical repetition of responses. When this theory is applied to the teaching situation, the learner is presented with the meaningful whole or final outcome. Where necessary, certain parts are practiced and then placed back into the context of the whole. The learner can then associate what is learned with other similar situations.

More recent theories (Piaget, 1950; Gagné, 1965; Bruner, 1966; Ausubel, 1968) consider the mental processes involved in learning. Their theories address the individual's readiness to learn, the way information is stored in the brain, and processes the learner uses to remember information. Attention is given to the way information is presented to the learner, to motivation and creativity, and to learning how to learn. In general, these concepts have become well known among adult educators.

From these theories, principles applicable to the educational design process have been derived. Among them are the requirements that learning be demonstrated as an observable change, learners be presented with situations similar to their actual situations to encourage application of learning, and information be presented in such a way as to stimulate problem solving.

Description of Educational Design

Educational design is the process of making decisions about the presentation of instruction. Though the process is presented in this chapter in a sequential order, planning involves consideration and reformulation all along the way. Decisions often run together as the planner strives to meet the learners' needs while making the best use of available resources.

The process of designing learning experiences, as presented here, includes setting goals, selecting the subject matter expert(s), establishing objectives, selecting methods and media, and specifying delivery approaches. Whether the planner is developing many activities for a broad CE program or providing periodic activities for a small service or department, the same process applies. The approach offers a means for considering a variety of alternatives for meeting an educational need and ensuring learning. It also contributes to developing an activity that is stimulating to the learners and that provides information they will be able to apply to practice.

When programs are being planned and developed, several different types of expertise should be represented: a planner who initiates a project and attends to schedules and logistics, a subject matter expert who helps develop the content to be taught, an educational designer who works with the subject matter expert to select and develop educational approaches, and a media specialist who selects or creates audiovisuals. Depending on the setting, all the jobs may be the responsibility of the CE planner or director, or there may be some combination of skills and responsibilities among the CE staff. When the development of an educational activity includes several people, a planning committee provides an excellent means of coordinating responsibilities, communicating progress, and making decisions. The committee should meet throughout the developmental process and should provide oversight during the implementation of the activity. The description of the design process in the following sections does not distinguish who does what, since that will depend on the specific CE provider unit, but rather it presents a general discussion of what should be accomplished.

Setting Goals. The goal or goals established for the CE activity define what the final outcome should be. The goal is based on the identified need and participants' interests, and all consequent planning serves to accomplish that goal. If, for example, a needs assessment indicates that physicians need more information about drugs relating to hypertension, the goal of the educational activity might be to provide guidelines for prescribing antihypertensive drugs. If the results of a needs assessment indicate that new staff members are not familiar with the hospital's inhalation therapy equipment, the goal of the educational activity might be that participants learn to operate all the inhalation therapy equipment in that hospital.

Though it seems obvious that there is an implicit goal or purpose for any educational activity, by explicitly stating the goal, the planner at least ensures that the stated expectations of the activity relate to the proposed outcome. In the example about hypertensive drugs, another goal of an activity might be that physicians learn the pharmacology of antihypertensive drugs. If the final outcome, however, is that the participants know prescription protocols, learning the pharmacology will not by itself lead to this outcome. Because the goal dictates specific objectives and directs the other decisions in the design process, it should be explicitly stated to reflect the desired outcome.

Selecting the Subject Matter Expert(s). The selection of the subject matter expert will depend on the role the individual will play in development and delivery of the activity. If the expert is to serve primarily as a content expert providing the subject matter that will be used to develop the activity, then the planner should seek someone who can (1) generate or provide content, (2) verify the completeness and accuracy of content, (3) review content in existing resource materials, and (4) review the final content of the educational activity.

If the experts also will be serving as faculty members for the learning experience, their teaching skills *must* be considered in the selection. When selecting a faculty member, the planner should determine whether the individual is a good presenter and has clear, organized, and interesting presentations; interacts well with learners; and uses teaching techniques that are effective with health professionals as adult learners. In an effort to attract participants, planners often invite well-known authorities to conduct a CE activity. However, many of these experts have a reputation for their research or practice achievements and not necessarily for their instructional skills. The knowledge an expert has may not be passed on to the learners because of the speaker's inability to communicate. Sometimes a lesser-known figure who is effective in working with adults is a greater asset than a prominent name.

Establishing Objectives. Learning objectives describe the desired accomplishments of the learner at the conclusion of the learning experience. The objectives provide the basis for developing the specific content of the activity and for deciding how the content will be presented. The use of learning objectives is not a new concept to any educational planner, but many do not realize the broad applications of objectives. Learning objectives serve to:

- communicate the specific learning outcomes so the learner knows what is expected
- allow prospective learners to decide whether or not the educational activity will meet their needs
- provide a link between the identified need and the outcome of the learning experience
- help faculty decide what to teach
- provide a basis for evaluating the outcome

In the considerable literature on objectives, recommending a variety of formats and components (Mager, 1962; Varges, 1972;

Gagné and Briggs, 1974), three attributes are shared by almost all types of objectives. Wherever possible, the objective should be *stated as a specific learning outcome*. It should specify what the learner is expected to be able to do after the learning experience. Though objectives sometimes do not reflect the abstractions that influence learning, they are used to guide the program development and therefore should be written to match as closely as possible the actions desired as a result of the education. Specifying objectives that state that the learner will be able to "know" or "understand" something provides a challenge in determining if learning was accomplished. These expectations may be appropriate for a general goal of a learning activity, but objectives should be defined as an outcome that can be assessed. For example, if the goal of a program were that the participants learn how to perform uncomplicated molar endodontics, the objectives for the learning experience would specify the particular actions expected of the learner, such as identify the uncomplicated situation requiring molar endodontics, perform the treatment successfully, and describe postoperative management. The objectives then provide a basis for assessing whether the educational activity accomplished what was expected.

Each objective should *represent an achievable and practical amount of learning*. Unfortunately, there is no rule as to what is achievable and practical. It must be the best judgment of the planners. The objectives should represent an amount of learning that can be accomplished in the time available. At times neglect of this basic tenet is the downfall of well-intended programs, and the expectations of an activity are overly ambitious. The learner has no time to learn or process what is presented and leaves the activity feeling dissatisfied. Involvement of faculty members and prospective learners can contribute to developing realistic objectives. In addition, changes in the rate of learning (described in Chapter Two) that occur with increasing age should be taken into consideration when defining the objectives and expectations of the activity.

There should be some *means of assessing whether learning was achieved*. Not all outcomes in continuing education can be measured, but they can be assessed in some form. Observations of geriatric patients who are no longer depressed after health professionals' training in geriatric counseling may be difficult to quantify;

however, qualitative methods of observation or a case study approach can be used to assess the relationship of patients' status to the outcome of the CE activity. Stating objectives so that the outcomes can be assessed increases the chances of obtaining the desired result. It is of primary importance that the planner understand the purposes and uses of objectives. Format or style of objectives are much less important than the appropriate application of the statements.

A planning committee provides a resource for establishing objectives and contributing to the planning of the activity. In addition to those mentioned earlier—a subject matter expert, an educational planner, and a media specialist—a representative of the target audience can be a valuable member of the committee. The committee can make decisions about development of the program and can provide an internal means of validating the activity's expectations. The subject matter expert may indicate that all necessary outcomes are not covered in the objectives, while the target audience representative can emphasize what the learners need most. The planner and media specialist can determine which aspects are most important and how they will influence the decisions about presentation. A planning committee can increase interest and commitment for the learning activity and avoid the shortcoming of developing a program in isolation from those who will be involved as learners.

Methods and Media. The art of creating an effective educational activity culminates in the selection of methods and media for accomplishing the objectives. There are a wide variety of methods and media available to program planners, though one often finds in CE an established set of approaches such as lecture and panel discussion. Planners sometimes hesitate to incorporate other methods for fear they might be too expensive or too time-consuming to develop. However, methods not usually used may actually be more appropriate for certain learning outcomes, and the old favorites may be more effective when used selectively. As planners begin to explore the alternatives, they may find that development is not overly labor-intensive, that there are numerous existing resources available, that certain alternatives are more compatible with learners' preferences, and that the results can be more appreciable.

The following is a brief description of some of the instructional methods that are appropriate for continuing education activities for groups. Table 1 summarizes the salient features of each method.

The *lecture* is the most commonly used educational method, though it is often used where other methods would be more appropriate. Some studies have shown that 80 percent of the information delivered in a lecture is forgotten within eight weeks (McLeish, 1968). However, when used properly for the appropriate purposes, the lecture can be very effective.

A lecture is particularly useful in providing an overview or disseminating general information to a large number of learners. A lecture can also be an efficient method for participants to determine the value and credibility peers place on certain topics or to confirm that what they are doing is appropriate. A well-planned lecture can emphasize key points and synthesize a large amount of information. Particularly dynamic speakers can influence participants' attitudes and motivation. The effectiveness of the lecture can be enhanced by a brief question-and-answer period. The difficulty with the lecture is not the weakness of the method, but its use when other methods would be more effective.

Discussion sessions actively involve the participants in the educational process. This method allows for free exchange of ideas and is particularly useful for problem solving, correcting misconceptions, or examining controversial issues. Discussion gives the learners an opportunity to clarify information and increase their understanding of concepts. Because of the participation and interaction of the learners, discussion may also be effective in changing attitudes; as a follow-up to a lecture, this method can increase the effectiveness of the lecture.

Discussion is usually more appropriate for small groups, with no more than twelve to fifteen people, but it can be successful with larger groups when there is someone responsible for keeping the discussion moving and for ensuring the participation of many learners. A seminar is a specific type of discussion but may be focused more on dissemination and clarification of content and may require preparation by participants.

Panel discussion, where several people express their viewpoints on a particular subject, is especially useful for presenting and comparing various sides of an issue and often can influence attitudes. The learner is not usually actively involved with this method, but a question-and-answer period allows for some interaction.

Demonstration, where the learner is shown a procedure or skill, allows learners to see the process and, in many cases, the final outcome of the procedure. The learners can also see the level of expected performance. Demonstrations are particularly effective for teaching skills but are sometimes difficult to use for large groups unless there is supportive viewing equipment.

Observation and practice under supervision, where learners observe an experienced practitioner and practice under supervision, is an excellent method for acquiring both skills and judgment. The experience provides the learner with a role model, as well as an opportunity to observe and practice in the real situation. An effective observation experience requires deliberate planning and a significant amount of teaching time.

Reading, of course, is a long-established educational method. It is the most frequently used means of continuing education selected by the individual health professional. Among others, journals, monographs, and texts are extremely effective means of acquiring information on an individual basis and can provide in-depth information. Learning experiences planned for groups may include reading assignments as preparation for the activity or as follow-up. Reading often is, but need not be, a passive means of instruction. For instance, the seeking of answers to specific questions or the preparation of a presentation to fellow learners can greatly enhance the effectiveness of reading. It should be noted that extensive reading assignments can be a time-consuming burden to busy health professionals; they may prefer a shorter, more direct, interactive experience.

Computer-assisted instruction (CAI) offers a flexible method of providing information, giving the user an opportunity to apply learning in simulated situations and to receive feedback on learning. Many commercial computer programs are available that present subject matter and practice problems, allowing the learner to practice decision making on a simulated case and then giving instant responses to the learner. Computers also allow users to learn at their own pace. Newly available data bases such as the American Medical Association/General Telephone and Electric (AMA/GTE) provide relatively inexpensive access to medical information and may prove to be valuable support to the learner. The initial investment in computers and the required software can be expensive. Each terminal reaches only one learner at a time; therefore, when CAI is used in group programs, arrangements must be made to assure learners' access to the computer.

As travel and the cost of meetings become more expensive, the *teleconference* is becoming popular in continuing education for health professionals. By using conference telephone equipment and commercial telephone lines, this method provides an opportunity for a presenter at one site to conduct educational experiences with participants at many other sites. *Satellite television* allows for transmission of visual and vocal information. Teleconferences and satellite television enable learners to participate in two-way communication. They are especially effective for reaching more remote locations. Early and detailed planning is essential for these methods to work well. All such presentations must be well organized, and learners must receive in advance any necessary material. To take full advantage of this approach, the program should include an opportunity for participant interaction.

Role playing involves learners in acting out parts reflecting real-life situations as they might occur in a particular set of circumstances. Role playing is effective in learning and practicing skills such as patient interviewing, supervising, and counseling. This method can also be useful in examining attitudes, because role playing gives learners an opportunity to express their feelings or the feelings they perceive in others.

Simulations replicate real-life situations and provide hands-on experience performing a skill or technique, such as practice on the Resusci-Annie doll used for cardiopulmonary resuscitation. Simulations may present an example where the learner must make decisions or apply what has been learned. This method provides an excellent means for learners to practice and demonstrate the final outcome of the learning experience. In creating simulations, individuals trained to act as patients can be used to replicate real situations. Simulations, however, may be costly or hard to create.

Games are a type of simulation restricted by rules. Here the learner interacts with others and puts into practice knowledge and

Table 1. Features of Instructional Methods.

Method	Characteristics
Lecture	• Reaches large group • Good for presenting general information or overview • May be effective in changing attitudes • Limited interaction with learners • Content often forgotten in short periods of time • Effectiveness dependent on presenter
Discussion Sessions	• Actively involves learners • Enhances understanding and knowledge of learners • Can be effective in changing attitudes • Better for small group • May require facilitator
Panel Discussion	• Presents various sides of an issue • May influence attitudes • Limited learner involvement
Demonstration	• Particularly effective for teaching skills or techniques • Allows learners to see what is expected • Better for small group
Observation and Practice Under Supervision	• Provides learners with a role model • Provides opportunity for practice of skills and techniques and for feedback • Learners can receive experience in real situations • Reaches few learners at one time • Requires much time
Reading	• Provides in-depth information • Allows for individual work and individual pacing • Passive form of learning • May be time-consuming
Computer-Assisted Instruction	• Involves learners • Effective for application of learning, practice, and feedback • Reaches few learners at one time • May be expensive
Teleconference and Satellite Television	• Reaches learners at other sites • Relatively inexpensive (compared to travel and meeting arrangements • Must be well planned)
Role-Playing	• Can be effective in changing attitudes • Involves learners • Provides opportunity to practice what is learned

Table 1. Features of Instructional Methods, Cont'd.

Method	Characteristics
Simulations	• Involves learners in hands-on experiences • Excellent opportunity to practice what is learned • Can demonstrate learning outcome • May be hard to create
Games	• Involves learners • Learners practice and apply what is learned • May be effective for changing attitudes • May be hard to create • Time-consuming

concepts that have been learned. Effective games may be difficult to develop (although commercial ones are available), and they take time to carry out.

Selecting Methods and Media. Media are the means of communicating knowledge, demonstrating skills, or influencing attitudes through graphic, photographic, or electronic means. In other words, they are audio or visual material. Media can be used as the sole means of providing instruction or can be combined with any of the methods already discussed. No medium is inherently better than another. The choice is based on the medium's suitability for presenting the specific content and leading to the desired learning outcomes, as well as on learners' preferences.

Attributes that should be considered when selecting appropriate media include motion, still picture, time-lapse, sound, color, self-pacing, and the need for immediate feedback. By deciding which attributes are important to conveying the subject matter, the planner can select the medium or media that incorporate those features. For example, color may be necessary to indicate skin rashes, or motion may be required to demonstrate a surgical technique.

The use of media is much more common today than it was eight or ten years ago. Now planners must avoid the temptation to use media where they are not needed. If motion is not required, slides are more appropriate than videotape. Often printed handouts are better instructional aids than crowded overhead transparencies displaying the content.

Although most media can be used as the primary means of learning, they are more often used in combination with other instructional methods. The selection of methods and media should be considered together, blending their application to promote the desired outcomes. Some questions to consider when selecting methods and media are as follows:

- Which method, medium, or combination of both, is best suited to meet each objective? For example, a sound slide show may be used to present general information, followed by a discussion to clarify understanding and enhance problem solving. Or a lecture may be used to present principles followed by videotaping of role playing to provide learners with practice and feedback.
- Can the objectives be achieved by the learners themselves, or is interaction required with other learners, with the teacher, or both?
- What sense or senses are involved in the learning outcome? What will the learner be expected to see, hear, touch, or smell in order to accomplish the learning objective?

The characteristics of each method or medium should be considered when making a selection, as well as the expense and time required. Some additional questions include:

- How many will participate in the educational activity? Some methods or media are better for individuals or small groups, while others are more appropriate for large groups.
- Does the program address a recurrent need, resulting in frequent repetition of the program? In such cases, methods or media might be selected that do not require a live instructor or that can be easily replicated.
- How much time do intended learners have available? The choice of methods and media may be dependent on learners' available time for participation in the experience as well as for any preparation or follow-up.
- Can all the material be covered in one meeting, or will it require a series of meetings? Sometimes a two-hour lecture will accomplish the desired outcome; in other cases, a course or workshop may be needed.

It is the process of putting it all together, by selecting the appropriate methods and media for presenting specific information or providing practice of a particular technique or skill, that results in the final product—the learning experience. The decisions during this phase of the planning are influenced by available resources, practice settings, and the participants' needs and preferences.

Selecting a Delivery Approach. The way in which the instructional methods and media are presented to the learners is referred to in this chapter as the delivery. It is the experience or activity that is often called the program. In the orderly process of educational design, a delivery approach is chosen to accommodate the methods and media selected. For example, if a lecture is presented and is followed by learners working in groups to apply the information from the lecture, a workshop might be the choice of delivery. However, because of the nature of the educational problem, a delivery approach is sometimes apparent or decided on first. If a small group of individuals are to learn a new therapeutic procedure, a miniresidency may be selected as the approach, even before extensive planning begins. The specific factors that influence the selection of a delivery approach for a group include proposed methods and media, participants' needs, the expected learning outcomes, and the available resources.

Many times, based on the content to be taught, a *single activity* is sufficient for meeting the educational need. A single activity usually ranges anywhere from one hour to half a day. It may present one format or medium such as a lecture or videotape or include a combination such as videotape and discussion. If the amount of content to be covered requires more than one meeting, it can be presented in a series of activities, a *course.* In this case, activities are offered within a specified period of time, at regularly scheduled intervals or on consecutive days.

A *miniresidency* usually occurs in the health care setting. It involves a single individual or a small group receiving training in a specific content or skill area under the supervision of an expert. It provides an excellent opportunity for intensive instruction and practice and can be individualized to meet the needs of a small number of people. Although miniresidencies are relatively easy to plan and implement, they require a large time commitment on the part of a facilitator or instructor. Programs may last from a few hours to a few days or even weeks.

A frequently used delivery approach in continuing education is the *workshop*. People who provide CE may refer to anything from a single lecture to any combination of activities and experiences as a "workshop." However, it most accurately refers to situations where learners participate in activities, usually problem solving, and receive feedback on their progress. A workshop should be designed so learners accomplish a particular task under guidance and in combination with a presentation of relevant information. Under these circumstances, a workshop can be extremely effective in providing information, giving learners an opportunity to practice, and providing them with feedback. A variety of formats and media can be used within a workshop situation. Workshops can be used for small or large groups and may range from half a day to four or five days.

Conference usually refers to an approach that covers several days, with activities throughout each day. Professional or association meetings exemplify the conference approach, where a variety of methods and other approaches, ranging from lecture to small group, panel discussion, and workshop, are offered. This approach can accommodate a large number of people, with participants having the opportunity to select the activities they want to attend. A conference is usually a large undertaking, expensive and time-consuming to plan.

Often objectives can be accomplished through independent learning, whereby learners acquire information on their own at their own pace. The use of media can be particularly appropriate in this situation, and a plan can be developed for learners to follow independently. Educational experiences can also be planned where the professionals identify their own learning needs, develop learning objectives, select and use methods for meeting the objectives, and then evaluate their success. (See Chapter Eleven for more information about self-directed learning.)

Developing Effective Activities for Health Professionals

Any plan for developing a learning experience and for selecting educational options should be directed throughout the planning by what is known about how adults learn. In continuing education, practicing health professionals bring with them unique backgrounds and experiences concerning both the health care practice and past learning experiences. By considering some general principles of learning when designing the activity, the planner increases the chances that learners actually accomplish the desired outcomes. The following are some general principles that can serve as guidelines when designing a learning experience. The principles demonstrate the implications of various learning theories and their application to developing programs (Gagné, 1965; Ausubel, 1968; Kidd, 1973; Houle, 1972; Knowles, 1980; Knox, 1980).

Learners should be involved in planning the educational experience. Most practicing health professionals have specific ideas about their own problems and practice-related needs. In their day-to-day practice they often identify areas where they feel additional learning would be beneficial, and the health professional may be the best judge of the appropriate level of complexity of information to be presented. Therefore, whenever possible, representatives of the potential learner audience should be involved in developing objectives and selecting learning opportunities. Including learners on a planning committee, for example, increases their commitment to the learning experience being planned and can affect the learning outcome.

Learners should know what is expected of them. Learning is more likely to occur if participants are aware of what they are expected to be able to do at the conclusion of the experience. Learning objectives are one means of communicating the expected outcomes. Objectives or expected outcomes for an experience should be listed in any publicity for that activity. This gives the learners an opportunity to decide if the activity will meet their needs and if it is relevant to their practice. Those participants who select to attend the course or to be involved in the activity have a commitment to learning the information being taught. Knowing what is expected at the end of an experience also helps the learner strive toward meeting those objectives.

Learners should have the opportunity to be active participants rather than passive observers in the instructional experience. Wherever possible, interaction should be built into the learning experience through discussion, questioning, or case examples, providing an opportunity for learners to become active in the educational process. There should also be opportunities for learners to express their thoughts on the learning experience, providing feedback for improvement even while the program is in progress. Interaction can be designed into the use and development of learning materials. Questioning, exercises, workbooks, audiotape, videotape, or computer can facilitate interaction by giving the learners feedback to their responses.

Learners should have an opportunity to practice using the knowledge and skills they have learned and to receive feedback on their performance. Gaining all the necessary knowledge only through listening or observing someone demonstrate what is expected does not guarantee competence. Health professionals should have an opportunity to practice what is being taught and to receive feedback to assess their performance in applying the knowledge or skill.

The planned learning experience should actually lead to the desired learning outcome. For example, if the learning outcome is to improve attitudes about treating geriatric patients, a learning experience that involves presentation of the medical problems of the geriatric patient will probably not result in changed attitudes. A small group discussion, role playing, or interaction with a geriatric group may be more effective.

Learners should be assisted in applying learning to practice. Because most health professionals participate in CE activities to enhance their professional performance, the activity should include strategies for, or actual practice in, applying what is learned in the work setting. In cases where administrative or environmental factors will influence the learners' ability to use new knowledge or skills, efforts should be made to obtain support in the work setting whenever possible.

Planners should consider the learning style preferences of the participants. A formal or informal survey can help identify the kind of learning experiences that the potential participants prefer. Participants may prefer after-hours lecture sessions or feel they learn best from small group workshops. Responding to learners' preferences and learning styles can increase participation and enhance learning.

Implementing the Educational Activity

The creation of an educational program should not be considered complete without attention to its implementation. The activity should be implemented as planned, and there should be a continuous effort to respond to the needs of the learners.

The way in which an activity is implemented is as important as the way it is designed. An effective learning activity is not only designed using the principles of adult learning but also includes these principles during the actual learning experience. The participants usually represent varied backgrounds, practice and educational experiences, and reasons for attending the CE activity. The learning experience should create a supportive environment for the participants to interact, feel comfortable, and meet their educational needs. Following are suggestions for facilitating learning during the activity.

Environment. The physical environment is an important aspect of learning. The room where activities take place should have adequate space and comfortable seats. The room setup should be appropriate for the types of activities planned and should also be conducive to informal conversations among participants during breaks.

A supportive atmosphere should be created. Adults appreciate sharing experiences and insights. Supportive relationships that can enhance learning can be encouraged in the group and may be valuable to participants after the activity is over. The first part of the educational activity can include an opportunity for the individuals to become acquainted and comfortable as a group. Introductions, discussions of backgrounds, or short group exercises help create a tone of informality and mutual respect, without being threatening or condescending.

Faculty. An enthusiastic and flexible instructor who responds to the learners' needs and assists the participants through the learning process is as much a contributing factor to the success of the program as the specification of appropriate objectives and selection of formats and media. Often the faculty member is a peer or colleague of the participants. That person's ability to create a responsive rapport with participants can be a deciding factor in the effectiveness of the program.

If the faculty have not been closely involved in the program planning, they should be oriented to the goals and expected outcomes of the activity and to the learners' needs and interests. The faculty should be contacted before the program to review what will take place and, if possible, should meet with the planner just prior to the program to clarify approaches. This orientation is particularly important where more than one faculty member is involved so that presentations can be correlated to complement one another.

Expected Outcomes. An important part of the implementation of an educational experience is making sure the right audience is there. A well-organized and appropriately presented program on physical therapy for sports injuries will have little impact if the participants in the program are primarily from geriatric care institutions. Publicity for programs should describe the goals or objectives of the experience and define the level of content being presented. Mailing lists, announcements in journals, and distribution of publicity material should be specifically focused on the selected audiences in order to notify and attract those most interested and those who will benefit the most.

Once the appropriate audience is gathered, the learning objectives are one means of letting participants know what is expected. Learners should also have an opportunity to express their expectations. At the beginning of the activity, the faculty and participants can discuss the plan or agenda. If it becomes apparent that the activity will not match the expectations of the majority of the participants, an effort should be made to modify the program plan, reaching a consensus among those involved. If a planning committee is used, the group should meet throughout the activity in order to respond to any need for changes in the program. Though modifying the program may be easier said than done, learners will respond to a conscientious effort to meet their needs more than they will to a rigid plan that is implemented, though inappropriate.

Learner Involvement. A balance should be sought between the contribution of the instructor and that of the learners. The faculty member can present the content and facilitate the learners' understanding. Learners should be given an opportunity to use the information, relate the content to past experience, and consider the application of the content in carrying out future responsibilities.

A variety of educational experiences should be used. Often busy health professionals are not accustomed to spending time in structured learning situations. The use of various methods and media can help maintain the participants' interest. For example, a discussion can be followed by a demonstration or case example. The program should be well planned but not scheduled so tightly that the participants feel rushed or pressured. Because individuals do not learn at the same pace, the program leader or faculty members should periodically assess the participants' progress and clarify any problems they may have.

Teaching Techniques. Whether the presentation of new content is accomplished through print, videotape, faculty presentation, or any other method, there are several principles of teaching that can enhance the learners' ability to understand and apply the information. When faculty members are involved in presenting the program, the CE planner should take time to review these principles with them.

- Provide the learner with an overview of the content that will be discussed and relate new content to familiar problems and issues, allowing learners to draw on past experiences. This helps learners relate the new information to concepts they already understand.
- Discuss the value of the new information and how the information will be applied. This helps increase the relevance and potential usefulness of the information and helps motivate the learners.
- Use examples when explaining the content. Examples help the learner understand the new information and see how the concepts can be applied in specific situations.
- Provide an opportunity to practice using the new information, which is, as mentioned earlier, a key component to learning. Whenever possible, this opportunity should be part of the learning experience. It is relatively easy to identify means for practice when the new information relates to skills or techniques. When the content focuses primarily on decision making or attitudes, written case studies or other simulations provide opportunities for practice and increase the potential for the information to be retained and applied.

- Because individuals learn differently, present information in more than one way. By using a verbal description as well as an illustration, for example, the information is more easily understood by both visually and verbally oriented learners.
- Provide feedback to learners about their progress during the educational activity or about their success in a practice situation. This will assist learners in judging their progress and can increase their understanding of the content.
- During the learning experience, provide encouragement to participants and assist them in meeting the goals and obtaining a sense of satisfaction from that accomplishment.

Conclusion

No matter the size or setting of a continuing education program, an educational design process based on learning theory and the principles of adult learning can help the planner develop activities that will be appropriate and valuable to the participants. The design process provides a means of considering a variety of options for accomplishing an educational goal and selecting the approach most appropriate. Though educational design is presented as a sequence of discrete events, in practice, the process of planning and analyzing is a combination of rigor and artistic intuition. The interrelationship of the components means that decisions at one point influence choices at another. Often such decisions as finances, schedules, or available expertise are predetermined, and all other considerations must be made in terms of those.

This chapter has briefly explained some of the major concepts behind designing educational programs, with the assumption that through an understanding of the important considerations, the planner can make the appropriate decisions that will lead to an educational program that will meet the needs of both the learners and of the health care setting.

References

Ausubel, D. P. *Educational Psychology: A Cognitive View*. New York: Holt, Rinehart and Winston, 1968.

Bruner, J. S. *Toward a Theory of Instruction.* Cambridge, Mass.: Harvard University Press, 1966.

Gagné, R. M. *The Conditions of Learning.* New York: Holt, Rinehart and Winston, 1965.

Gagné, R. M., and Briggs, L. J. *Principles of Instructional Design.* New York: Holt, Rinehart and Winston, 1974.

Guthrie, E. R. *The Psychology of Learning.* New York: Harper & Row, 1935.

Houle, C. O. *The Design of Education.* San Francisco: Jossey-Bass, 1972.

Kidd, J. R. *How Adults Learn.* Rev. ed. New York: Association Press, 1973.

Knowles, M. S. *The Modern Practice of Adult Education: From Pedagogy to Androgogy.* Rev. ed. Chicago: Follett, 1980.

Knox, A. B. "Helping Teachers Help Adults Learn." In A. B. Knox (Ed.), *New Directions For Continuing Education: Teaching Adults Effectively,* no. 6. San Francisco: Jossey-Bass. 1980.

Koffka, K. *The Growth of the Mind.* 2nd ed. New York: Harcourt Brace Jovanovich, 1928.

Kohler, W. *Gestalt Psychology.* New York: Liveright, 1929.

Lovell, R. B. *Adult Learning.* New York: Halsted Press, 1980.

McLeish, J. *The Lecture Method.* Cambridge, England: Cambridge Institute of Education, 1968.

Mager, R. F. *Preparing Instructional Objectives.* Belmont, Calif.: Fearon, 1962.

Piaget, J. *The Psychology of Intelligence.* London: Routledge and Kegan Paul, 1950.

Skinner, B. F. *The Behavior of Organisms: An Experimental Analysis.* New York: Appleton-Century-Crofts, 1938.

Thorndike, E. L. "Animal Intelligence: An Experimental Study of the Associative Processes in Animals." Monograph Supplement. *Psychological Review,* 1898, 2 (4) (entire issue).

Tolman, E. C. *Purposive Behavior in Animals and Men.* New York: Appleton-Century-Crofts, 1932.

Varges, J. S. *Writing Worthwhile Behavioral Objectives.* New York: Harper & Row, 1972.

Wertheimer, M. *Productive Thinking.* New York: Harper & Row, 1945.

Evaluating
Continuing Education
Activities and Outcomes

Harold G. Levine
Donald E. Moore, Jr.
Floyd C. Pennington

This chapter provides a thorough treatment of the basic concepts involved in evaluation to close the loop for the educational development process as described in Chapter Seven. It suggests a systematic approach aimed at evaluating continuing education (CE) projects by determining the most critical evaluation issues as viewed by the key audiences for the evaluation. The discussion includes an extensive list of questions that can be used to focus the evaluation effort and describes a plan for conducting the evaluation process.
—Editors

The ultimate criterion for judging the effectiveness of a CE provider unit is the extent to which the continuing education activities of the unit contribute to improved health care of the public.

Evaluation is a basic function of the CE provider unit to assess its success or failure in meeting that criterion. Much evaluation focuses on monitoring the unit's educational projects, addressing issues related to the instructional effectiveness of individual activities, products, or services. Evaluation serves as a tool throughout the planning process to improve projects and close the loop between project design and outcome.

This chapter is divided into three major sections. The first two sections review many of the important concepts underlying evaluation and describe a systematic process for carrying out an evaluation. The third section suggests a diversity of issues that can be examined by evaluation throughout the planning process—during the planning stages, while the projects are being conducted, and at the conclusion of the project. Most CE provider units ask some of these questions routinely, while others address them at varying time intervals. Still other issues are rarely addressed by many units, and, even when the questions are raised, the data needed are often collected ineffectively or are used inappropriately. The following discussion is intended to assist CE provider units in generating a broad set of evaluation questions and gaining insight into the application of evaluation for improving the impact of projects on the health care setting.

Formal CE plays an important role in bringing about change in professionals' practice. As Stein (1981) indicates, well-planned CE projects directly influence practice performance. However, it is often difficult to document how an individual's CE experience influences medical practice because health professionals have a variety of educational resources available and because those who do not attend formal CE use these alternative resources (Goldfinger, 1982). Furthermore, those who attend formal CE projects often serve as resources to those who do not.

However, lack of evidence of impact should not discourage CE providers from evaluating the other elements of CE projects. The ability of health professionals to deliver quality care relates partly to the quality of the CE system. Improvements in individual CE projects can influence quality of care.

Basic Concepts

Disagreement is not uncommon among conclusions drawn about the reported merit or value of specific educational projects. The arguments may occur because of disagreements or misunderstandings about the data, which may lack reliability or validity (discussed later), or may arise from disagreements about the criteria and standards for evaluation.

Criteria and Standards. Simply stated, *criterion* is defined as an attribute selected for judging an object. *Standards* are agreed-upon levels for assessing specific criteria. For example, an evaluation criterion established for a CE activity might be that learners' needs are satisfied. Two standards specified for determining the level of success might be that 80 percent of the participants are able to apply the new information in their daily responsibilities and that one year later the original need no longer exists.

At times, however, the criterion used for making the evaluative judgments may be inappropriate or the standard invalid, rendering the evaluation unsatisfactory. For example, a CE project director may plan a project and give a pretest and a posttest on knowledge. If the mean of the pretest is sixty and that of the posttest is sixty-five, then the project director might try to state that the project is a success. The criterion in this case may be deceptive for two reasons. The test may be inappropriate, that is, the project could have focused on methods of interviewing but the test focused on knowledge of facts about interviewing; or the standard may be defective since a 5 percent gain may not be meaningful and 65 percent performance may still be inadequate.

Some of the criteria used to evaluate CE projects include evidence that identified needs were used in the selection and design of educational projects; evidence that participant needs were satisfied; evidence that participant performance deficiencies were reduced or performance goals were achieved; evidence that project objectives were met; comparisons that demonstrate that the projects followed established practice based on similar CE provider units; comparisons that indicate that the participants' performance met normative standards based upon scientific research or expert judgment; evidence that the project followed established principles of educational development—for example, the project should attend to participants' level of current functioning, the faculty should be oriented, and the information included should be correct; adherence to the criteria and standards of accrediting agencies; and evidence of concern for cost-benefit issues.

In evaluation, the decision maker seeks data to support decisions about the development, organization, promotion, and conduct of instructional activities. Data about changes in participants are important parts of evaluation but are not the only data needed.

Learning Outcomes. While project evaluation requires looking at all elements of the instructional system, it is necessary to be particularly clear about the purposes of the CE project and the methods used to assess programmatic outcomes. Planners often use goal statements such as "upgrading the physician's competence in the area of congestive heart disease" to define the purpose of a project. Such statements inform potential participants about the instructional purposes or intentions of the educational project but are not specific enough for planning instruction or for evaluating it. Objectives are then developed to describe behavior or the desired learning outcomes (Gronlund, 1970), such as "the learner is able to indicate the proper management of a typical infant with heart disease." The specific learning outcomes are indicators of project effect because they represent the level of achievement of the objectives.

However, these specified outcomes are only a subset of the possible outcomes that can indicate progress toward the goal. Consider a workshop where an objective is "participants will list the steps to be used in the emergency treatment of a burn caused by hot oil." During the workshop the participants may get the name and phone number of a burn facility, and after the activity they may call the burn unit to ask for advice in certain situations. These types of outcomes are often called *unanticipated outcomes* since they are rarely among the project expectations but nevertheless are important indicators of effectiveness. In order to draw conclusions about project effectiveness, evaluators should study both the anticipated and unanticipated outcomes.

The American Board of Pediatrics (1974) reports five types of abilities or learning outcomes that probably apply to all health professions. *Attitudes* are attributes such as concern, thoroughness, and healthy skepticism manifested through the activities of health professionals. *Factual knowledge* is the ability to recall and use appropriate information. *Interpersonal skills* are required for interacting effectively with patients and their families and with fellow members of the patient care team. *Technical skills* describe the ability to carry out technical procedures. *Clinical judgment* is the ability to derive appropriate conclusions from patient data presented in different forms and to reach conclusions in developing plans for management. These five outcomes indicate the changes that are usually embodied in the goals and objectives of most CE projects and help provide a focus for areas of evalution.

Evaluation Design. In the past, project evaluation has met with criticism because of the lack of scientific rigor used in the design of the evaluation. The weaknesses in evaluation in CE, however, have not been due solely to the incompatibility of scientific control and project evaluation; the inadequate or inappropriate use of evaluation techniques (Bertram and Brooks-Bertram, 1977) has greatly influenced the validity of the findings.

One of the challenges of those responsible for and involved in evaluating CE projects is to determine the causal effects of the education on some practice-based performance of the health professional. As McCall (1923) points out in his work entitled *How to Experiment in Education,* the task of the evaluation is to do the best possible job of studying the effects of educational intervention in real-world settings while controlling as many intervening variables as possible. Because education (and especially CE) does not occur in a tightly controlled laboratory, the most that can be expected from evaluation results is to be able to state that a given CE project will "most likely" lead to an increased level of knowledge or skill. What is unrealistic is to assume one can prove that A (education) caused B (change in performance).

A variety of evaluation procedures are available to the CE planner for conducting realistic and sound program evaluation. An evaluation design that involves use of comparison groups with random assignment of participants is called an experimental design. In some CE settings this approach can be accomplished, providing the most unbiased estimates of program results. However, in most CE settings the option of random assignment or comparison groups is not available due to the voluntary nature of continuing education. Quasiexperimental designs provide alternative methods (Cook and Campbell, 1979; Campbell and Stanley, 1963). Quasiexperimental designs include, for example, use of nonequivalent comparison groups or time-series approaches.

It is important, however, that educational researchers and evaluators be cognizant of possible explanations for identified changes other than the educational treatment itself. Ruling out other plausible explanations for changes in performances becomes a critical task. There are a number of these "other plausible explanations" that should be understood by CE professionals (Cook and Campbell, 1979). *History* is the term used to describe those other events that are occurring simultaneous to the educational intervention that might also potentially influence behavior change (such as new drug literature arriving in a physician's office the day of a workshop). *Testing* refers to the effect that occurs when a learner's responses are measured a number of times by the same instrument. (A posttest score increase may be due to having learned the material or having remembered the correct answer during the second testing.) *Instrumentation* occurs when detected increases can be caused by changes in the measuring instrument between pretest and posttest (such as when observers become more sensitive to subtle changes on a second measurement). *Selection* of different types of individuals into experimental and control or comparison groups might cause a difference in performance measures, as opposed to the existence or nonexistence of the educational intervention. *Mortality* is a problem because different types of individuals might drop out of the treatment and comparison groups, leaving the two groups potentially different, with resultant changes caused by this difference. One means of control for these "other explanations" is through the use of standard procedures and instruments.

Another concern for CE evaluators is the generalizability of the results of the evaluation. At the heart of this issue is the distinction bewteen educational research (testing hypotheses) and educational evaluation (assessing the value of education). The goal of the former is to produce knowledge and facts that will generalize broadly; on the other hand, the aim of the latter is to assess the effectiveness of an educational intervention. This evaluation effort focuses on a particular project, with a specific set of learners, objectives, and instructors. There is usually little concern with whether the same project would be as effective if held elsewhere with different learners or instructors. The evaluator's emphasis is on determining the total effect of the activity, not (as with a researcher) sorting out the different effects of the program (vis-a-vis the instructors) input to that total effect. CE evaluation can focus on assessing the impact of CE on the health professional's competence or performance or even on patient care outcomes; to do so, however, will probably require moving toward the quasiexperimental or experimental designs needed to rule out other sources of causality or to generalize to a wider audience.

For those involved in CE evaluation, it is important to understand these concepts so as not to overgeneralize or otherwise misuse the results of evaluation efforts. The primary benefit of most evaluation is to provide CE decision makers with valuable information to improve their CE processes so as to increase the chances that the CE will have the desired impact within the health care setting.

Data Requirements. Effectively implemented project evaluation is the process of identifying the essential questions, gathering the best available data, applying standards and criteria to the information collected, and then making judgments based upon the data. Most people consider evaluation to be a complex process of collection and analysis of numeric information, called *quantitative data.* However, *qualitative data* collection techniques used by anthropologists and ethnologists are equally relevant to CE evaluation. Case studies, self-reports, and interviews, for example, result in narrative information that can give depth and perspective that often cannot be acquired through quantitative data alone. Collection of qualitative data can result in findings that would not otherwise be revealed and is sometimes the most effective way of determining unanticipated outcomes. As with quantitative data, there are specific methods of analysis for ensuring reliable and valid conclusions (see Guba, 1978; Smith, 1978). Often a combination of both quantitative and qualitative data will provide the most valid information needed to answer the evaluation questions.

In current practice, much of the data about project implementation are obtained from participants. Pennington and LaScala (1978) have collated sample items to illustrate some of the ways participant reaction data can be gathered. Three types of data may be collected—*participant satisfaction data, administrative information,* and *attitudinal feedback.* Participant satisfaction data do not necessarily indicate that participants learned anything or that they will apply what they have learned to the way in which they deliver care. Nonetheless, "happiness" data do provide insight into the effectiveness of project execution. Administrative information refers to information about what has transpired during the activity; for example, could the slides be seen and the speakers heard? Participants can indicate whether they have received promotional material and whether they understood it. Attitudinal feedback reflects participants' changes in attitudes that are often appropriate objectives of educational projects. This type of change may be revealed on participant reaction forms.

This type of opinion data is relatively easy to collect. However, because the project evaluator can be overwhelmed with such data, the data should be collected with the following purposes in mind: to test the assumptions made during the planning phase in order to facilitate the planning of more effective projects, to discover how well the planned project actually was implemented, and to identify project weaknesses in order to correct them, sometimes while the project is going on. Chapter Eight contains an in-depth discussion of methods for collecting other types of data.

It is not always cost-effective or possible to obtain direct measures of changes in behavior such as changes in delivery of care. Evaluators, therefore, may gather indirect evidence of project success, for example, participants' self-reports. In order to make judgments about the effectiveness of a project, whether from direct or indirect measures, data-gathering instruments are used. If these instruments are inappropriate or badly designed, the results of the data-gathering process may be useless or even harmful (Cronbach, 1949; Ebel, 1972).

The decision maker seeks to make valid and reliable decisions. *Validity* relates to the accuracy and appropriateness of the judgments made as a consequence of the information-gathering process. Judgments may lack validity for a number of reasons. One of the most important is that the decision makers may make unwarranted assumptions about the relationship between two types of behavior. For example, tests of factual knowledge may be used to decide about examinees' clinical judgment. Although the ability to recall information and the ability to make clinical judgments may be related to one another, the relationship is by no means close enough to draw conclusions based exclusively on the knowledge test. Another common error is to make judgments that are not justified by the instrument's precision of measurement. A CE director may decide that participants failed to achieve an objective, without realizing that the test used to make that judgment does not adequately relate to the specified learning outcomes.

Reliability is the likelihood that, if the data-gathering process were repeated using another appropriate sample of questions, behaviors, or observations, the results would be similar. Because most data-gathering involves a sampling process, the reliability of a measurement procedure is strongly influenced by the number of samples of data gathered and the representativeness of the sampling process. Another common source of unreliability is situations in which human observers or raters are used. Unless data collection is systematically structured, raters may concentrate on different aspects of performance, have different criteria for making judgments, or may be inconsistent in applying judgments. In these cases, the measurements contain more error than measurements that are more objective in nature, such as counting the number of correct answers in a multiple-choice test.

Feasibility relates to all aspects of the evaluation. At times, for example, the most desired data-gathering methods cannot be used for reasons of practicality or cost-effectiveness. The size and scope of an evaluation, including the number of people involved, the issues addressed, and the amount of data collected, are influenced by the feasibility of obtaining the required resources and expertise. When considering the feasibility of an evaluation, the evaluator should also consider the appropriateness of the plan. There is the temptation to overevaluate, using elaborate techniques on projects that may be too small to warrant the resources or that require only simple methods of evaluation.

Another feasibility issue affecting evaluation planning is the reluctance of many participants in CE activities to engage in evaluation activities. Participants often are concerned that inappropriate judgments may be made based on inadequate samples of data. Although it is possible to provide anonymity in data gathered for evaluation purposes, evaluators of CE usually avoid gathering performance data because of the sensitivity of participants. However, careful planning and consultation might allay such sensitivities, allowing collection of more direct measures of performance.

When drawing conclusions from the data collected, the evaluator should recognize the fact that the actual process of evaluation may influence the behavior of those participating in the process. For example, if some health professionals are involved in establishing standards for practice, members may be influenced to change behaviors as a result of participating in the standard-setting process. Therefore, the effect of the evaluation on participants must be an important consideration in conducting evaluations.

Systematic Approach to Evaluation

CE providers can use the tools of educational evaluation without necessarily being experts in evaluation, though collaboration and consultation with evaluation experts may greatly enhance the efforts. One of the simplest methods of organizing evaluation is to pose a series of questions. The questions should be raised during project planning, implementation, and at some periods of time after the conclusion of the project. The role and activities of the evaluator will vary from project to project. The role and activities will also vary according to whether the entire yearly program of the CE provider unit is being assessed or some individual project during that yearly program.

When evaluators approach the task of project evaluation, they should develop a systematic plan that outlines the process that will be used to focus the evaluation, collect the data, analyze the data, draw conclusions, and report the findings (Groteleuschen, Gooler, and Knox, 1976). Though the plan need not be elaborate, it should be precise enough to ensure that the appropriate data will be collected to answer the issues raised by the evaluation. The plan should address the following considerations.

What types of evaluation decisions must be made? Information from evaluation is usually used by project directors to make improvements. Plans for how the evaluation results will be used focus the decisions about data requirements and data-collection techniques. Depending on the purposes of the evaluation, data will be needed about project selection, project changes, resource development, staff development, and project justification.

Who is the audience for the evaluation data? The chief consumer of evaluation data is often the project director who has discretion in making many programmatic decisions. However, there may be others who have an interest in the issues raised by the evaluation. To increase the likelihood that decisions affecting the CE programming and resources are based on relevant data, the evaluator should identify any other users of the results and determine their information needs. The audience may include those who implement the project, faculty, funding agencies, or accrediting bodies.

What evaluation issues are most pressing? One key to carrying out an effective evaluation is the formulation of the issues that will be examined by the evaluation. Specification of evaluation questions is usually a consensus process among those who have information needs (the audience described in the previous paragraph). Usually more issues are identified than can be successfully studied within available time and resources. Therefore, priorities must be established that have been agreed upon by all information users. Because the identification of key questions is so crucial to the effectiveness of evaluation results, a major portion of this chapter is devoted to a discussion of potential issues and their implications.

What criteria and standards will be applied to the evaluation? Once the evaluation issues have been selected, some implicit or explicit criteria must be established. The relationship of the criteria to project effectiveness should be justified and specific standards should be set. Data collection can then focus on gathering information that will allow the comparisons called for within the evaluation.

What resources are available for the evaluation process? The availability of resources directly influences the scope of the evaluation. The most important resources are time and personnel expertise. Before decisions about data collection or analysis are made, the availability of necessary expertise, time, and financial resources should be considered. The collection of data may require highly sophisticated techniques and instrumentation. Limitations of resources generally require that simple techniques using logic and understanding of the educational process be employed before more complex methods are adopted. If this is the case, it is better to make this determination in the beginning so the plan does not involve an elaborate evaluation that cannot be carried out.

What kinds of evidence should be collected to answer the key questions? Once the issues for study have been decided, the evaluator should seek the information from the most reliable sources to address the questions relating to these issues. An extremely wasteful procedure is to gather evidence to answer questions no one asked or to gather data that do not address the issues. If the purpose of an evaluation is to assess the extent of changed attitudes, data about technical capabilities will not supply valid information.

What data-gathering procedures should be used? Because judgments are made from the information gathered, it is most important that the measures used to collect the data are appropriate. If data about performance are required, the instruments must focus on that information. If the instruments collect data on participants' knowledge rather than what they actually do on the job, inaccurate judgments and assumptions will be made. Decisions about data collection should take into consideration the type of data required to answer the evaluation issues, the available resources, the feasibility of using particular methods, and the implications of data analysis. Chapter Eight describes data-collection methods that can also be applied in evaluation.

How should the data be analyzed? Data analysis can be highly technical or very simple. Questions about the complexity of the data analysis depend upon the nature of the issues, the type of data collected, and the availability of resources. Analysis procedures should be selected at the time decisions are made about data collection. Often, huge amounts of data, impossible to analyze quickly and efficiently, are gathered. If in-depth analyses are required and a consultant is necessary, the person should be involved in the planning stages to assure that the appropriate data are collected in the most usable form.

What is the best way to report evaluation findings? A report of findings should be tailored to the issues requiring decisions and to the target audience. Reports crammed with data may please evaluation specialists but may be incomprehensible to those receiving the evaluation results. Most importantly, the results should be made available. Evaluation information cannot be used in decision making if the results are not reported.

Evaluation Issues

Formulation of the evaluation questions is one of the single most important components of a systematic evaluation. Whether evaluation results are applied is directly related to how relevant the issues were to the audiences for the evaluation. Evaluations that ask questions that cannot be answered or that provide answers that no one is interested in are of little benefit and are a waste of resources. On the other hand, simple evaluation of the accomplishment of course objectives overlooks the other influences that affect project success. The following sections will stimulate CE planners' awareness of the diversity of questions that can be raised about program effectiveness. Depending on the purpose of the evaluation, the issues may focus on project planning, project implementation, or outcomes occurring sometime after the project. Some issues may require collection and examination of information throughout all three phases. The questions discussed below are not exhaustive; however, they suggest most of the major issues involved in CE evaluation. Many of the ideas in the following sections were influenced by Stake (1967).

Does the planned activity clearly relate to identified community health needs? Often the community health needs that the project is attempting to meet are vague and ill-defined. Sharpening the definition of needs helps to establish the education and evaluation issues to be addressed during project design and implementation. Focusing on community health helps one to recognize that there may be several ways of solving the same problem. For example, Kattwinkel and others (1979) used a variety of means to improve the quality of care provided to infants and mothers at risk in community hospitals.

Is there some logical relationship between the planned educational project and the identified needs of participants in relation to their practice responsibilities? Because participants attend educational activities for a variety of reasons, it is important that their needs be clearly identified and analyzed before making project design and evaluation decisions. Are the participants interested in changing or improving their skills, their knowledge, or their clinical judgment? If so, in what ways? Are they interested in increasing their awareness rather than changing their abilities? Learners often want to discover whether they are doing things correctly. CE evaluators should be aware of the diverse needs that learners bring to CE programs and consider how to gather data about unexpected outcomes and their meaning for program development.

What evidence is there that the program actually attended to the learning needs of participants? One strategy for addressing this question is to repeat the needs assessment activity to see if the educational needs have been reduced for the target population. One should realize that the short-term objectives of instruction may not necessarily correspond to the clients' needs. Sometimes, the clients may fail to reach the short-term objectives, though the instructional activities may still lead to reduction of learning needs. For example, a posttest given after a three-day activity on the treatment of rheumatoid arthritis may indicate that many of the participants were unable to distinguish various types of arthritis treatments. Such a finding might indicate failure to achieve one behavioral objective. But if the project were aimed at improving the ability of the participants to treat rheumatoid arthritis, the findings do not indicate participants' failure to actually respond to rheumatoid arthritis in an improved fashion in practice. If the project resulted in increased referrals of difficult arthritis cases and in an increased demand for arthritis clinics, the activity would have to be considered successful, regardless of the impact on the participants' specific knowledge or skills.

What evidence is there that clients perceived the intended relationship between the project and their learning needs? Sometimes CE planners assume that the relationship of their projects to the activities of health professionals is self-evident. Interviews or questionnaires at the conclusion of the workshop may help answer this question.

Are the projects' goals and objectives stated appropriately? Objectives stated in behavioral form are usually considered optimal by educators. Subject matter specialists, however, are often content to describe their objectives in terms of what they will do—"introduce the audience to the latest approach in the management of rheumatoid arthritis"—rather than in terms of what learners will gain as a consequence of instruction. In order to improve the statement of objectives, the project is best planned in terms of possible impacts on performance.

It is often advisable to let project objectives evolve out of the interaction between the perceived needs of the potential learners and the interests and proficiencies of instructors (Knowles, 1975). Project goals and objectives are most effective if stated ahead of time and described with indicators of project success. Assessment of project impact and instructional improvement are difficult if objectives are vague or nonexistent.

What evidence is there that the goals and objectives of the project have been achieved? The clearer the goals and objectives, the more feasible it is to gather data regarding project success. Sometimes it is necessary to use indirect approaches, such as gathering data on the enrollment of participants in other projects or counting the number of referrals. Sometimes it is possible to use more direct measures, such as administering inventories or pre- and posttests of knowledge and clinical judgment. An important issue in assessing achievement of course objectives is whether or not the changes in attitudes or abilities persist over time. Often, without a supportive environment that provides continuing reinforcement and feedback, older patterns of behavior reassert themselves. In addition, much learning is latent and will only become apparent over time. However, in order to conclude that learning has taken place, some behavioral evidence must be available, and the statements of expected learning should be linked to some behavioral indicators.

Are the selection, orientation, and motivation of faculty effective? The most important resource for CE is the faculty conducting the projects. If a project fails to have an impact on the behavior of learners, the problem may be caused by poor use of faculty. Some of the factors to be assessed are whether sufficient attention has been paid to rewards for faculty participation, the success of faculty orientation, and faculty ability.

Did the faculty demonstrate appropriate instructional and interpersonal skills in conducting the activities? Information about faculty effectiveness in the teaching of skills and knowledge and their ability to relate to the participants can be obtained from end-of-course questionnaires. Often CE provider unit staff or other faculty need to participate or observe instruction to gain insight into faculty abilities.

Did the practitioners who attended the project have the background and experience that were anticipated when the project was planned? This information may often be obtained by preproject questionnaires, either at registration or before the start of the activity.

Did any side effects occur as a result of the project? Projects are designed to meet specific intended outcomes. The designers should be aware that all human activities have side effects. For example, the participants in a workshop on using new methods may demand that their hospital buy new equipment. The project evaluator should be aware of these possible side effects and try to gather data about their impact (Scriven, 1974).

Are the planned instructional activities based on logic and on the principles and generalizations of management and educational psychology? Planners must be realistic about what objectives can be accomplished by typical instructional experiences of limited time and scope. Educational projects that take into account the diversity of needs, interests, abilities, and situations of the clients are apt to be more successful than those that do not allow for such diversity.

Did the intended instructional activities operate as planned? During the conduct of instruction, things may occur differently than planned with respect to physical elements, the faculty, or the participants. For example, the room may be too small or too large, the sound system can be weak, the sight lines may be blocked by obstacles, the slides may be unreadable, the equipment may fail to work, or the handouts fail to arrive. The faculty may misunderstand instructions or alter presentations unexpectedly. Participants may have more diverse interests than expected, be reluctant to participate in certain types of activities, or have different needs than expected, which can lead to changes in instruction.

What evidence is there that the rationale for designing and implementing the project was appropriate? What reasons are there for successes or failures? The process of project planning and implementation might be conceived of as similar to a rigid experimental design. The data are the evidence that one uses to ascertain the success or failure of the experiment. For example, if a project objective was to increase the knowledge of participants about antihypertension medications, small group sessions where participants could interact with program faculty and fellow participants might be employed as part of the project design. Some evaluation data might indicate that the sessions were highly interactive and that the participants enjoyed them. Posttest data might reveal no change in knowledge. Analysis might indicate that lively discussion left the participants confused rather than enlightened. An unanticipated outcome of the project might be increased interest in hypertension, but the project (experiment) would probably be judged as only partially successful. Other methods might prove move effective for achieving the particular project objectives. Each element of project design should be tested in some fashion. Activities that work with one group of participants in one setting may fail with other groups in other settings.

Are the planned physical facilities appropriate? Although impressive auditoriums especially designed for CE may be available in some instances, usually multipurpose facilities are being used. The effectivenes of formal activities can be influenced greatly by a setting that is compatible with the educational situation and has a good sound system, adequate sight lines, seating comfort, temperature control, ventilation, nearby restrooms, easy access to coffee and other refreshments, and the availability of small meeting rooms.

Do the instructional materials meet accepted criteria and standards of the art and science of instructional materials development? Many CE activities distribute or make use of print or audiovisual materials. Do the instructional materials have clear, explicit goals and objectives? Are they at an appropriate level of complexity and detail? Have steps been taken to assure that the information in the materials is correct? Are the materials grammatically and editorially consistent and correct? Are the figures organized in a fashion that facilitates their use for reference purposes? Are practice exercises and feedback included when appropriate? Is the material appropriately concise, yet complete in terms of the objectives? If visual aids are used as part of the instructional materials, are they technically polished? If slides or overheads are used, are they legible to everyone in the room and are they easily understood or do they contain too much information? Have the materials been evaluated to confirm that they teach what they are designed to teach? Have the materials undergone some type of peer review to assure that they present information and concepts considered important in the field of study?

Were the instructional materials used as planned? At times instructional materials that are carefully designed are not used properly. They may be inserted in the presentation at the wrong time, used with too small or too large a group, or in general not applied well.

What was the impact of the evaluation? Evaluation methods can be powerful instructional tools with considerable impact on behavior. Often, the identification of deficiencies that practitioners genuinely accept as being related to their practice effectiveness can result in efforts to modify and change the practice procedures. Similarly, changes could occur in program planning and administration, marketing, or cost-benefit analyses. Because behavioral impact data can be costly to obtain, it is advisable to have a thorough understanding of the questions to be answered by the data being collected. The collection of data without any meaningful purpose, so-called orphan data, should be avoided (Nelson, 1976).

Is the project cost-effective? The basic principle of cost-benefit analysis is that resources are used in ways that will maximize progress toward meeting the project's goals and objectives.

Is the promotion of the project effective? Marketing is often not a high priority for staff of CE provider units whose main experience may have been in teaching and patient care. Yet low attendance at activities may not indicate that the project is failing to meet professionals' needs, but rather that marketing has been ineffective.

Conclusion

In many situations, the CE director also functions as the evaluator. In other situations, the CE provider units will have several staff, some of whom can assume the role of evaluator. The evaluator has considerable discretion in deciding what questions to ask and in explaining and interpreting the findings (House, 1980). To the extent that the evaluator can focus on issues of programmatic effectiveness as they relate to the improvement of health care, the evaluation can gain credibility. Since program directors are emotionally and professionally involved with the success of their efforts, it is desirable that the CE management functions and evaluation functions be separated. On the other hand, the evaluator must be sufficiently involved with the project to have access to key data. Furthermore, it is important from the standpoint of the use of resources that the evaluator communicate effectively with the program director and address issues that are important to those who have decision-making power. Stufflebeam and others (1971) have emphasized the importance of evaluation as a method of judging decision alternatives. Since evaluation can be costly, evaluators should focus their efforts on the aspects of the project where alternative actions are still possible.

References

American Board of Pediatrics. *Foundations for Evaluating the Competency of Pediatricians.* Chicago: American Board of Pediatrics, 1974.

Bertram, D. A., and Brooks-Bertram, P. A. "The Evaluation of Continuing Medical Education: A Literature Review." *Health Education Monographs,* 1977, *5* (4), 330–362.

Campbell, D. T., and Stanley, J. C. *Experimental and Quasiexperimental Designs for Research.* Chicago: Rand McNally, 1963.

Cook, T. D., and Campbell, D. T. *Quasiexperimentation: Design and Analysis Issues for Field Settings.* Chicago: Rand McNally, 1979.

Cronbach, L. J. *Essentials of Psychological Testing.* New York: Harper & Row, 1949.

Ebel, R. L. *Essentials of Educational Measurement.* Englewood Cliffs, N.J.: Prentice-Hall, 1972.

Goldfinger, S. E. "Continuing Medical Education: The Case for

Contamination." *New England Journal of Medicine*, 1982, *306* (9), 540–541.

Gronlund, N. E. *Stating Behavioral Objectives for Classroom Instruction*. New York: MacMillan, 1970.

Groteleuschen, A. D., Gooler, D. D., and Knox, A. B. *Evaluation in Adult Basic Education: How and Why*. Urbana-Champaign, Ill.: Office for the Study of Continuing Professional Education, College of Education, University of Illinois, 1976.

Guba, E. G. *Toward a Methodology of Naturalistic Inquiry in Educational Evaluation*. Los Angeles, Calif.: Center for the Study of Evaluation, Graduate School of Education, University of California, 1978.

House, E. R. *Evaluating with Validity*. Beverly Hills, Calif.: Sage, 1980.

Kattwinkel, J., and others. "Improved Perinatal Knowledge and Care in the Community Hospital Through a Program of Self-Instruction." *Pediatrics*, 1979, *64* (4), 451–458.

Knowles, M. S. *Self-Directed Learning: A Guide for Learners and Teachers*. New York: Association Press, 1975.

McCall, W. A. *How to Experiment in Education*, New York: Macmillan, 1923.

Nelson, A. R. "Sounding Board: Orphan Data and the Unclosed Loop: A Dilemma in Professional Standards Review Organization (PSRO) and Medical Audit." *New England Journal of Medicine*, 1976, *295* (11), 617–619.

Pennington, F. C., and LaScala, E. *The Evaluation Sourcebook*. Office of Continuing Medical Education, Department of Postgraduate Medicine and Health Professions Education, University of Michigan Medical School, 1978.

Scriven, M. "Evaluation Perspectives and Procedures." In W. J. Popham (Ed.), *Evaluation in Education: Current Applications*. Berkeley, Calif.: McCutchan, 1974.

Smith, L. "An Evolving Logic of Participant Observation, Educational Ethnography, and Other Case Studies." In L. Schulman (Ed.), *Review of Research in Education*, no. 6. Itasca, Ill.: F. E. Peacock, 1978.

Stake, R. E. "The Countenance of Educational Evaluation." *Teachers College Record*, 1967, *68* (7), 523–540.

Stein, L. S. "The Effectiveness of Continuing Medical Education: Eight Research Reports." *Journal of Medical Education*, 1981, *56*, 103-110.

Stufflebeam, D. L., and others. *Educational Evaluation and Decision Making*. Bloomington, Ill.: Phi Delta Kappa, 1971.

Facilitating Self-Directed Learning

David M. E. Allan
Sarina J. Grosswald
Robert P. Means

𝔁𝔁𝔁𝔁𝔁𝔁𝔁𝔁𝔁𝔁𝔁𝔁𝔁𝔁𝔁𝔁𝔁𝔁𝔁𝔁𝔁

Self-directed learning has its foundation in theories of learning, educational psychology, and adult development. This chapter builds on the learning theories and principles reviewed in Chapter Two, focusing on their relationship to self-directed learning and describing a new paradigm for education. The chapter provides an excellent practical approach to the process of self-directed learning. A plan for designing self-directed learning projects is described, as well as specific suggestions for assessing needs, selecting activities, and evaluating outcomes. The chapter offers recommendations on how continuing education (CE) provider units can foster self-directed learning and assist individual health professionals.

—Editors

Once health professionals complete basic and specialized training and enter practice, they must assume the major responsibility for the continuing learning necessary to provide optimal, up-to-date care. Professional education unfortunately provides little preparation for meeting this responsibility. More often than not, the curriculum orientation of formal, professional training reinforces institution-centered rather than learner-centered approaches to education. Decisions regarding what to learn, how to learn, and how to demonstrate competence are made by the faculty rather than by the student. Consequently, health professionals enter practice somewhat unaware of their resources and capabilities for planning their learning.

Health professionals who attend formal continuing education activities throughout their career continue to encounter CE offerings that reinforce the institution-centered or teacher-oriented approaches to learning. Conditions in the practice setting create additional obstacles to health professionals' continuing learning. Work loads that restrict the professionals' ability to devote extended periods of time to CE, increasingly high costs associated with formal CE, and the magnitude of CE from which professionals must choose constrain professionals' efforts. In addition, a considerable number of CE activities focus on highly specialized or unique practice problems and fail to address the more prevalent practical needs of many practitioners.

In their daily work, however, health professionals are frequently confronted with clinical practice problems or issues that often need quick resolution. As discussed in greater detail in Chapter Four, professionals select a variety of ways for obtaining the information to resolve their problems—such as which journal or book to purchase, which article to read, which audiotape to review, or in which conference to invest their time, money, and energy—and thus make decisions about their continuing education. Unfortunately, professionals at times seem to opt for what is most convenient and entertaining rather than what is most effective and thus fail to resolve their problems.

Among providers of CE for health professionals, there is an increasing awareness that individual professionals learn better and translate that knowledge into behavior change more readily if the professionals are actively involved in the learning process and in making decisions about what they learn, how they learn, and when they learn. The self-directed learning (SDL) process establishes the learners as the decision makers and planners for meeting their own unique needs.

Definition

In response to professional needs and a rapidly increasing body of scientific knowledge, health professionals are becoming more aware of and adept at assuming the primary responsibility for directing their own learning. Self-directed learning represents a nontraditional approach to learning, sometimes referred to as self-initiated, self-planned, or individual learning. This form of learning involves the individual learner's initiative and responsibility to (with or without assistance) identify, assess, and set priorities for learning needs; define goals; select and organize learning activities; and evaluate outcomes in terms of performance (Knox, 1973).

The self-directed approach to learning provides significant benefits to the professional. It provides an opportunity for professionals to resolve their specific practice problems, generally within their own practice setting. It is responsive to the autonomy, flexibility, and convenience so important to practicing professionals; it allows the professionals to select the content and learning method and to control the pace of learning. Even more importantly, self-directed learning increases the professionals' capability to respond rapidly to the frequent changes in health care expectations and delivery (Allis, 1980).

The concept of self-directed learning must be distinguished from independent learning. Independent learning is an instructional method in which the professional works alone. On the other hand, self-directed learning is a process encompassing a wide range of methods and approaches to meet different needs and preferred learning styles within the constraints of existing resources. In one situation, self-directed learning can be achieved independently, with the learner defining deficiencies in knowledge, setting precise learning objectives, identifying a journal, book, or other resource to obtain the knowledge, applying the new knowledge to patient care, and assessing the change in performance or in the patients' responses. In a different situation, self-directed learning may involve the aid of a tutor or facilitator and include the selection of workshops or seminars that meet the learner's objectives, satisfying the preferred style of learning. Peer group support may be used to help apply the new knowledge in practice and to evaluate defined changes in performance. In either case, the learning process is centered around the learner. A teacher or facilitator may or may not be included, a variety of human and nonhuman learning resources can be utilized, and the learning process meets the practitioner's needs in terms of time, finances, and access to resources.

Theoretical Foundations

The concept of self-directed learning is based on the research underlying the principles of adult learning, including the theories of personal growth and development, the theories of learning and educational psychology, and the tenets of the individual-centered approach. These principles are described in detail in Chapter Two. This section synthesizes those theories and principles that have direct implications for self-directed learning. Following that is a suggested paradigm for learning that applies these theories and the capabilities of information technology in a general approach to continuing education.

Theories of Learning. Theories of learning identify many concepts that contribute to the principles of self-directed professional learning. These concepts recognize the need for the learner to grow and to acquire experiences by reaction to different environments and situations (Piaget, 1952) that can be used as a basis for future problem solving. Learning is nurtured by curiosity, a desire for competence, and a sense of social responsibility (Bruner, 1961). Wisdom and experience increase with maturation, compensating for the decline in the neurophysiologically based fluid intelligence, and enabling problem-solving skills to be maintained and even enhanced (Horn and Cattell, 1966).

The work of Carl Rogers (1969) provides additional perspectives on self-directed learning. Rogers argues that much more significant and lasting learning can take place when the learning is integrated with work or is acquired through active involvement by placing the student in direct experiential confrontation with problems. Learning is facilitated when the learners define their own problems, discover their own learning resources, decide their own course of action, and recognize the consequences of their decisions. The most lasting, pervasive learning results when learners identify the learning as their own personal initiative. Self-evaluation of performance, rather than evaluation by others or denial of deficiencies, will strengthen independence and the self-reliance of the professional. Self-directed learners consider change a necessity and are comfortable with adapting their professional performance in response to new knowledge.

The research and writings of Knowles (1975), Tough (1978), and Houle (1980) reinforce the importance of positive attitudes and self-concepts for the self-directed learner. In addition, Knowles states that "there is convincing evidence that people who take the initiative in learning (proactive learners) learn more things and learn better, than do people who sit at the feet of teachers passively waiting to be taught (reactive learners) . . . they also tend to retain and make use of what they learn better and longer than do the reactive learners" (p. 14). Knowles points out that in a world in which the half-life of many facts and skills may be ten years or less, where rapid change will be the only stable characteristic, "the basic human competence of the ability to learn on one's own has suddenly become a prerequisite for living in this new world" (p. 15).

Personal Growth and Development. From the perspective of humanistic psychology—the study of personal growth, development, and motivation—self-directed learning is a self-discovery process. Rogers (1969) defines the process as having the qualities of complete personal involvement, being self-initiated and persuasive (changing the behavior and attitude of the learner), and using self-evaluation and feedback to reinforce the appreciation of self-growth as a total experience. Rogers states that human beings are curious, with a natural potential for learning. Continual learning is necessary to meet the inner needs of living and working and leads to the adventure of change that is the core of self-directed learning. Personal growth must continue and be rewarded both by the individual and by society. Personal change is initiated by an attitude of accepting responsibility for oneself to function as an internal change agent.

Adult Learning. Principles of adult learning, which have their basis in theories of learning and development, espouse the concepts that as people mature, they move from dependent personalities to becoming self-directed human beings; they have growing reservoirs of experience that are resources and bases for learning; they become increasingly motivated to learn developmental tasks oriented to their social and professional roles; and they gradually focus learning on immediate application, shifting from a subject to a problem orientation (Knowles, 1980).

From studies of adult development and learning and from research in the biological, social, and behavioral sciences, a better understanding of how adults learn has emerged. Knox (1977) summarizes the physiological changes that take place that enhance or inhibit the ability of adults to learn and to learn how to learn (see Chapter Two). Some of these changes are especially relevant to the concept of self-directed learning.

Trends in learning are influenced by the physiological changes caused by aging (Knox, 1977). However, the ability to learn can be kept constant by controlling the pace of the learning activities. Self-directed learners can choose educational methods that allow them to control the speed at which they learn. Intellectually able and stimulated adults maintain stable or increasing learning ability throughout their working life. The continual process of assessment and definition of practice deficiencies accomplished through self-directed learning can help foster educational development and personal growth.

Self-Directed Learning and A New Paradigm. The key concepts that consistently arise from the theories described, providing the basis for self-directed learning, are that significant learning should take place as close to the work setting as feasible, as close to the time of need in a professional-patient encounter as possible, and should provide the learners with immediate feedback to enable them to recognize the need for further information. In patient care today, there is a vast amount of rapidly changing medical and health knowledge that potentially bears on the care of a patient. Professionals have to learn to apply modern technology of information management that supports optimal professional performance, high-quality patient care, and constant self-evaluation.

Weed (1976) has redefined the premises on which medical education should be based to enhance the use of information. These premises about medical education also provide the springboard for moving traditional continuing education into the future, providing both the rationale and the challenge for supporting self-directed learners. Weed compares the old premises of education to new ones in what he refers to as a new paradigm for education.

Old premise— *A core of knowledge should be taught.*
New premise—*A core of behavior should be elicited [Weed, p. 79].*

For the practicing health professional, the concept of a manageable core of knowledge has been destroyed by the knowledge and technology explosion of the last thirty years. Human memory requires help to organize and retrieve information at the moment of need so that practitioners can be consistently reliable and efficient in their analytical, diagnostic, and therapeutic actions. The continuing education for practitioners should include the use of the computer for information, answers to problems, and evaluation of perform-ance in the real world of practice.

Old premise— *Faculty, research facilities, extensive clinical facilities,*
　　　　　　 and teaching facilities are the principal resource of a
　　　　　　 medical school.
New premise—*The principal resource is the student's natural capac-*
　　　　　　 ity to learn and solve problems on his own in an en-
　　　　　　 vironment that allows and encourages him to do so
　　　　　　 and provides essential feedback [Weed, p. 81].

The major function of continuing education should be to develop the health professionals' capacity to solve problems on their own and to produce "individuals with resourceful, independent minds who will naturally turn to books and modern computer tech-niques and all the other sources of information and skills that abound in our society" (Weed, p. 82). A self-directed learner will become more concerned with problem solving than with knowledge and will place increasing value on the patient encounter as a resource for learning and as assessment of professional competence.

Old premise— *Students should learn given facts and understanding in the absence of real work and responsibility.*
New premise—*Real work with real responsibilities should form the basis of all educational activity right from the beginning* [Weed, p. 85].

Self-directed continuing education, carried out by the learner and arising from a concern during patient care, becomes immediately relevant and linked to performance. Performance outcome is documented and can be reviewed and used by the professionals to reassure patients and their public representatives about their competence.

Old premise— *Time and number of courses covered should be the constant, and achievement the variable in medical education.*
New premise—*Achievement should be the constant, and time and number of tasks the variable in medical education and medical practice* [Weed, p. 86].

For continuing education, the old premise is that there is a core of knowledge that can be acquired by sitting for hours in a formal educational setting. By placing education into the work setting and by using the modern tools of education, such components of professional performance as problem solving can be enhanced and evaluated. Mandatory hours of continuing education will become irrelevant, the need for formal, distant programs of continuing education would be reduced, and millions of dollars of the health professionals' and patients' money would be saved.

Old premise— *A person should take examinations at points in his education to qualify for practice.*
New premise—*A person's performance should be audited at random throughout his career and according to rules for medical practice, clearly defined and used, from the very beginning of medical education* [Weed, p. 87].

For self-directed learners, this means an assessment of their performance at frequent intervals, in their practice environment. Performance can be measured against that of peers on the basis of previously defined standards. This removes the need for unrealistic proposals for relicensure and recertification based on hours of formal education or examinations of knowledge.

Facilitating the Self-Directed Learner

Several variables influence one's ability and readiness to learn and have particular significance to self-directed learning. All individuals have their own style of processing and organizing new information that influences the effectiveness of different educational methods. By assessing the ways in which the professional prefers to learn and learns most effectively, the professional can select means of meeting educational needs that are most likely to be successful and stimulating. Individuals' self-concepts influence their acceptance of new experiences and learning. The professionals' skills of self-assessment, questioning, problem solving, and self-evaluation affect their capabilities to compare realistically current levels of competence to desired levels. The role of the CE provider unit is to assist the professionals in this assessment process and to provide resources to facilitate their learning.

Chapter Four describes research that identifies criteria for the selection, organization, and determination of the value of various sources of information used by a group of family physicians as they pursue their continuing education. These same criteria can apply to choices made by self-directed learners and indicate areas in which a provider of continuing education can assist self-directed learners. The criteria include the clinical relevance of the information, the familiarity with the sources of information, the availability and accessibility of the information at the time and place it is needed, the stage of information seeking, and the opportunity for active involvement in the learning process.

Some general implications for supporting self-directed learning can be drawn from these criteria. The CE provider can assist professionals in identifying their learning needs and in identifying and using those resources that are accessible in the practice settings.

A variety of resources should be available to assist the professional at various stages of information seeking, including immediate access to journals and books, consultation opportunities with peers, and formal CE activities. CE activities should build on the professionals' experience, demonstrate and encourage new learning methods, and include opportunities for practicing new skills in order to encourage the application of learning in the work setting.

Self-Directed Learning and the CE Provider Unit

The self-directed learner is characterized as one who uses a planned learning process to assess educational needs through self-evaluation, choose specific learning resources, and translate and apply new knowledge into specific practice situations. Providers of continuing education wishing to facilitate self-directed learning should ensure that health professionals possess the skills to carry out these plans and should help them locate the resources they need.

The theoretical and practical foundations described earlier in the chapter provide the framework for the design and implementation of self-directed learning. The process closely parallels the systematic design of any learning experience. It includes the identification and analysis of needs, the setting of goals and objectives in relation to defined needs, the selecting and organizing of learning experiences, and the evaluation of outcomes in practice.

Identifying Problems and Concerns. The primary motivation to learn for health professionals arises from problems or issues in their daily practice. Frequently, professionals select "interest areas" for the focus of their continuing education rather than "need areas." While "interest areas" can provide stimulation and are part of a well-rounded program of learning, the cornerstone of self-directed learning is the planned process of identifying problems or concerns in the practice setting. Often, however, professionals lack the skills for accurately assessing their educational needs. Even those professionals who do assess their own needs may be confronted by questions about where to begin and how much to do. To reduce some of the confusion and increase the professionals' capabilities to assess needs, the CE provider can show practitioners how to focus on needs associated with major areas of their practice, areas in which the greatest number of patients are seen, or gaps in performance that may represent the greatest threat to patient health. Identifying needs not only improves the practitioner's ability to select educational activities but also establishes a base for determining changes that occur following an educational intervention.

The professional's practice provides a storehouse of sources for identifying needs. However, this information is usually difficult to retrieve because the practitioner's records system is not constructed to provide the data. A crucial role for the CE provider is assisting professionals in learning how to organize practice data and how to use new technologies to make information more accessible and usable for identifying educational needs. Specific sources of data for needs identification include practice-related indicators, colleagues, self-assessment, the literature, and continuing education activities.

Practice-related indicators can be divided into four sets of data—the professional's own perception of performance, statistical data, standards of practice, and patient responses.

The professionals' *perceptions* of their knowledge and capabilities can give them the motivation and incentive to pursue learning. At times, however, the professionals' perceptions of daily practice are inaccurate because they are influenced by the most unusual occurrences rather than the most common. Nevertheless, their perception of learning needs may provide the impetus for more systematically evaluating problems and concerns.

As a starting point, professionals can gather *statistics* about their practice, considering the most frequent patient problems presented over a period of time, the most frequent prescriptions written, and the final diagnosis on patient charts. An informal method of collecting these data is a daily patient log on which the professional can record information about types of patients, diagnoses, and follow-up needs. Such a collection of practice data, which also can be achieved with a simple computer program, is frequently referred to as a practice profile. A practice profile may reveal, for example, that the proportion of patients with athletic-related problems has increased, indicating the professional's need to learn more about sports medicine or the need to focus on particular types of injuries.

A special organization of office records will make practice data more accessible. For example, patient records can be cross-filed by major complaint, identified problems, primary diagnosis, drug prescription, or referral. At periodic intervals, the data can be collected and analyzed to identify particular areas on which learning activities should focus.

Some professions have established *standards of practice*. These are often derived from a consensus of experts or from research data and usually include aspects ranging from the expected competencies of the professional (for example, American Nurse's Association, 1973; American Board of Pediatrics, 1974) to specific treatments for particular health problems. Established standards of practice are made available by professional and specialty societies or by the institution in which the professional works. These standards provide an excellent means for professionals to assess their level of performance or knowledge and to identify areas of need for continuing education. However, this is an area in which further development is needed as it provides a significant resource for more effective continuing education. CE providers can facilitate review of existing standards by providing copies for practitioners, by setting aside portions of regular CE activities to discuss these standards, or by developing small groups to discuss the standards and their implications for continuing study.

Another source of data is the *patients* themselves, reflecting the extent of satisfaction or dissatisfaction with the care they receive. Surveys can be conducted periodically with a selected patient population to yield data indicative of patients' reactions and concerns. The role of patients in the educational process will be increasingly important in the next decade as patients become more self-directed and less passive about their health care.

Colleagues can have a significant impact on the individual professional's performance, by creating an awareness of new information and procedures that should be explored for their applicability (Houle, 1980). The peer group establishes the norm for specific practice approaches, as well as for levels of performance and ambition. Peer interaction may include informal conversation, consultation, or journal and study clubs. A professional may ask another professional for feedback on performance or suggestions for areas of further study. Either individually or as a group, a consultation can be arranged where the professionals can discuss particular strengths and weaknesses in a specific area of performance.

Self-assessment programs developed by professional and specialty societies provide a straightforward method for identifying deficiencies in knowledge. The specialty societies often provide an examination that is either self-graded or graded by the organization. Professionals can use the self-assessment to obtain a profile of their knowledge in a variety of subject areas, to measure their own performance against the data collected from their peers nationwide, and to define areas in which continuing education may be appropriate. Patient management problems or simulations of clinical practice are another form of self-assessment that enables the practitioner to define educational needs (Storey, Williamson, and Castle, 1968).

Literature is one of the most common sources of identifying needs informally. Professional society and association journals allow the professional to gain new perspectives on the latest developments in patient care. Written material from drug and equipment companies can draw attention to new advances in technology, stimulating the professional to seek more complete information. The latest textbooks provide sources for comparing one's level of practice to new advances or standards of clinical practice.

Professionals are inundated daily with brochures and announcements about *CE activities*. Program topics reflect current and emerging developments in health care. A review of proposed course topics can identify potential means for meeting educational needs by incorporating the activity into a self-directed learning plan. Participation in formal CE activities may also result in the identification of information needs and areas for further study.

Analyzing Learning Needs. All the sources of information described can produce a list of possible educational needs. The needs may be the result of discrepancies in desired competence or the result of a desire to expand current knowledge. The professional must then select which needs or problems to address. CE providers can assist the professional in establishing criteria for a priority list or for long-term planning, where the professional identifies the order for meeting several needs or for concentrating on a single area in depth.

To analyze and choose the topics to pursue, several criteria can be considered: the extent of the problem, whether the problem can be solved, the available resources, and the individual's own considerations of time, money, availability, and interest.

The first step in analyzing an identified problem or concern is to determine the cause. The professional should establish whether the problem can be solved by education or whether it requires a change in the system or management of practice. The solution to the problem may be to add another staff member who can meet the need and eliminate the problem (systems or management solution) or to increase one's own capabilities to meet the need (educational solution).

Once the cause has been identified, several factors can be considered to judge the priority of the problem: the number of patients affected, the potential impact of solving the problem, the cost of the problem to the patient or professional, and the extent of the discrepancy between the present level of practice and the desired level of practice. The professional should consider whether the problem can actually be solved and whether the solution is within the control of the professional. The resources required, the cost of different solutions, the required time away from practice, and available resources will all influence the analysis of needs and the selection of priorities. The provider of CE should be prepared to facilitate the self-directed learners to assess these issues, to review the available options, and to establish priorities for solving the problems.

Professionals should assess their own degree of commitment and motivation to pursue a particular topic and to effect a change in their behavior. A key element in self-directed learning is the ability to seek and accept change; to that end, many self-directed learners will be able to use the process to develop a plan for their future career development.

Setting Learning Goals and Objectives. The ability to specify learning goals and objectives is a critical factor in solidifying the health professionals' commitment to improving levels of competence and performance. It is this step in any learning process that generates the most difficulty and most resistance. Many professionals do not possess the skills or experience to complete this stage of the self-directed learning process. Answering the simple question of "what do I need to be able to do at the end of the learning process?" enables learning to be focused and evaluated and the appropriate learning method or resource to be defined. CE providers can pose the question, facilitate the development of the response, and bring together people with similar objectives. Setting learning objectives is also essential in enabling the health professional to establish a benchmark or standard by which to measure the outcome of a learning experience.

Several objectives may be required to meet a particular learning need, and a single learning experience may address a number of objectives. To serve as guidance in the development of the learning plan, objectives should reflect two characteristics. They should state the need as learning outcomes, and they should provide a basis for evaluation by suggesting a means of assessing the extent to which learning was achieved.

Because setting learning objectives is essential to the health professionals' likelihood to engage and persist in the self-directed learning process, the CE providers' role in assisting a professional at this stage is critical. Objectives should provide enough challenge to sustain interest and stimulate further discovery, without overwhelming the learner. While care should be taken in the documentation of objectives, the professional need not become "bogged down" by the task, inhibiting the self-directed learning process.

Selecting and Organizing Learning Activities. Health professionals as self-directed learners make a firm commitment to some form of change to enhance competence or performance. These commitments are translated into objectives or intended outcomes. To fulfill such commitments, professionals should be knowledgeable about a range of learning activities, materials, and resources; possess the ability to select methods of learning appropriate for the learning objectives; and be able to organize learning activities in a way that encourages learning and sustains motivation (Knox, 1973).

The educational activities selected should have a high correspondence between the professional's learning objectives and the content of the learning activity, and there should be compatibility between the professional's learning style preferences and the method of the learning activity. The activity should include opportunities to practice using the new information via, for example, discussions, role playing, and problem solving. Whenever possible, the activity should be flexible enough to enable the learner to modify the pace and, if necessary, ask for help (Knox, 1974).

The health professional as a learner typically gains new knowledge and experience by selecting a variety of formal and informal learning activities that require reading, writing, listening, discussing, observing, and practicing (Richards and Cohen, 1981). CE providers can assist learners in identifying and using the available learning activities, as well as create learning opportunities for the self-directed learner.

Learning opportunities can be categorized into four broad groups: print material, interpersonal contact with colleagues, formal CE, and use of technology.

Health professionals prefer and use *print materials* more frequently than any other source of information (Richards and Cohen, 1981). While print materials are plentiful, the professional often has difficulty finding time to read all that is available. Sometimes materials are outdated or fail to address the specific clinical needs of the practitioner. For the individual professional, several strategies offer a partial solution to this dilemma. The use of traditional abstracting services and monthly or annual digests of specialty or subspecialty literature can reduce searching and reading time. The National Library of Medicine's Current Awareness System offers selective dissemination of information (SDI) bibliographic retrieval programs through MEDLINE, tailored to the needs of practitioners (Darling, Bishop, and Colaianni, 1982). Practitioners specify subject areas of interest as parameters for bibliographic searches and retrievals from a computer data base. Each month the practitioner receives a printout of new bibliographies within the specified subject areas that have been entered into MEDLINE.

The National Library of Medicine can also access information by disease entity, using existing Index Medicus and MEDLARS/MEDLINE data bases. Instead of system searches resulting in extensive bibliographic lists, the professional defines the problem area and chooses a limited number of sources from increasingly specific subcategories. Selected experts nominate major works representing a synthesis of the most current and comprehensive statements about the problem area. This eliminates the necessity for additional sorting of data by the practitioner and encourages use of the information on current diagnostic and therapeutic plans.

A "user-friendly" literature search system has been developed and introduced into the library of a major teaching hospital by Horowitz and Bleich (1981). This system, called Paperchase, is designed so that: the program permits self-service without a manual, the terminal is located in the hospital library, the program accommodates the references shelved in the hospital, and the user will not lose data even if called away during a search. Graham, King, and Whitney (1981) describe a relatively sophisticated yet low-cost bibliography retrieval system called Simultaneous Remote Search (SRS) that allows a rural practitioner to conduct and receive on-site delivery of bibliographic searches on a phone terminal linkup with the regional medical library and the MEDLARS system of the National Library of Medicine.

Clintworth and others (1979) and Manning and Denson (1979) have described an educational system whereby practitioners have their drug prescription records reviewed by a panel of physicians and clinical pharmacists. Print material (journal articles or medical texts) are selected and sent to the practitioner as a learning packet for those areas where deficiencies in prescribing are defined. As an alternative, the CE provider unit can define local faculty who will consult with an individual practitioner.

An effective complement to the use of print material, particularly journal articles, is journal clubs. Journal or study clubs provide a small group with a focus for reading. One or more articles on related topics are read ahead of time; the group then discusses the application of the information in a particular practice setting. To enhance the application of readings, Jeghers (1964) developed a model for a reference file system that provides easy access to personalized reading needs. Jeghers' example uses physicians' topics but can be adapted for any profession.

One of the informal ways that health professionals learn is through daily *encounters with colleagues.* Conversations and consultations with colleagues provide the immediate feedback, clarification, or confirmation necessary when addressing clinical problems needing immediate attention, problems that have gone unresolved yet periodically reappear, or problems that represent areas of broad interest. Unlike journal articles that may represent theoretical aspects of new findings, conversations with colleagues generally reflect the current and practical application of the information. Telephone dial-in systems, such as the University of Birmingham, Alabama MIST (Medical Information Service via Telephone) System (See "Statewide Outbreak: Medical Information," 1982), which have operated with varying degrees of success, allow a more formal mechanism for access to consultation with experts.

Small groups of peers can be used by the CE provider to facilitate the introduction into practice of new techniques or drugs and to evaluate the effects of these on professional performance and patient care outcomes. Tumor boards, mortality and morbidity committees, and audit committee meetings are sources of learning and can be planned so that the learning meets specific objectives and can be documented (Sandlow, Bashook, and Maxwell, 1981).

During formal CE activities, CE providers can plan opportunities for professionals to consult with one another and with course faculty, enhancing the sharing of resources and ideas. As part of a self-directed learning contract, the consultation between colleagues can be arranged to meet a specific need, including the development of educational objectives and evaluation of the outcome (Clintworth and others, 1979).

An innovative approach to interpersonal contacts is a learning exchange. Such a network of interpersonal contacts and consultation has been proposed by a state professional association of family physicians (Pennington, 1975). As part of a larger centralized continuing education network, a centralized data file system would be kept on persons seeking information and those individuals who have an interest in or who are experts interested in sharing information with others.

The component of continuing education that has received the most attention and energy has been *formal CE activities.* This includes short courses, conferences, workshops, or seminars, whether they be part of an in-service program, staff development series, professional society meeting, or programs conducted in academic settings. A common misconception is that formal CE and self-directed learning represent mutually exclusive approaches to learning.

Rather, formal CE is a resource for fulfilling a self-directed learning plan. To foster self-directed learning, the CE provider unit can incorporate in these formal courses opportunities for independent study that may then lead to a planned self-directed approach to the professionals' unique problems. These independent study options might include mailing syllabus materials to the professionals prior to a conference, allowing the professional to determine the base knowledge on which the conference will build, or acting as an early organizer for learners' thoughts on certain topics. Supplemental materials such as journal articles can be sent out after a formal activity as reinforcement for the learning that occurred at the conference. Self-directed learning can be stimulated by patient care simulations, in print or with computerized, interactive videodisc or other media that can be included in the formal activity.

With the exception of in-service programs that take place in the work setting, formal CE programs for large groups suffer from their inability to take the educational process through to application in practice. While these programs can transmit enthusiasm and knowledge, they are often ineffective as change agents for health professionals' practice behaviors. For a self-directed learner, formal CE activities can be part of a planned effort to meet defined needs. Self-directed learners selecting formal CE programs act as their own agents of behavior change and establish their own mechanisms for translating the newly acquired knowledge into clinical practice. The need to change, the objectives to enable the change to take place, and the tools to evaluate the effectiveness of the change are already defined prior to taking the CE activity. CE providers can assist learners by surveying participants prior to formal activities, asking them to define their objectives for attending the activity. The faculty can then set matching objectives to respond to participants' needs. The CE activity can include suggested methods for professionals to evaluate their learning and can facilitate the development of support groups at the practice setting to encourage the application of new information.

Miniresidencies, clerkships, intra- and interinstitutional exchange of staff are effective methods for professionals to acquire short-term intensive learning experiences designed to fit the educational needs of self-directed learners. These activities can be developed by the CE provider unit and become part of the overall CE program.

In recent years the use of *technology* such as nonprint media including television, radio, telephone, slide tape, video cassette, videodisc, audiotape, and computer-assisted instruction has experienced dramatic growth and enhanced sophistication. This technology has made consistent progress in capturing the attention of learners and in bringing education closer to the practice setting. Audiotape programs that were at one time only available through a few nationwide networks such as Audio Digest have multiplied in number with the entry into the market of many media producers, including pharmaceutical and other commercial companies, and specialty societies.

The cost of nonprint sources such as computer-assisted instruction and videotapes traditionally has been a prohibitive factor in individual use. The current state of technology is advancing quickly enough to reduce much of the excessive start-up costs for the hardware and software systems. The increased use of cassette recorders and playback systems has substantially reduced the costs of individuals owning their own system. The advent of the interactive, or "intelligent," videodisc makes educational programs even more adaptive to the individual professionals' needs. Intelligent videodisc represents the joining of branching capabilities, high-quality audiovisuals, rapid random access, and pictorial representation in an interactive learning format (Leveridge, 1982). Unfortunately, the preparation of these programs requires enormous manpower investment.

A generation of compact microcomputer systems is currently available at considerably lower cost than just a few years ago. These systems can be used in hospital and office settings for data bases, access to other data bases, clinical decision aids, and quality-control mechanisms to provide information at the time of the patient encounter. This technology is presently in place; the barriers are our own inexperience, hesitancy, professional time, and money.

Institutional and organizational providers of CE need to recognize the importance of nonprint materials as a means of augmenting health professionals' learning process. While cost and availability continue to limit widespread use of nonprint materials, providers of

CE could develop subscription services that would provide software such as tapes, films, computer programs, and hardware such as projectors, slide viewers, and recorders to individuals or hospital library systems at costs substantially lower than the price of purchasing such materials.

CE providers can educate health professionals in the use of nonprint materials and can assist them in finding answers to the questions "where to locate" and "how to use nonprint resources." These questions could be answered as part of a workshop or continuing education course, through an independent study center set up as a part of a hospital or clinical library and audiovisual program, or through periodic information mailings and samples sent to professionals, describing resources available in their community and how to locate and use them. Efforts should be made to develop programs on the latest information sources and retrieval systems in cooperation with university medical school libraries or regional medical library systems.

Evaluating Outcomes. As in each of the preceding steps in the learning process, health professionals assume the major responsibility for evaluating their efforts. Evaluation is a dynamic or continuing process that enables the professionals to collect data or evidence about the level of progress being made in order to enhance the chance that a learning experience will lead to positive outcomes. Evaluation requires the health professional and the facilitator with whom the professional may be working to describe and make judgments about what has transpired in the learning process (Knox, 1973). Comparisons are drawn among conditions or circumstances prior to learning, the professional's intentions, and what actually occurred. These descriptions and judgments include examination of input (materials used), resources and process (the methods used to accomplish learning), and outcomes (what actually happens as a result of the learning). The collection and examination of data focus on ways to improve or modify the learning experience to help the professional achieve the desired goals.

Evaluation for the self-directed learner may entail periodic checks to see that progress is being made toward completing the specified objectives. The evidence that such progress is occurring can come from self-assessment exams, completion of mastery-level tests, or comparisons with known standards of practice, In other cases the critical measures of achievement or success are reduction in the recurrence of a particular problem or its elimination. Evaluation methods that are available to the self-directed learner include audits, peer reviews, checklists, and computer technologies.

Evaluation is a major contributing factor to the professional's motivation and persistence in learning because it serves as immediate feedback concerning the value of the experience in terms of the professional's time, money, and energy. CE providers can encourage the self-directed learner to use evaluation as a means to measure progress periodically or alter the course of action to enhance levels of performance.

Conclusion

The concept of health professionals as self-directed learners departs from the traditional teacher- and institution-directed educational system. According to this concept, self-directed learners take the primary responsibility for learning, take the initiative to continually identify and assess educational needs, set goals and objectives, select learning activities, and evaluate their own performance.

The learning process provides an autonomous, individualized, convenient, and flexible means for professionals to identify and address issues in their practice setting. The benefits of self-directed learning are becoming increasingly recognized because of its relevance to the needs of health professionals and patients. Self-directed learning focuses on the unique needs of the professional and enhances the application of learning to improve performance.

References

Allis, E. "The Health Professional as Self-Directed Learner." Unpublished paper, North Central Regional Medical Education Center, Minneapolis, Minn., Oct. 1980.

American Board of Pediatrics. *Foundations for Evaluating the Competency of Pediatricians.* Chicago: American Board of Pediatrics, 1974.

American Nurse's Association. *Standards of Nursing Practice.* American Nurse's Publication, no. NP-41. Kansas City, Kans.: American Nurse's Association, 1973.

Bruner, J. S. "The Act of Discovery." *Harvard Educational Review,* 1961, *31* (1), 21–32.

Clintworth, W. A., Gilman, N. J., Manning, P. R., Biles, J. A. "Continuing Education and Library Services for Physicians in Office Practice." *Bulletin of the Medical Library Association,* 1979, *67* (4), 353–358.

Darling, L., Bishop, D., and Colaianni, L. A. (Eds.). *Handbook of Medical Library Practice.* 4th ed. Vol. 1. Chicago: Medical Library Association, 1982.

Graham, D. L., King, C., and Whitney, P. J. "Simultaneous Remote Research: On-Line Bibliographic Library Services For Practicing Physicians." *Journal of the American Medical Association,* 1981, *246* (10), 1115–1116.

Horn, J. L., and Cattell, R. B. "Refinement and Test of the Theory of Fluid and Crystallized General Intelligence." *Journal of Educational Psychology,* 1966, *57* (5), 253–270.

Horowitz, G. L., and Bleich, H. L. "Paperchase: A Computer Program to Search the Medical Literature." *New England Journal of Medicine,* 1981, *305* (16), 924–930.

Houle, C. O. *Continuing Learning in the Professions.* San Francisco: Jossey-Bass, 1980.

Jeghers, H. "Medical Care, Education, and Research: Philosophy and Technics of Self-Education of the Medical Student and Physician." *New England Journal of Medicine,* 1964, *271* (25), 1297–1301.

Knowles, M. S. *Self-Directed Learning: A Guide for Learners and Teachers.* Chicago: Association Press, 1975.

Knowles, M. S. *The Modern Practice of Adult Education: From Pedagogy to Androgogy.* Rev. ed. Chicago: Follett, 1980.

Knox, A. B. "Lifelong Self-Directed Education." In Project Continuing Education for Health Manpower, *Fostering the Growing Need to Learn: Monographs and Annotated Bibliography on Continuing Education and Health Manpower.* Rockville, Md.: Health Resources Administration, Public Health Service, U.S. Department of Health, Education, and Welfare, 1973.

Knox, A. B. *Adult Development and Learning: A Handbook on Individual Growth and Competence in the Adult Years.* San Francisco: Jossey-Bass, 1977.

Leveridge, L. "The Interactive Videodisc." Paper presented at University of Southern California conference on the Practical Impact of the Computer and Other Electronic Technology on the Future of Continuing Education, Palm Springs, Calif., 1982.

Manning, P. R., and Denson, T. A. "How Cardiologists Learn About Echocardiography." *Annals of Internal Medicine,* 1979, *91* (3), 469–471.

Pennington, F. C. "Proposal for Statewide Continuing Medical Education System for Family Physicians." Unpublished doctoral dissertation, University of Michigan at Ann Arbor, 1975.

Piaget, J. *The Origins of Intelligence in Children.* New York: International Universities Press, 1952.

Purcell, E. F. (Ed.). *Recent Trends in Medical Education.* New York: Josiah Macy, Jr. Foundation, 1976.

Richards, R. K., and Cohen, R. M. *The Value and Limitations of Physician Participation in Traditional Forms of Continuing Medical Education.* Kalamazoo, Mich.: UpJohn Company, 1981.

Rogers, C. R. *Freedom to Learn.* Columbus, Ohio: Merrill, 1969.

Sandlow, L. J., Bashook, P. G., and Maxwell, J. A. "Medical Care Evaluation: An Experience in Continuing Medical Education." *Journal of Medical Education,* 1981, *56* (7), 580–586.

"Statewide Outbreak: Medical Information." *Alabama Journal of Medical Sciences,* 1982, *19* (3), 237–239.

Storey, P. B., Williamson, J. W., and Castle, S. H. *Continuing Medical Education: A New Emphasis.* Chicago: American Medical Association, 1968.

Tough, A. "Major Learning Efforts: Recent Research and Future Directions." *Adult Education,* 1978, *28* (4), 250–263.

Weed, L. L. "A New Paradigm for Medical Education." In E. F. Purcell (Ed.), *Recent Trends in Medical Education.* New York: Josiah Macy, Jr. Foundation, 1976.

Leadership of Continuing Education: A Strategic Management Approach

Joseph S. Green
J. Morris McInnes

Chapters Twelve and Thirteen are tandem chapters that should be read together. At the beginning of Chapter Twelve several questions are raised that are typical of those faced by continuing education (CE) provider unit managers. These questions require decisions, which in turn require information. The two chapters offer a framework for CE managers to develop a management information system that will assist the decision making in their organizations. Examples and specifics on the management tasks involved in the typical day-to-day running of a CE provider unit are not discussed; rather, a rationale is advanced for rethinking the role of the manager of a CE provider unit in proactively shaping a desired future such as described in Chapter Six. The rationale and specifics that help

define this new "strategic management" approach are presented,
along with examples applicable to CE provider units. If the reader's
concern is more administrative in nature, several other books are
suggested that would be of assistance. The primary audience for the
chapters are those managers who have the major responsibility for
leading the CE provider unit. The content is relevant to those
responsible for a CE provider unit of fifteen to thirty professionals,
as well as to the more common case of CE provider units of two or
three full- or part-time staff members.—Editors

You have just been selected to become the new Director of
Continuing Education. Your background has been in the health
professions as a faculty member at the local university health science
campus where you were often involved in planning or teaching CE
courses. Now, however, your responsibilities will involve providing
the direction to the entire institutional CE program as manager of
the CE provider unit. Your staff includes professional educators, as
well as logistics and administrative personnel. Your organization is
located within the dean's office. This is the good news.

The bad news is that you are being asked to take a cut in your
allocation from the school because of a pending fiscal deficit. Your
office is a profit center within the school and you already share your
profits with other departments. Everyone seems to want more from
you and is willing to give less of their resources. Final fiscal decisions will be made shortly for the coming year and within six or
eight months for the ensuing year. Also, long-range plans are being
developed that will affect your organization for years to come. Your
job is to manage the CE provider unit. You are faced with a plethora
of problems and issues. You have limited time and dwindling
resources. You must provide the leadership. How should you proceed? Which decisions must you make and which can you defer to
the future? What information is available to help you in making the
decisions?

Those individuals who have been assigned the "responsibility for deciding the direction an organization will take, and who
hold the authority to move it toward its goals, are the single most
important ingredient in determining the organization's success or
failure" (Robbins, 1976, p. 7). This chapter will examine manage-

ment philosophy, research, and practice in order to prescribe a management approach to improving the function of CE within the health professions.

Management within a CE provider unit includes not only top-level, executive decision making but also operational functions aimed at directing and controlling resource allocation, personnel supervision, production of educational projects, and logistical support. Regardless of the organization's size or the specific function of management, certain decisions are required. Some of these decisions are more important than others and they all require information. Typical decisions faced by managers in CE provider units might include:

- How much money can be charged per contact hour before participants will stop using our service or go elsewhere?
- How much of our resources would it be worthwhile to spend on assessing learner needs or evaluating impact?
- Do we need to upgrade our data processing equipment to assist in our administrative tasks?
- Should we be providing learners with alternative educational methods, such as computer-assisted instruction?
- What kind of person do we need to fill the vacancy we have on our staff?
- What measures can we take to assure that our educational activities, products, or services are of the requisite quality? (see Chapter Thirteen)
- Is our budget soundly based to reflect current priorities and is it realistic in terms of available resources? (see Chapter Thirteen)
- Would a reorganization of staff assignments enhance the unit's efficiency or its effectiveness?
- What steps can be taken to improve the relationship to the other units of the parent institution?
- Do we need to be doing something different now in order to develop the capabilities to meet the future needs of our constituents?

What is the essential role of management within a CE provider unit? It includes deciding on the organization's mission and strategic plan; setting goals that reflect this mission; establishing attainable but demanding long- and short-term objectives for reaching these goals; organizing the CE provider unit to accomplish the objectives; matching the allocation of resources with resource needs; establishing procedures to assure that the necessary tasks are carried out appropriately; monitoring the accomplishment of the tasks; providing a work environment that fosters growth, development, and task accomplishment within the organization; and monitoring the external environment in order to sense the need for adapting the organization to projected changes in external conditions.

Context

There is tremendous diversity of CE provider units within health care (see Chapter Six for a more detailed description). Almost all health professions and specialties within a profession are involved in providing formalized CE to its members. Many professions now mandate CE for recertification or relicensure and for membership in professional associations. The size of CE provider units varies from one-person units to centers with fifteen to thirty professional and administrative staff. In some cases none of the staff has had formal training in education, while in other cases professional educators are involved in research aimed at improving the CE process.

Each CE organization is involved in providing a variety of types of continuing education. The outputs of any CE provider unit include educational activities, products, and services. The management principles discussed in this and the next chapter are considered to be applicable regardless of the type of organization, the health profession involved, or the size of the organization. The critical decisions and appropriate managerial approaches are no less relevant for a single-person CE provider unit than for a large CE organization. The difference is the number of individuals over whom the management functions are distributed.

In managing a CE provider unit, certain political realities concerning CE have to be understood. Effective managers must become students of the system within which they operate, "partly because they often operate from a power-poor position and therefore require a detailed and accurate understanding of relations with the parent organization" (Knox, 1980, p. 260). In almost all cases CE is not the primary function of the parent organization and, therefore, does not automatically command the support of resources that might be deemed ideal.

The location of the CE unit within the parent organization thus becomes very important. If, for example, the CE provider unit is separate from the departments within a health professional school, it is often politically advantageous to be within the dean's office. CE provider units within university health science campuses fall into one of two basic organizational patterns—a centralized or a decentralized system (Moore, 1982). In the decentralized pattern, programming responsibility is distributed among individual schools or even departments according to academic content, and the departments make the fundamental decisions about the frequency, timing, and content of CE activities. In the centralized pattern, a single unit is established to plan, administer, and staff all continuing education programs throughout the health science center and its component schools. The organizational form has significant implications for the means and mode of influence exerted by the CE manager.

To the degree the leader of the CE provider unit has succeeded in making CE an integral part of the mission of the parent organization, necessary support and appropriate resources may be more readily available. Unfortunately, this is not often the case; instead CE is frequently seen as a somewhat unrelated activity and is required to pay its own way by collecting fees and obtaining research grants. This constant, yet necessary, concern with survival on "soft money" can lead to episodic, crisis management that tends to displace attention to the long-term picture. Based on a survey of practice, Moore (1982) concludes that "the picture on continuing education that emerges is an institutional form that has developed without conscious planning and as the result of short-term adaptions to external pressures" (p. 5).

This chapter and the chapter that follows are written for and about top-level leadership within CE provider units. The role of the leader in shaping the organization focuses on having a vision of the present and future, being able to translate that vision into day-to-day priorities and decisions, and motivating those with whom the leader works to help shape that vision and creatively carry out the tasks necessary to meet the present and future goals of quality CE. Shaping the values of the CE provider unit is of paramount importance to the leader of the organization.

As a manager of a CE provider unit, a relevant concern must be a determination of the information necessary to assist in making the kinds of critical decisions outlined in the first section of this chapter. Another concern must be how to determine which decisions are the most critical for the success of the organization. The remainder of this chapter deals with a rationale for effective management of a CE provider unit. To accomplish this, several important developments in management theory are discussed, leading up to the concept of strategic management. In the description of strategic management, implications for successfully managing a CE provider unit are presented. Finally, four management functions critical to the success of a CE provider unit are identified and described. These management functions provide the basis for developing a management information system, which is the subject of Chapter Thirteen.

Evolution of Management Systems

This section is based on an article by Ansoff (1977). It traces through time some of the major developments in management systems and identifies the fundamental assumptions underlying them, providing a perspective for understanding the rationale of "strategic management."

Operational Planning and Financial Budgeting. Early management theory focused on the development of financial budgeting systems on the one hand and operational planning systems on the other. Financial budgeting was principally concerned with ensuring that the organization could meet its fiscal responsibilities of "living within its means." Operational planning was oriented toward increasing the efficiency with which the organization conducted its work. Efficiency was seen as stemming first from the specialization of work and then from a successful coordination of the work into a functioning entity. The bureaucratic theory of organization provided the management principles for this coordination. All these systems—financial budgeting, operational planning, and coordination—were impersonal. Indeed, they were actually concerned with designing and regulating the organization to minimize the unpredictability that might otherwise arise from the idiosyncrasies of individual behavior.

Management by Objectives. Around 1950 there emerged the notion of management-by-objectives (MBO). McConkie (1979) provides a comprehensive and succinct appraisal of the MBO literature. The MBO movement began from the perspective that organizations are comprised of people. In order to avoid alienation and the subversion of the rational design and functioning of organizations as specified by the preceding systems, it was posited that it was necessary to achieve a congruence between the goals of the organization and the individual goals held by the members of the organization. MBO was proposed and widely implemented as a means for achieving goal congruence. These systems—financial budgeting, operational planning and coordination, and MBO—were all designed to operate within a short planning horizon and implicitly assumed a high degree of predictability in the conditions affecting the organization's operations.

Several writers (Knox, 1980; Knowles, 1980; Votruba, 1981) have dealt with CE management and administration and can be consulted for details of specific management tools and their application to CE provider units.

Long-Range Planning. With the concentration of the size of organizations and the emergence of production technologies requiring substantial commitment of resources for their implementation, there emerged the realization that longer planning horizons were necessary in order to provide a framework in which to work through the consequences of major decisions. Thus, around 1955 an emphasis on long-range planning systems appeared. Long-range planning was, however, implemented principally as an extension of financial budgeting, simply conducted in a multiperiod context. It was extrapolative and internally oriented in its approach. It was based, in other words, on the supposition of a stable external environment.

Strategic Planning. Around 1960 the concept of strategic planning began to evolve. Strategic planning was motivated by a recognition that the external environments of organizations are not stable. They are changing, frequently in unpredictable ways in terms of the direction and timing of change. Further, it was recognized that parts of the external environment are not neutral and passive to the organization but react to the strategies of the organization either in a supportive manner or in a manner designed to thwart the organization in the pursuit of its goals. It was these assumptions about the external environment that fundamentally distinguished strategic planning from the earlier long-range planning systems and, indeed, from the planning and budgeting systems conducted in shorter planning horizons.

The rationale for formal long-range planning derives from the context of large organizations. As such, this kind of management system may not be of much relevance for most CE provider units. The same is not true for strategic planning. Since the rationale for strategic planning stems from the dynamic and uncertain nature of the organization's external environment and since these conditions are characteristic of the environments faced by most CE provider units, effective strategic planning is likely to be an extremely critical ingredient of CE provider unit management.

Capability Planning. Around 1975 capability planning emerged as a formal planning approach. Its content is concerned with defining the necessary capabilities to support the organization's future mission, comparing these with an assessment of existing capabilities and formulating strategies for upgrading and maintaining capabilities. Capability planning is concerned with maintaining and enhancing the particular skills, knowledge, and technologies that are central to an organization's continued effectiveness. Strategic planning, as it was initially implemented in practice, shifted managerial attention to the external environment, especially to opportunities and threats to the demand for the organization's primary outputs, the products and services produced for customers and clients. This was desirable in the sense of redressing the previous preoccupation with internal matters in the planning and resource allocation processes. However, there emerged a tendency to "overcorrect," in essence to overlook the continual need to assess strengths and weaknesses of the organization's internal capabilities and to invest in correcting identified weaknesses. In other words, management appeared to take for granted the organization's core capabilities. Methods for developing and maintaining critical capabilities of a CE provider unit in the area of ensuring educational quality are discussed in detail in Chapters Fourteen and Fifteen. Chapter Thirteen discusses the development and maintenance of critical capability with respect to the managerial competence of the unit.

Strategic Management—An Emerging Concept

The current vanguard of management theory and practice focuses on the idea of strategic management (Ansoff, 1979; Gluck, Kaufman, and Walleck, 1982). Strategic management is an emerging idea, not yet fully articulated as a managerial system. It reflects a widely held belief that strategic planning has by and large failed to realize the potential that its advocates once held for it. Two reasons can be identified to explain this failure. First, strategic planning has tended to be practiced as an analytical activity; for example, in larger organizations strategic planning units have often been formed and have placed greater concern on planning methods than on the effects of the planning decisions made in the organization. Secondly, and in a similar vein, strategic planning has tended to be conducted as a periodic exercise rather than as an ongoing and continual managerial concern. Current thinking does not question the potential value of strategic planning; the need is real enough. Rather, it addresses the difficult issues of effective implementation.

Strategic management is, above all, a philosophy about management and leadership. It recognizes that each of the management systems enumerated in the preceding paragraphs has emerged to fulfill a need. Successive systems do not displace previous systems since the needs that gave rise to them have not disappeared. Each is additive, complementing and extending the capabilities of the systems already in place. To be sure, with the addition of a new system the existing managerial systems cannot continue totally unaffected; they have to be modified to accommodate innovations in managerial methods as these are implemented. Strategic management is simply seeking an effective way to integrate the various pieces into a coherent, functioning managerial approach. The power of strategic management may well be that it comes "empty-handed," unburdened by any new techniques. Its purpose is to make sense of, and more effective use of, what we already have—no more than that, but no less. Its message and relevance is not particular to large organizations; to the contrary, it is as applicable to an individual as to a large organization.

The central proposition of strategic management is that strategy and operations should be conducted both simultaneously and continuously in an ongoing manner. This inevitably means that managerial decision making involves a complex cross-walking between consideration of current operating objectives and the mandate of the longer-term mission of the organization as expressed in its strategic goals. Within a CE provider unit, this joint concern with both current objectives and strategic goals involves, for example, preparing for an increasing use of mediated, individualized educational materials, while continuing to develop and market traditional, group-oriented workshops. If the latter concerns predominate at the expense of developing the future capabilities, the CE provider unit's future viability could be jeopardized.

Planning and the Management Process. The first aspect is a simple, yet fundamental plank in the philosophy of strategic management. It reflects the proposition that management is centrally concerned with decision making to affect the future. Further, it advocates a shift from a reactive, crisis-responding style of management to a purposeful and proactive posture. A proactive approach is characterized by the belief that a vision of a desirable and feasible future for the organization can be created, shared, and, through the collective action of management and staff, achieved. A proposal for a new, modified role for CE provider units was described in detail in Chapter Six. However, it can only come about if the managers of CE provider units have the vision to see the need to adapt and have the means to lead the organization toward that future. One of the most powerful tools at the disposal of CE management to bring about these changes is the information system used to support decisions about the current and future critical priorities agreed upon in the planning process.

Integration. The second aspect stresses integration. There are several important dimensions of this. First, the planning and control of the organization must deal with integrating the different valid perspectives of the organization's key strategic resources: its *human capital* and technologies, its *financial capital,* and its *political capital.* These are not different sets of resources; they are simply different ways of viewing—describing and explaining—the same set of resources. CE provider unit managers must integrate all available resources, including staff and faculty, budget allocations and potential revenues from products and services, and political influence in order to help move the CE unit toward its goals.

Next, the needs and demands on the organization arising from its *external* environment have to be reconciled continually with its *internal* resources and capabilities. This implies the creation of an outside-in mode of planning to exist alongside the more typical inside-out mode. For instance, in addition to planning what the CE provider unit will offer in the way of educational activities based on the interests and capabilities of staff and faculty, the CE manager must develop the mechanisms to determine the demands (both content and process) of external clients and develop the organization to meet those demands. If physicians in a given area, for example, are demanding self-directed CE for credit and the CE staff have never developed such educational activities, staff development may be necessary to meet the demand.

Thirdly, the *long-term* and *short-term* demands on the organization have to be reconciled; that is to say, the planning that supports the organization's decision making should embody future-to-present planning as well as the present-to-future extrapolations that commonly constitute planning. Decisions made in planning by CE provider managers must take into account the effect that goals for the future have on current operating objectives. For instance, to develop the capability to provide self-directed learning packages for the future, current operating dollars may have to be diverted to staff development or to the hiring of an expert in this particular educational mode.

Fourthly, *change* and *continuity* have to be reconciled. Philosophically, we are used to equating change with progress. Since progress is idealized in our ideological view of the world, change is often likewise valued for its own sake. But change can be destructive, since it typically involves replacing the present order of things with a new, and perhaps better, order. The key consideration is the rate of change that is tolerable in an organization, such as to allow orderly progress without destroying the sense of the organization's stability and confidence in itself. Changing the role of a CE provider unit will almost certainly entail changing the competencies needed by staff to fulfill the new role. If the CE staff have been competently developing CE workshops for several years but suddenly have to develop self-directed learning activities for individual health professionals or develop materials for broadcast over a cable television network, the new demands may be perceived as being very threatening. The role of the CE manager has to be to move toward the new future by facilitating needed internal changes in such a way as to preserve the organization's confidence in itself.

Finally, an integration between *total organization* and *localized* perspectives is necessary for effective planning and decision making. For a CE provider unit, the localized perspectives may be the smaller subunits of education and logistics staff within a larger CE organization or the self-interests of a small group of constituents. The CE manager's role is to keep the best interests of the total organization in mind without slighting any subgroup within or external to the CE provider unit. This oftentimes will require considerable political sensitivity and negotiating skills.

Integration does not imply dominance of any one dimension over another. The missionary zeal with which strategic planning was promulgated during the 1970s, for instance, tended to suggest the strategic perspective as having more intrinsic validity and value than an operational perspective. This is not the case, and strategic management is consciously attempting to redress the emphasis. The existing reality of the organization and the traditions stemming from its past provide the grounded reality from which to build change, expand the mission, and link these to the organization's sense of its identity.

The integrating task—integrating the various perspectives about the organization's key resources, the external with the internal demands, the long-term with the short-term requirements, the needs for and risks associated with change and stability respectively, and the needs of the total organization with localized interests—presents a considerable challenge to the intellectual and interpersonal skills of a leader. The task can never be made easy. However, it can at least be facilitated by the provision of relevant information.

Sharing Strategic Responsibility. This addresses the need to vest the managerial process with relevant authority and, in particular, to create a shared responsibility for establishing and carrying out the strategy of the organization. Management, to be sure, is never impersonal; it relies on the motivating force of personal leadership. Nevertheless, in creating an organizational process, perceptive leaders realize that they must empower the process by vesting it with some of their own authority. This means that personal power and discretion must in some degree be relinquished to the process. The effective executive has to be prepared to acknowledge the collective will and usually needs to abide by that, even if not always directly engaged as a participant in shaping it. Of course, in exceptional circumstances personal preferences may override the process. But if the exceptions are so frequent as to become the rule, the process is likely to fall into disrepute.

An important consideration for CE managers is to be congruent in their leadership style. To profess an open, democratic view of management, while consistently ignoring input from staff, is to invite low morale and alienation. This is not to suggest that some autocratic decision making may not be necessary or at times desirable. The important point is to be open about how input from staff will be obtained and decisions made and then to be congruent in the manner in which that is carried through.

Measures and Incentives. The foregoing has significant implications for the measures and incentives used in organizations. Drucker (1964) points out that the real control in an organization centers on how people perceive themselves as being evaluated and rewarded. Naisbitt (1982) decries the use of short-term performance measures, reinforced by incentives, which he sees as being endemic to American organizations and undermining their future vitality.

Strategic management, with its emphasis on the integration of strategy and operations and the extension of a strategic concern throughout the management group, clearly requires careful attention to performance measures and rewards. In the first place, the measures need to be aligned with the strategy and goals of the organization. And, since an organization typically has goals on multiple dimensions, this implies multiple measures. Some of these will reinforce the needs for current performance, while others will relate to goal-paths leading the organization in the direction of a revision or expansion of its mission. Further, some performance dimensions may be readily quantified in an objective way—for example, by the use of accounting data—while others may require considerable ingenuity to arrive at a measure. The latter is especially true of the effects being created by the organization among its external constituencies. And yet, these effects are ultimately of the greatest importance to the organization's long-term position. The seemingly "soft" measures may in fact be the most important indicators of the hard reality the organization has to cope with in terms of its strategic viability. For each of the areas of measurement, decent, acceptable— and accepted—standards of performance are required. Finally, the measures and the performance standards associated with them should be motivating and rewarding, in and of themselves; they should be demanding and interesting to the members of the organization in that they represent the whole range of activities critical to the organization's strategic progress and to the professional stature of the group jointly and individually.

To the extent that a reward structure is explicitly used to reinforce the performance measures, three points are of particular importance. The first is so obvious it seems hardly to require saying were it not for the fact that it is so commonly ignored in practice. It simply is that outstanding performance should be rewarded. The corollary to this is that mediocre performance should not be rewarded. Secondly, the incentive system should be used to acknowledge and reward outstanding *individual* performance. Finally, since the organization's performance must inevitably be greater than the sum of the performance of the individual members (otherwise there would be no good reason for the existence of the organization as an entity), the incentive system should reward *cooperative and collective* performance.

CE managers need to establish evaluation systems and incentives for staff to perform in a way that leads to accomplishing the current mission and future goals. For example, faculty need to be given incentives to improve their lecturing techniques, staff need to be motivated to learn more about meeting the educational needs of self-directed learners, staff development needs to be provided to upgrade individual's knowledge and skills related to using emerging computer and word processing technologies, and individual health professional learners need to be given incentives to study their own practices as a basis for determining their educational needs. Rewards and incentives may be financial, or they may be indirect such as allowing opportunities for staff development, travel, and variety of assignments. Motivating individuals through the use of a variety of incentives, these in turn being based on the intended direction in which the unit is headed, is a critical leadership task.

Analysis of the Managerial Process

How might a CE provider unit manager benefit from this encapsulation of management theory? How might the CE director obtain information necessary to answer the previous list of questions? In order for a CE provider unit to develop quality CE activities, products, and services, the management of that organization needs to have a system for making critical decisions based on relevant information. The purpose of this section is to set the stage for a description of a management information system (MIS) that provides critical information to CE managers as they make decisions that affect the short- and long-term viability of their CE organizations. The theoretical perspective provides a logical structure within which the design of the MIS is formulated.

In his seminal framework, Anthony (1965) proposes an analysis of the management process into three relatively distinct processes or functions: *strategic planning*, concerned with the overall organization as an entity, its direction, and strategic goals; *management control*, concerned with acquiring and using resources effectively and efficiently in accomplishing the goals of the organization; and *operational control*, concerned with carrying out designated tasks in an efficient manner.

Subsequently, Anthony divides management control into two processes. One, which he refers to as programming, is concerned with the development of plans that are feasible within the organization's resources and capabilities and are justified in terms of the accomplishment of the organization's mission as defined in the strategic planning process. The second is the budgeting and authorization of resources within the organization. This function is concerned with mapping the decisions and priority emphases arrived at in the programming function into the structure and procedures used by the organization for translating plans into action. It focuses on the coordination of the work in the organization to ensure that it is directed toward achieving program plans, and it addresses specific resource allocation to activities through the budgeting mechanism.

These four functions—strategic planning, programming, budgeting and coordination, and operational control—are relevant for analyzing the managerial task in a CE provider unit.

Four Functions of CE Provider Unit Management

Before beginning the topic of this section, it is important to point out that the four functions do not refer to different levels of management. Indeed, the functional analysis does not necessarily have any direct correspondence with organizational structure. For instance, in a one-person operation the individual involved may be setting direction one minute and taking care of the logistical support for a workshop the next. In other words, the individual would have to perform all four managerial functions. In larger CE organizations with two or three levels of management, the functions could correspond closely with managerial levels. The leader, for example, might carry principal responsibility for the strategic planning and programming functions, while others in the organization carry principal responsibility for fulfilling the other two functions. The point is that all four functions are essential to the efficiency and viability of any CE provider unit, regardless of size. It should not be thought that any one of the functions is more important or essential than any of the others. To the contrary, failure or neglect of any one function will eventually cause a deterioration in the unit's viability.

Strategic Management of the Unit. This function deals with setting direction for the CE organization as a whole and assuring that the total program fulfills the mission and goals of the organization. It includes such responsibilities as establishing a mission, strategic planning, setting goals and policies, exception monitoring,

dealing with external organizations, and meeting external accountability requirements.

Program Management. This function involves establishing
the overall program (the totality of projects to be undertaken) to
meet the goals of the unit and to reflect priorities identified in the
strategic planning process and allocating resources to projects comprising the program. It also involves establishing procedures and
monitoring systems to ensure that the overall program is carried out
effectively.

Project Coordination and Control. This function is directly
concerned with assuring the quality and quantity of projects specified by the program and with coordination among projects. It also
involves assuring efficient resource utilization, a good image among
the unit's various client populations, and the timely completion of
tasks.

Project Development and Implementation. This final function involves accomplishing the variety of tasks embodied in approved project plans in a timely and efficient manner and in
accordance with defined policies and procedures.

These four functions can be related to the managerial systems
discussed earlier in the chapter. The function of strategic management of the unit relies directly on strategic planning and monitoring systems. The program management function entails operating
planning and financial budgeting, but at a highly summarized level
of detail; it also directly entails capability planning, MBO, and
design of incentives to achieve congruence between program goals
and the goals of the individual faculty and staff of the unit. The
project coordination and control function relies on operating planning and financial budgeting to ensure that resource commitments
are coordinated across projects. And the project development and
implementation function requires detailed operating, planning,
and monitoring systems. The philosophy of strategic management
provides a leadership perspective for ensuring that the four functions and the managerial systems used to support them are effectively integrated around the strategic themes comprising the unit's
overall strategy.

As an example, within a CE provider unit, the manager may
have decided that the new or modified role outlined in Chapter Six

is a viable and desirable one. This vision corresponds to one aspect of the function of strategic management of the unit. To move the organization in that direction, however, requires constantly making planning decisions to facilitate progress in the desired direction. In the development of management information to support these decisions, it is important to look at the other three functions of management. In this example, decisions will need to be made concerning priorities for the overall CE provider unit program, and these are part of the program management function. New directions in using the microprocessor in physicians' offices as a tool for studying the practice and identifying educational needs require some higher priority be given to these activities than has been typically the case in the past. Perhaps the CE provider unit manager will decide to dedicate some specified portion of this year's operating budget to pursuing computer-based learning efforts. Chapters Fourteen and Fifteen provide mechanisms for assuring the quality of educational activities. In order to assure that the project coordination and control function is supporting this quality goal, specific criteria for the evaluation of staff must be included that relate directly to acquiring the skills to assist physicians to use computers to profile their practice. Finally, in the project development and implementation function, the CE manager must have specific criteria, perhaps in the form of planning checklists, that require encouraging potential learners to make available to the CE provider unit practice-related needs assessment data.

Conclusion

The foregoing illustration indicates both the need to consider each function separately to ensure its individual effectiveness and the need to integrate strategic themes through the four functions in a coherent and coordinated manner. The integration of strategic themes can be accomplished by personal supervision and intervention, and indeed this mode will always be important. However, it can also be greatly facilitated by a systematic provision of information designed for the purpose, which is addressed in Chapter Thirteen.

This chapter began by describing a number of pertinent decisions typical of those that the manager of a CE provider unit faces.

In the next chapter it is demonstrated how the design of an MIS can help to provide a regular flow of information to facilitate making these decisions.

References

Ansoff, H. I. "The State of Practice in Planning Systems." *Sloan Management Review,* 1977, *18* (2), 1–24.

Ansoff, H. I. *Strategic Management.* New York: Wiley, 1979.

Anthony, R. N. *Planning and Control Systems: A Framework for Analysis.* Boston: Division of Research, Graduate School of Business Administration, Harvard University, 1965.

Drucker, P. F. "Controls, Control and Management." In C. P. Bonini, R. K. Jaedicke, and H. M. Wagner (Eds.), *Management Controls: New Directions in Basic Research.* New York: McGraw-Hill, 1964.

Gluck, F., Kaufman, S., and Walleck, A. S. "The Four Phases of Strategic Management." *Journal of Business Strategy,* 1982, *2* (3), 9–21.

Knowles, M. S. *The Modern Practice of Adult Education: From Pedagogy to Androgogy.* Rev. ed. Chicago: Follett, 1980.

Knox, A. B. "Future Directions." In A. B. Knox and others (Eds.), *Developing, Administering, and Evaluating Adult Education.* San Francisco: Jossey-Bass, 1980.

McConkie, M. L. "A Clarification of the Goal-Setting and Appraisal Processes in MBO." *Academy of Management Review,* 1979, *4* (1), 29–40.

Moore, D. E., Jr. "The Organization and Administration of Continuing Education in Academic Medical Centers." Unpublished doctoral dissertation, University of Illinois at Urbana-Champaign, 1982.

Naisbitt, J. *Megatrends: Ten New Directions Transforming Our Lives.* New York: Warner Books, 1982.

Robbins, S. P. *The Administrative Process.* Englewood Cliffs, N.J.: Prentice-Hall, 1976.

Votruba, J. C. (Ed.). *New Directions for Continuing Education: Strengthening Internal Support for Continuing Education,* no. 9. San Francisco: Jossey-Bass, 1981.

Information Systems That Meet Management Needs

J. Morris McInnes
Joseph S. Green

※※※※※※※※※※※※※※※※※※※※※※※※※

This chapter flows directly from Chapter Twelve and discusses specifically the process of designing a management information system (MIS) to support the continuing education (CE) manager in decision making and monitoring. A combination of the decision analysis and the critical success factor methods is suggested as an approach to defining management information needs of CE provider units. The chapter describes in some detail the critical success factors that have been developed for a CE provider unit. These are expected to have considerable generalizability to CE provider units, regardless of size or type. This management information system is in

The authors of this chapter wish to acknowledge the contribution of the following individuals to the conceptual development of the CE management information system: Donald Cordes, Sarina Grosswald, Kenneth Lawrence, Gregg Seppala, Emanuel Suter, and David Walthall.

the process of being developed for the Regional Medical Education Centers within the Veterans Administration Health Care System by the members of the Continuing Education Systems Project (CESP). In the beginning of Chapter Twelve several questions were listed that are typical of those faced by CE provider unit managers. This chapter will attempt to show how two of these typical decisions can be made by CE managers with the assistance of the proposed MIS.—Editors

In the previous chapter a framework was developed for understanding and analyzing the total managerial task of a CE provider unit. In this chapter the analysis is extended to propose a design for an information system to support the key managerial decision-making and monitoring activities.

People are the key ingredients—the strategic force—in organizations. People get things done. They set directions and priorities and decide what should and should not be done. People are motivated to action, and they in turn motivate others to act. In the course of this, much of the essential communication and information flow in an organization occurs in an informal and highly interactive manner.

Having said this, it is nevertheless evident that some degree of formalization is essential for coherent, purposeful, and efficient action. Especially as the organization grows in size, it becomes a challenging and vital managerial task to provide a design and a procedure for information gathering and use in the organization. Even for a single-person unit the task is vital, for the information system design ensures the best use of the organization's scarcest resource, namely, the time and energy of the person involved.

The problem confronting managers is usually not a lack of information (Ackoff, 1967). On the contrary, it tends to be the opposite—too much information, haphazard in its content, availability, and presentation, to the extent that important messages are obscured. Managers are busy, pressured people, moving rapidly from one incident or encounter to another (Mintzberg, 1980). In such circumstances they do not have the time to sift carefully through files and reports seeking the heart of the matter or trying to extract the right information for a particular purpose at hand. It is the task of the information system to do much of this selective sifting, highlighting, and underlining for the manager.

A manager's effectiveness is inevitably, and to a large degree, dependent on the quality of the management information system (MIS). This chapter sets out the important concepts for guiding the design of an MIS and then proceeds to the application of these to the information requirements of a CE provider unit. It may well be that in small CE units the MIS consists solely of a file drawer, the contents of which are organized and administered by the manager's secretary. In large units there may be a full-time person concerned with running the MIS, supported by access to sophisticated computer-based data management and processing. In either situation the principles guiding the design and use of management information are basically the same. It is true, of course, that advances in data processing technology—both the increasing power and easy application of software and the decreasing cost of hardware—enable solutions to the problems of information provision that could hardly have been imagined ten years ago. For instance, microprocessors put considerable data processing power comfortably within the reach of even a single-person unit. Even so, the analysis and prescriptions put forward in this chapter make no assumptions about either the data processing technology to be used or the size of the organization.

Since a manager's effectiveness is dependent on the quality and availability of information, it follows that the manager should pay careful attention to the design of the MIS. It is important in this regard to distinguish between two commonly used and seemingly similar terms, *management information system* (MIS) and *information management system*. They have, in fact, different meanings. The former refers to the design of information to support the managerial task; as such, it is an area of central concern to managers. The latter refers to the principles and methods of managing the work entailed in running the data processing and information-producing activity itself, to support all the information requirements of an organization. This is not an area that is usually of great concern to managers, particularly in large organizations where a specialist in information systems typically is available to handle the activity. It may, however, occupy some attention of a manager in a small CE provider unit, who does not have the benefit of such staff support.

Information Systems—An Overview

Design philosophy in information systems has, following Scott Morton's (1971) influential work, emphasized the need to tailor information to the characteristics of the process for which the information is being developed. In an extension of Scott Morton's work, Gorry and Scott Morton (1971) drew on Simon's (1960) classification of decisions based on their degree of programmability and Anthony's (1965) analysis of the management process into strategic planning, management control, and operational control to derive a matrix to guide the design for information systems. For the purpose of this chapter, these three management functions have been extended to four to be more responsive to the realities of CE provider units. These four include strategic management of the unit, program management, project coordination and control, and project development and implementation.

In approaching the topic of information systems, the first question to address is: What kinds of demands for information arise from the organization? And hence: What capabilities should the information-providing activity ideally have in order to satisfy these demands? The following generic sets of demands can be identified in most organizations. Each is sufficiently different in its characteristics to require its own design emphasis.

- operating information for logistics, task, and project control
- external reporting to satisfy information provision to outside parties and to support external accountability
- management information for strategic planning, program management, project coordination, and project planning and implementation
- analytical capabilities to respond to nonroutine information needs

Each of these sets of information is important to the effectiveness and viability of an organization, but they are not equally critical to immediate survival. The focus of the present discussion is on management information. However, the discussion assumes that the operating information and external reporting systems are already in place and functioning effectively. A CE provider unit that cannot reliably track the tasks and costs of its primary activities is likely to experience severe problems in carrying out and coordinating its operations. By the same token, if it cannot meet its external reporting requirements, it is likely to dispel the goodwill of its sponsors, putting its continued viability in jeopardy. Thus, these two sets of information must be accorded top priority. Moreover, by no means being complete, these two information sets are significant sources of input to meeting the information needs of management.

Beyond these basic information requirements, the next priority in enhancing the unit's managerial capability is to ensure that management information needs are identified and provided for. Finally, the need for an analytical capability to support ad hoc information gathering and analysis can be important, especially for larger, well-established CE provider units. These units are likely to be proactive in their strategies and may be involved in ongoing research into such things as the effects of CE on the provision of health care. An established analytical capability can provide valuable support to strategy formulation and to research. Smaller CE provider units may of necessity be more reactive in their strategies and are likely also to face greater stringency in the resources that can be commited to information providing. For these units, the analytical capability perhaps should be accorded the lowest priority among the four sets of information identified. Each of the information sets is discussed in turn in the following sections.

Operating Information. Operating information is largely intrinsic to the organization's primary work (Hax, 1973). Consequently, the design of the data collection and processing to provide operating information can be appropriately treated in a technical manner, in much the same way that a hospital administrator would approach the design of a patient care information system. The key design emphases are accuracy, timely information output, and data processing efficiency. The data themselves are largely generated by the activities and transactions that occur as a result of the organization engaging in its primary tasks. Examples of operating information in a CE provider unit include: logistics information, to track the physical availability in terms of time and space of key resources such as faculty, staff, classrooms, and teaching equipment; personnel and payroll, to ensure that people are paid appropriately according to contract; payables and receivables, to track the creation of obligations and their fulfillment; and cost accounting, to accumulate costs and revenues in relation to activities.

Operating information can be visualized in general terms as a matrix, having on one dimension line items of costs and revenues—and a record of the physical attributes and events giving rise to these—and on the other dimension the distribution of these among the organization's primary activities. Cost-accounting information should in theory be designed to distribute all costs to activities, including staff costs. However, this would necessitate a routine recording of staff time to activities, something that CE provider units, in common with many other kinds of professional organizations, seldom undertake as a matter of standard procedure. In the absence of this, it is necessary periodically to estimate the staff input into the various activities in order to build a full cost for each activity. This is essential information input to planning, resource allocation, and subsequent evaluation of the efficiency with which operations have been conducted, a subject that will be addressed later in the chapter.

Alongside the transaction-based data in the organization's operating information system, other data bases are typically created to capture and store descriptions of a flow of events or of states of the relevant environment judged to be useful in guiding operating decision. Examples of these in a CE context would include specific needs assessments, course evaluations, educational quality monitoring, and reasons for staff turnover.

External Reporting. It is not necessary to dwell at length on the external reporting demands on the organization's information-providing activities. To a large extent, these are stipulated by parties external to the organization, for example, by the parent organization, other funding sources, or accrediting bodies. The CE provider unit manager may have some influence on the definition of the timing and format of external reporting requirements. Nevertheless, once defined, it is imperative that these requirements be met in a consistent and reliable manner.

Management Information. In contrast to the operating and the external reporting information, there exists a considerable degree of managerial discretion with regard to timing, content, and format of information to support the managerial functions. In some organizations, for instance, no conscious effort is given to designing information specifically to meet the needs of management. Instead, management information is treated, in essence by default, as a by-product of operating and external reporting information. In other organizations management information is regarded as a key resource. Considerable effort is devoted to assessing the information needs of management and to designing and implementing systems to meet the needs.

In a fully developed MIS there are four interdependent, but nevertheless distinct, information flows: goal-centered information, monitoring of the external environment, operations monitoring, and monitoring of the internal environment.

Goal-centered information refers to a disaggregation of the mission and strategy of the total into unit subgoals, operating objectives, and performance standards. Its purpose is to disperse throughout the organization the essential direction and priorities contained in the unit's mission and goals. It provides a normative and evaluative framework that shapes the managerial judgment that goes into planning and ongoing, day-to-day decision making. The CE manager must ensure that the vision of where the unit is headed is translated into specific goals and objectives and carefully communicated throughout the organization. These goals and objectives make explicit and reinforce the expectations of management and ultimately facilitate the accomplishment of the unit's mission. Curiously, small organizations tend more than large organizations to give insufficient attention to this information flow. Perhaps the assumption is that the smallness of the organization allows communication of goals to occur by some kind of osmosis. Such is not the case, and interpersonal conflict and diminished operating effectiveness will usually result from neglecting this part of the MIS.

The *external environment* is a key source of information for formulating the mission and strategy of the unit. Moreover, it provides the real test of whether the unit, in pursuing its mission, is effectively meeting the expectations and demands of its external constituents. Thus, it is necessary to monitor the organization's external environment in order to be informed about trends and conditions within and among important constituencies, including, of course, the organization's client population.

An important flow of information concerns an aggregation of the unit's *operating data*. The project development and implementation function is primarily concerned with this, in considerable detail. But the other management functions are also concerned with operations, at least on an exception-reporting basis. The key to a good design for this flow of information is the reduction of complexity and detail, while at the same time providing for a timely identification of exception that might signal the need for higher-level intervention. This approach is widely used and is referred to as management by exception (MBE). MacKintosh (1978) provides a guide to the design and implementation of MBE systems for reporting operating information to management.

It is necessary to monitor the *internal environment* of the organization itself. This is quite distinct from the transaction and task-generated data of the operating information system. It is, rather, concerned with monitoring the organization's infrastructure—its morale, its ability to communicate effectively and to resolve conflicts as they arise, and its capabilities to support existing and future missions and the operations implied by these.

Analytical Capabilities. For all but the most stable organizations, it is virtually impossible to anticipate all future information needs and to provide for these in a formalized, routine manner. Responding to change requires continual learning, which implies new sources of information and new ways of interpreting existing information—hence, the need for an ad hoc information gathering and analysis capability, such as the occasional input from an ad hoc multidisciplinary advisory group describing implications of new technologies. While this is not commonly thought of as being an intrinsic component of an MIS in the conventional meaning of the term, its importance is increasingly being reflected in practice and in the literature (see, for example, Rockart and Treacy, 1982).

It is not the intention to imply any sharp distinction, either conceptually or in practice, between a manager and the formal information system. To the contrary, a more constructive view is to consider them together as an information-processing and decision-making entity. The degree to which the information system is formally structured can be left as a secondary, albeit important, concern. It will depend on such things as the level of resources that can be committed to the formal information system and the personal preferences of individual managers.

Defining Information Needs

An excellent review of the literature on information requirements analysis is provided by Davis (1982). He summarizes the principal approaches that have been proposed and followed in practice. The primary approach selected for the present purpose is based on the decision analysis (also referred to as activity analysis) method. However, to deal with the problem of information overload referred to in the introduction, a second approach, a modification of Rockart's (1979) critical success factor (CSF) method, is used in conjunction with the decision analysis method.

Decision Analysis Method. This approach entails an analysis of the total work of an organization into its discrete tasks and the sequencing of these in flow diagrams. The information required to carry out each task is specified in detail. This is then used as the basis for defining sources of data, files, data processing, and the provision of information to support each task (Martin, 1980). There are in practice many variations on the basic method. One variation focuses on managerial roles in the organization rather than on the total organization. The work allocated to each role—including the primary work of the role, the supervisory content, and the requirements for coordination with the work of contiguous roles—is specified and becomes the basis for defining the information requirements to support the role. Another variation focuses on specific kinds of decisions, for example, the commitment of monetary resources in the budgeting process.

In the CE context, project planning and implementation provides a good example. The method would require a detailed flow diagram for sequencing all the tasks involved in designing and carrying out an educational project, from the initial formulation of a project proposal through to the final evaluation of whether or not the project accomplished its objectives. Another example, at a higher level of management, might be an analysis of all the steps required to establish a new CE provider unit in a medical center. For more detail about flow diagrams concerning CE project development and the establishment of a new CE provider unit, see Chapter Sixteen.

In the previous chapter a characterization of management as a decision-making process embedded in an organizational context was adopted in identifying the four management functions. From this perspective, the analysis of information needs, defined by reference to the decisions assigned to each function, and the design of formal information systems to provide at least part of the information needs, recommends itself as a logical approach.

Critical Success Factor Method. The decision analysis approach has a number of limitations. First, it appears to work well for decision making that is fairly well structured and can, therefore, be programmed into clearly defined protocols, but it is less successful in its application to decision making that is more ambiguous and intuitive in its content. Thus, for example, it is difficult to use in the area of strategic planning. Secondly, the method does not discriminate between decisions on the basis of how important they are to the overall mission of the organization. Finally, the method is essentially impersonal. It deals with tasks, decisions, and roles; it does not address individual managers, their personal styles, and the information they bring to bear on their jobs from their backgrounds and previous experience.

The CSF approach was designed specifically to address these shortcomings of the decision analysis method. Rockart's CSF approach proposes that the individual manager should be the center of attention in designing and developing information systems. The approach requires the development of answers to the question: "Given the managerial task I am responsible for, what factors are critical to my success?" The CSFs then provide a design focus for the development of monitoring systems to support the manager. In Rockart's philosophy, the monitoring requirements are a function of two things: the background, experience, and personal style of each manager; and the particular strategy and operating situation faced by the organization of which the manager is a part.

Rockart describes CSFs as follows: "Critical success factors thus are . . . the limited number of areas in which the results, if they are satisfactory, will ensure successful . . . performance for the organization . . . . As a result, the critical success factors are areas that should receive constant and careful attention from management. The current status of performance in each area should be continually measured and that information should be made available" (1979, p. 85).

Framework for Approaching MIS Design

This section describes the approach that was used to develop the proposed MIS for CE provider units, while the next section describes the MIS. The goal of the approach was to arrive at a generic proposal for an MIS, that is to say, a proposal that would have a large measure of applicability to every CE provider unit. The design approach that was followed is illustrated in Figure 1.

The first step (denoted (1) in the figure) was the analysis of the total managerial task into the four functions, as described in Chapter Twelve. Dealing with functions rather than with managerial roles allowed a specification of information needs to be made in a manner independent of the size or organizational structure of any specific CE provider unit.

The second step (denoted (2) in the figure) involved the application of the decision analysis method to each of the four functions. This resulted in very detailed documents diagramming the flow of tasks, decisions, and related information needs. The CSF method was used to reduce this level of detail and to focus on the salient tasks and decisions embodied in each function.

Since the CSF method as proposed by Rockart places an individual manager at the center of the information design process, a means had to be devised for modifying the method to the purpose at hand. A field study was undertaken involving a number of experienced CE managers in the health field. Each manager was asked in the course of one or more interviews to specify a set of functions critical to the successful management of CE provider units. These were then collated and merged into one set of factors. This set was

Figure 1. MIS Design Process.

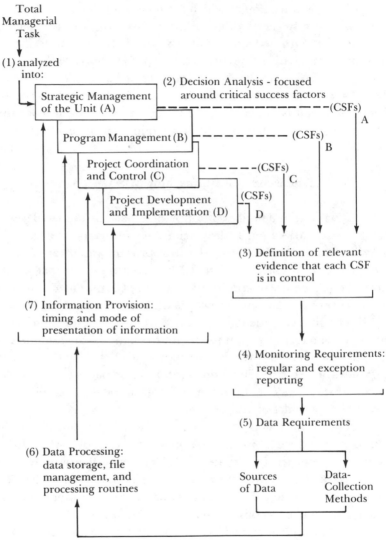

Total
Managerial
Task

(1) analyzed
into:

Strategic Management
of the Unit (A)

(2) Decision Analysis - focused
around critical success factors

(CSFs)
A

Program Management (B)

(CSFs)
B

Project Coordination
and Control (C)

(CSFs)
C

Project Development
and Implementation (D)

(CSFs)
D

(3) Definition of relevant
evidence that each CSF
is in control

(7) Information Provision:
timing and mode of
presentation of information

(4) Monitoring Requirements:
regular and exception
reporting

(5) Data Requirements

(6) Data Processing:
data storage, file
management, and
processing routines

Sources
of Data

Data-
Collection
Methods

analyzed and mapped into the four management functions. Thus, the CSFs discussed in the next section represent a distillation from many years of managerial experience in CE in many different types of CE provider units. Accordingly, their general relevance is likely to be high, even though they do not refer to one particular CE provider unit. At the time of this writing, their validation, by implementation in the design of an MIS for a CE provider unit, had been started;

however, the work is expected to require approximately two more years to complete.

This was followed (step (3) in the figure) by an analysis of the relevant evidence that would satisfy a manager that each CSF is within some satisfactory range. For example, if a CSF for the strategic management of the unit related to the progress of the overall educational program, the following questions might be posed: What *minimum evidence* is needed and *how frequently* is it needed to ensure that the program will satisfactorily meet the planned goals? The frequency of the provision of information is determined by a judgment about the stability (or the converse, the volatility) of the factor in question and the time required for corrective intervention, should this prove to be necessary.

The answers to these kinds of questions for the total set of CSFs assigned to each function provided a specification of the monitoring requirements (step (4) in the figure) that would be ideal for supporting each function. This led to the next step (denoted (5) in the figure) of the analysis, namely, the definition of sources of data to support the monitoring requirements and consideration of data collection methods. Some of the data may be readily available from sources such as the unit's operating information system. Other data, for example, the opinions and attitudes of defined client populations toward the CE provider unit, would be likely to require careful design of the data collection.

The next step (denoted (6) in the figure) is largely technical and addresses the choice of data storage and processing methods. This choice in practice would depend on the size of the CE provider unit concerned and the resources available for commitment to the data processing activity. As was mentioned earlier in the chapter, this might entail a manual system of folders in file drawers or it might entail a computer-based system. Finally (step (7) in the figure), there is a choice of methods for making information available to managers. This choice depends on the preceding choice of data processing methods; in addition, however, it depends on the preferences and management styles of the particular managers who are to receive and use the information.

The design sequence as depicted in Figure 1 and described in the text did not, in fact, proceed as smoothly as appears to be suggested. There were, as would no doubt be expected, many false starts and many iterations and reiterations through the process. Nevertheless, the figure captures the essence of the logic and sequencing that was followed.

MIS for a CE Provider Unit

The total set of CSFs for a CE provider unit and the evidence necessary to ensure that each factor is within satisfactory limits are presented in the Appendix at the end of this chapter. They are presented in relation to the four functions of management. These, along with the design framework described in the previous section, should provide useful guidance for readers when they are reviewing the management information systems of their own CE provider units or when undertaking the task of designing an MIS for their units, if one does not already exist.

In Chapter Twelve, several decisions typically faced by CE managers were listed. An MIS should assist the manager in obtaining the information necessary to make effective decisions. Several of these decisions deal with two basic issues: determining the quality of the educational activities, products, and services; and assessing the allocation of resources and the efficiency of resource usage. In this section, two CSFs, along with the related monitoring of the factors, are selected and used to illustrate how the MIS can provide the relevant information. General aspects of the MIS are also discussed.

Educational Quality. "What measures can we take to assure that our educational activities, products, or services are of the requisite quality?" The analysis of the CSFs tracking "Educational Quality" is presented in Table 1. The factor statements that have direct bearing on educational quality are presented alongside the respective management functions. The figures following the statements in the second column provide a reference by which they can be located within the total set of CSFs by function as detailed in the Appendix at the end of this chapter. The evidence necessary to ensure that each factor statement is holding true in practice is set out in the third column of the table. The MIS should be designed to supply the manager or managers of a CE provider unit with this evidence.

The first function, strategic management of the unit, is concerned with whether the unit can, as a matter of ongoing procedure, address educational quality as an element within the overall mission

Table 1. Critical Success Factors Corresponding to Educational Quality.

Function	Factor Statement	Relevant Evidence
Strategic management of the unit	CE provider unit has an effective quality assurance and assessment program. (A5)	A quality assurance and assessment plan, which conforms to CESP QEs, is established. A system for review of projects to assure conformance to quality assurance and assessment program is established. Staff competencies necessary to achieve quality assurance and assessment programs are defined, and a system for developing these is established. Program evaluation indicates that program is contributing to improved health care delivery.
Program management	Education quality assurance system is established and is effectively supporting the goals. (B4)	Educational quality assurance system exists. Output plans embody quality assurance criteria. Quality criteria are met. Sample audits of quality assurance system show system to be working.
Project coordination and control	For each project a plan is developed which . . . meets quality criteria . . . . (C1)	There exists a plan for each project. Project plans are approved by program manager.

**Table 1. Critical Success Factors
Corresponding to Educational Quality, Cont'd.**

Function	Factor Statement	Relevant Evidence
Project development and implementation	Project is implemented according to approved plan. (D3)	Plan and authorization for implementation exists. There is an evaluation plan and subsequent monitoring, covering quality assurance criteria.

and strategic plan. The relevant evidence pertaining to the factor statement is appropriately broad. It includes ensuring that planning and review procedures are in place to allow the requirements stemming from educational quality to be managed in a delegated mode. It also addresses the requisite knowledge and skills of the unit's staff to deal creatively and in a professional manner with the demands of the quality elements. Where deficiencies in expertise are identified, a staff development program to correct these would be necessary. Finally, it is suggested that information be gathered to assess the impact of the CE program on the delivery of health care, with a view to judging whether the quality elements built into the program are contributing to improvements in health care. Chapter Ten provides an in-depth treatment of evaluation.

Program evaluation should involve focusing on three possible, and increasingly difficult, measures of impact: first, the subjective opinions of learners as to the likelihood of desirable behavior changes resulting from their immediate experience of CE activities; second, observation of health professional performance; and finally, direct measures of improved health care outcomes within the health care system. The difficulty in obtaining unequivocal evidence concerning the effects that the unit's activities are having on its defined client populations certainly has to be acknowledged. To derive significant correlations between CE provider unit activities and behavior patterns in the related health care system is difficult enough; beyond that, an attribution of causality may require a leap of faith.

A social scientist might justifiably shrink from such an undertaking, but managers cannot afford to be so cautious. The most important information that managers need may simply not be obtainable in a form that would satisfy the demands of a scientist. But that does not diminish the need for the information, nor does it excuse managers from the responsibility of giving their best efforts to ensuring the information is developed. It simply says that an appropriate degree of judgment, even a healthy skepticism, must be applied in the managerial use of such information, in recognition of the limitations of the methods of data collection and analysis that were used in its development.

The program management function has the responsibility of ensuring that an educational quality assurance program is developed and implemented and that it is effectively supporting the program goals. The evidence of this includes ensuring that a quality assurance system is in place and that it is understood and accepted by all members of the unit; it also includes the observation that plans embody quality criteria appropriate in light of the program goals and the monitoring of whether these criteria are being met. This monitoring should include a mechanism for periodically sampling that the reported information is accurately describing what is actually going on. This is not to suggest an absence of trust or a questioning of professional standards in the organization. Nevertheless, assurance of the integrity of the information system is simply a matter of sound managerial practice. Professional staff should not object to this; on the contrary, they should realize the importance of safeguarding the standards within their areas of professional practice.

The project coordination and control function has the responsibility of ensuring that each educational project is soundly planned with a view to meeting the quality criteria. This function is also responsible for ensuring that all project plans are approved by the program management function. The approval process is presumed to provide a check that the planned criteria at the project level are consistent with the overall program goals for quality.

Finally, the project development and implementation function generates the project plans and, after proper review and approval, carries them out. Project planning and implementation should be guided by procedures and checklists, some of which specifically address quality assurance. Part of the evidence about quality will come from project evaluations. These evaluations can serve a very worthwhile management purpose. They can assist those directly involved in project planning and implementation to improve their procedures. CE management, in turn, can use summarized evaluation data to allow all the unit's staff to benefit from the collective experience and to establish plans and goals aimed at improving the relevance and client acceptance of the quality elements of CE activities.

Resource Allocation and Efficiency Assessment. "Is our budget soundly based to reflect current priorities and is it realistic in terms of available resources?" Resource allocation and the evaluation of the efficiency with which resources have been used in operations are important aspects of the responsibilities assigned to the strategic management of the unit and the program management functions. One CSF statement addresses resource allocation in a long-term planning mode as follows: "Given current goals and goals for the future, there are sufficient quantity and quality of resources" (A9). In greater detail but still in a planning mode, another CSF states: "The defined program is feasible within known and estimated resources" (B1). Two CSF statements refer to ongoing monitoring and after-the-fact assessment of resource utilization as follows: "Personnel utilization is effective" (B7); "Resource utilization is effective" (B8).

A useful method for both planning and assessment of resource allocation and use is illustrated in Figure 2.

The method, an input-output matrix, requires a complete listing of all categories of activity that give rise to resource use. These include the primary outputs of the unit, such as courses, seminars, and other educational products and services. Also included would be such things as research and publication, development projects aimed at enhancing the capabilities of the unit's staff to produce future primary outputs, and the management and administration of the unit. These comprise the output dimension of the matrix; illustrative outputs are shown as the column headings in the figure.

The framework also requires a listing of all line items of resources, categorized in a manner useful from a managerial stand-

Figure 2. Input-Output Matrix.

Inputs / Outputs	Primary Outputs			Secondary Outputs			
	Activities	Products	Services	Program Planning and Evaluation	Staff Development	Unit Administration	System Support
Staff							
Needs Assessment							
Program Design							
Evaluation							
Logistical Support							
Media Support							
Management Support							
Clerical							
Faculty							
Permanent	$x_{ij} / \$x_{ij}$						
Consultant							
Facilities							
Office							
Meeting							
Work							
Equipment							
Production							
Office							
Implementation							
Supplies							

point. That is to say, the basis for categorizing line items of resources should reflect the way the manager is accustomed to thinking about resource allocation in the unit. These comprise the input
dimension of the matrix; illustrative inputs are shown as the cap-
tions to the rows in the figure.

Current estimates of the resources needed to produce a unit of
each output are entered into the cells in the body of the matrix.
These estimates are entered in both physical terms and in their corresponding dollar amounts. For instance, the coefficient x_{ij} shown
in the matrix might be an estimate of permanent faculty hours
required for a particular type of seminar and the full dollar cost of
these hours. These are referred to as the resource coefficients. The
sum of the resource coefficients for each column is a current estimate
of the resources and costs required for a unit of each of the organization's outputs.

In the planning phase, the total planned output is quantified
in resource and cost terms by multiplying the planned output
volumes by their respective resource coefficients. This is then compared with the resources that are anticipated to be available during
the period being planned for. If the estimated resource requirements
exceed availability—in aggregate or in terms of a specific line item
of resource—the output plan may have to be modified. Alternatively, strategies for obtaining more resources may be devised to fill
the anticipated gap. If the reverse is true, a more demanding output
plan can be developed.

In assessing efficiency, the same process is applied. However,
in this case the *actual* outputs that were produced during the period
under review are used. They are multiplied by their resource coefficients to derive an estimate of the level and mix of resource usage
that should have been incurred to produce the outputs. This is compared with the resources that were, in fact, available and used. If the
resource usage exceeded the estimate of what should have been used
again—in aggregate and in terms of each line item of resource—
there is evidence of inefficiency that should be investigated further.
If the reverse is the case, there is evidence of efficiency gains.

This method requires sound, current estimates of resources

required and their related costs per unit of each of the primary and secondary outputs of the organization. If the cost accounting system and the operating information system cannot provide these directly, then additional analysis will be necessary. The estimates should be developed at least once each year, in preparation for the planning and budgeting process.

It takes a considerable amount of effort to develop an input-output matrix the first time; however, its ongoing maintenance is less demanding. The matrix is extremely useful in planning, resource allocation, budgeting, and monitoring the efficiency of operations. In addition, since it enhances the precision and rapidity of planning and resource allocation, it greatly facilitates the revision of plans and budgets if this should prove to be necessary during the progress of the operating year.

General Features of the MIS. It should be clear that a very broad interpretation of the term *information* has been used in the formulation of the proposed MIS, much broader than that typically used in the information systems field. A considerable part of the evidence suggested for monitoring the CSFs derives from the knowledge and skills of the person or persons fulfilling the four management functions. For instance, the "face validity" of procedures and plans is accepted as relevant evidence with regard to several of the CSFs. This kind of judgment depends on the experience of the managers involved. This was alluded to earlier in the chapter when an organization was referred to as an information-processing and decision-making entity. From this perspective, the accumulated knowledge residing in the managerial organization is explicitly viewed as an important source of information. The formal monitoring system simply extends the base that is supporting managers as they exercise their judgment in the decision-making process.

As organizations develop, they continually experience new problems requiring analysis and solutions. The ensuing question concerns whether a procedure should be specified to take care of the problem if it is encountered again. Some observers of organizational practice decry the tendency to reduce managerial activity to a set of formalized procedures supported by routinized information flows; they interpret this as a bureaucratic encroachment on managerial discretion. Another perspective, however, views the organization's formal information systems and procedures as a repository of past learning about how to deal with particular managerial tasks and problem situations. From this perspective, formal specification can be viewed as releasing managerial time, allowing it to be directed to new problems as they arise. The proposed MIS is put forward in this latter spirit. It is intended to be supportive of constructive managerial action, not a constraint on the professional creativity that is an essential ingredient of effective CE in health care.

     A second important point is that each CSF is interconnected with the total set. This becomes evident, for example, in the discussion of educational quality. There, the point was made that the strategic management of the unit function should be concerned with ensuring that the staff members of the unit possess the requisite skills and knowledge demanded by the quality goals. Were this not the case, a staff development program would be necessary. Staff skills, development needs, and the organizational climate to support staff development are all contained in other CSFs. Further, since staff development absorbs staff time and probably also budget dollars, development programs have direct implications for resource allocation, the focus of yet another CSF. Thus, while each CSF has its own differentiated focus of concern, around which is generated a flow of procedures and monitoring for ensuring that its requirements are met, the interdependence among CSFs also requires attention. The appropriate integration of the CSFs around specific strategies is an important leadership responsibility, a theme that was stressed in Chapter Twelve.

     The sources of information input to the MIS are broad and varied. They include external and internal sources, and they include data that are relatively "hard" and objective in nature, along with data that are "soft" and intuitive. The different functions rely on different mixes of information. The strategic management of the unit function depends heavily on external sources of information. Further, because the decision making assigned to this function is relatively unstructured, the pertinent information is typically of a subjective and intuitive nature. It is also highly summarized since the concern here is with issues affecting the total unit over a long time period. By contrast, the project development and implementation function is more focused, more detailed, and tends to be more dependent on internal data sources, such as the unit's operating information and cost accounting systems. Accuracy and timeliness of information are of greater importance to this function. Furthermore, since the underlying structure of the tasks embodied in this function are typically well understood, the information requirements and operating procedures supporting the function can, in large part, be defined in advance. Indeed, much of it can be specified in the form of precise algorithms and checklists to be followed. The nature of the information to support the program management and the project coordination and control functions lies between these two extremes. They are principally internally oriented, but they rely on more summarized data, and they use a greater amount of judgmental, rather than objective, data.

Finally, the MIS has been described principally in terms of monitoring, that is to say, the provision of an ongoing flow of descriptive information to keep the manager informed of what is, or what has been, happening. In the management process, forecast information is also required, that is to say, a description of what is likely to, or what may, happen in the future. Forecasting methods to develop future-oriented information have not been addressed in this discussion. Further, the management process requires prescriptive or normative information as well as descriptive information. In a future context, this information expresses the decision making that translates forecasts into goals, strategies, and plans, that is, statements of managerial intent. In a retrospective context, this information has an evaluative purpose; it is concerned with saying what should have happened, to provide a basis for appraising what actually did happen. This appraisal process supports the evaluation of managerial performance as a basis for allocating rewards and for learning about how to improve future performance. Again, methods for constructing normative information, for example, the organization's goals and the levels of performance contained in the goal statements, have not been addressed directly in the course of the discussion. Techniques for developing forecast and evaluative information are clearly important, and their exclusion from the discussion was not intended to suggest otherwise. Nevertheless, the initial step of developing and making explicit the basic information structure, within which these techniques can be effectively applied, should take precedence. The basic information structure was the thrust of this chapter.

Getting Started and Keeping Going

There is no doubt that a demanding task has been outlined in this chapter, one not likely to be achieved in a short time frame. It will never be achieved, of course, if a start is not made, and it will never approach completion (if, indeed, there even is such a thing) if the effort is not sustained.

The key to getting started is to avoid being overwhelmed by the magnitude of the total task. Instead, management should focus on a CSF that is particularly relevant to their CE provider unit and to the circumstances it currently faces. This is used as a focus of an information system development project, a project that can be defined, planned, and accomplished in a specified, reasonably short time period. This incremental approach has the merit of contributing usefully to managerial decision making fairly quickly and therefore of building and sustaining motivation to the overall effort. There is nothing as effective as success for building enthusiasm to continue, and this success has to be demonstrated pragmatically in the realm of managerial action and decision making.

A comment on data processing technology is perhaps appropriate at this juncture. As has been stressed throughout the chapter, the required data for monitoring the CSFs can readily be assimilated and used in a traditional manner, relying on project folders and manually maintained data files. However, there is much to be said for minimizing the degree of manual data handling and paperwork in an MIS. Beyond the question of efficiency, automation can greatly enhance the ad hoc analytical effort referred to previously in the chapter. New questions, or ways of viewing and interpreting phenomena of concern, are continually occurring to managers as they deal with strategy formulation, resource allocation, and evaluation of performance. These naturally give rise to a demand for additional analysis. If the data are maintained in computer files in a system that allows ready access to packages for statistical analysis, this kind of inquiry will be greatly facilitated.

The annual planning cycle is the time to address information systems projects, alongside all the other concerns of mission, educational activities, products, and services. Improving information, with a view to enhancing managerial capabilities, should have a legitimate claim on the organization's resources. Management must ensure that the claim is seen to be necessary and legitimate and is given adequate representation in the resource allocation process.

Summary

This chapter has outlined a framework, based on decision analysis and the CSF method, for designing information systems to meet the management needs of a CE provider unit. The information requirements were related to the four managerial functions identified in the previous chapter. A proposal for an MIS was described.

The proposal would obviously entail significant costs to implement properly, and it is only worth doing if done properly. It would claim a considerable commitment of managerial resources and related expenditures of financial resources. In common with any course of action aimed at major organizational change, it has attendant risks. The top manager of the unit must take an energetic and proactive position in support of the effort in order to enhance its chances of success. Thus, the prestige of the leader within the unit and perhaps beyond the unit will inevitably be identified with the success of the MIS development. This cannot be avoided; it is simply a fact of leadership.

But what of the potential benefits? Among these are the likelihood of achieving a better-informed and more effective allocation of resources to the unit's activities, the maintenance of a longer-term, strategic thrust alongside the concerns stemming from the immediate pressures of current operating problems, and an improved capacity to handle risk and uncertainty in responding to unexpected contingencies arising in the unit's environment. These are the rational benefits, and there are no doubt others that could be claimed. Just as important, however, is the possibility that designing and meeting the management information needs of the unit are activities that involve intellectual challenge and intrinsic satisfaction. The fun and personal reward of responding to the managerial challenge of the task should be at least as compelling as the rational benefits that are promised to lie at the end of the information-systems rainbow!

Appendix: Functions, Critical Success Factors, and Evidence

Function A: Strategic Management of the Unit

This function deals with setting direction for the organization as a whole and assuring that the total program fulfills the goals and mission of the organization. It includes such responsibilities as establishing a mission, strategic planning, setting goals and policies, exception monitoring, and dealing with external organizations and meeting external accountability requirements.

Success Factors and Evidence

Factor A1: CE provider unit has appropriate mission and strategic plan.

Evidence

- Mission statement defines purpose, scope, domain, and general potential educational needs of target population
- Mission reflects relevant expectations of parent organization and/or significant external groups and individuals
- Strategic plan forecasts future directions and events that could influence CE provider unit's mission

Factor A2: CE provider unit has goals that meet the parent body's expectations, respond to the general demands of the target population, and are consistent with the mission and strategic plan.

Evidence

- Goals fall within scope and domain of CE provider unit as defined by mission statement and strategic plan
- Goals have face validity of mission and strategic plan that they are fulfilling
- Goals appear to be achievable
- Goals address identified client demand

Factor A3: CE provider unit has policies and procedures that contribute to development of programs to accomplish goals.

Evidence

- Policies and procedures set the operational parameters for each critical function of the CE provider unit as defined by top management
- CE provider unit policies and procedures do not violate parent body policies
- Policies and procedures do not place undue constraints on program development and implementation
- Policies and procedures are applied appropriately
- There is a mechanism for review and revision of policies and procedures

Factor A4: CE provider unit's authority is commensurate with its responsibility.

Evidence

- Proper placement of CE provider unit on parent body organizational chart
- Authority is defined in the position description of CE provider unit leader
- CE provider unit plans are authorized by parent body
- Important persons, such as service chiefs, acknowledge CE provider unit authority
- Parent body has policies that enable accomplishment of CE provider unit's mission and goals
- Resource commitments by parent body are commensurate with CE provider unit plans

Factor A5: CE provider unit has an effective quality assurance and assessment program.

Evidence

- CE provider unit has a quality assurance and assessment plan that conform to CESP quality elements (QEs)
- CE provider unit has a system for review of projects to assure conformance to quality assurance standards

- CE provider unit has defined staff competencies necessary to achieve quality assurance
- CE provider unit has a system for assuring necessary staff competencies
- CE provider unit program evaluation indicates that program contributes to improved health care delivery

Factor A6: Program output and enrollment are sufficient to maintain CE provider unit's economic viability.

Evidence

- Activity enrollments and revenues match fiscal plans
- Number and mix of enrollments match plan
- Product sales match fiscal plans
- Number and mix of products match plan
- Cost of outputs matches fiscal plan
- Service revenues match fiscal plans
- Number and mix of services matches plan

Factor A7: Significant institutional and external relationships are appropriate and expectations are met.

Evidence

- CE provider unit maintains a list of institutional and external groups with whom relationships are critical
- CE provider unit has defined expectations of significant internal and external groups
- CE provider unit periodically assesses current relationships and expectations and decides which ones are satisfactory and need only periodic monitoring and which ones are unsatisfactory and need a plan for change and frequent monitoring

Factor A8: CE provider unit program leads to fulfillment of goals.

Evidence

- CE provider unit management agrees that long- and short-range program plans appear to accomplish CE provider unit goals

- Short-range program plans apportion this year's resources appropriately
- Progress reports indicate that program plan is being carried out or needed changes are being made and justified
- Projects carried out fulfill the program plan

Factor A9: Given current goals and goals for the future, there are sufficient quantity and quality of resources.

Evidence

- See Figure 2 in this chapter

Factor A10: CE provider unit staff is organized and managed to facilitate efficient accomplishment of the goals.

Evidence

- Delegated authority is commensurate with assigned responsibility
- Responsibilities are explicitly defined
- Formal channels of communication are defined and used as appropriate
- Management periodically assesses staff morale
- Mechanisms are implemented to facilitate supportive environment
- CE provider unit performance standards exist and have been negotiated with staff
- Performance review is carried out in a timely and effective manner
- Staff turnover is not the result of nonsupportive environment
- Management communicates with staff

Factor A11: The organizational environment supports growth and development of staff.

Evidence

- CE provider unit management and staff develop and fulfill plans for growth and development
- CE provider unit staff development plans respond to both personal and organizational needs

Factor A12: CE provider unit's resources are managed efficiently.

Evidence

- There is a plan for utilization of resources that leads to accomplishing the goals and maximizes output of the CE provider unit
- There is an accurate and timely resource monitoring system
- Timely changes are made to resource utilization plan as a result of monitoring

Function B: Program Management

This function involves establishing the overall program to meet the goals of the unit, allocating resources to projects comprising the program, and establishing procedures and monitoring systems to ensure that the overall program is being effectively carried out.

Success Factors and Evidence

Factor B1: The defined program is feasible within known and estimated resources.

Evidence

- Output plan (description of projects) defines required resources
- There are strategies for matching available resources with required resources
- Strategies are developed for obtaining additional resources needed

Factor B2: Program outputs are relevant to the needs and concerns in the health care setting.

Evidence

- Program is based on defined needs and concerns
- Program is responsive to "total" client population needs and concerns (quantity, intensity)
- Program outputs meet needs and concerns as planned

Factor B3: The total program outputs meet the stated goals.

Evidence

- Top management approves program plan
- Top management approves program accomplishments in relation to plan

Factor B4: Educational quality assurance system is established and is effectively supporting the goals.

Evidence

- Educational quality assurance system exists
- Output plans embody quality assurance criteria
- Quality assurance criteria are met
- Sample audits of system shows quality assurance is working

Factor B5: Administrative procedures are established and effectively support the goals.

Evidence

- Administrative procedures are established
- Staff knows the procedures and why they exist
- Procedures that require documentation of compliance are documented
- External reports are produced when needed to satisfy accountability requirements of parent body
- Personal review process is established and operational
- System for monitoring compliance is established and in operation

Factor B6: Information and control system is established and effective.

Evidence

- System architecture is defined
- Information system supplies the data needed to meet criteria factors
- Information system identifies problems
- Information is timely, accurate, complete, retrievable, and anticipates departures from plans

Factor B7: Personnel utilization is effective.

Evidence

- Things are getting done as planned
- Interpersonal conflict is minimized
- There is high morale/high job satisfaction/appropriate turn-over
- Delegated authority is commensurate with assigned responsibility
- Individual development plans reconcile program needs of CE provider unit with individuals' aspirations
- Development plans are facilitated and monitored

Factor B8: Resource utilization is effective.

Evidence

- Books remain balanced

Factor B9: Organization has a positive image among constituency and clients.

Evidence

- Clients are satisfied with CE provider unit activities
- Constituency supports the CE provider unit
- Any research completed is published and publicized

Function C: Project Coordination and Control

This function deals with assuring the quality and quantity of projects as specified by the program and coordination among projects. It also involves assuring efficient resource utilization, a good image among the unit's various client populations, and the timely completion of tasks.

Success Factors and Evidence

Factor C1: For each project a plan is developed that is congruent with program intent, meets quality criteria, and conforms to administrative procedures.

Evidence

- There is a project plan
- Plan is approved by program manager

Factor C2: Adequate resources are made available to each project according to the approved plan.

Evidence

- Recurring conflicts for access to certain fixed resources are identified and corrected
- Required space, equipment, personnel, faculty, and monies are committed for each project
- Actual space, equipment, personnel, faculty, and monies for each project are available in a timely manner

Factor C3: Each project is implemented in an acceptable manner.

Evidence

- Actual project activities are consistent with the plan
- Deviation from the plan had prior approval or was justifiable

Factor C4: Each project creates a positive image with clients.

Evidence

- Clients are satisfied
- Constituents are supportive

Factor C5: Projects stay within budget.

Evidence

- Project budgets are within acceptable limits
- Actual project costs are consistent with budgeted costs
- Equipment utilization meets defined standard
- Space utilization meets defined standard
- There is an effective scheduling system for space and equipment
- There is an accurate inventory system that defines space and equipment capability

- Resources are available when needed

Factor C6: All projects within the CE provider unit are coordinated.

Evidence

- There are no conflicts in access to resources
- Duplication of effort is minimized
- There is an overall scheduling plan for projects

Function D: Project Development and Implementation

This function involves accomplishing the variety of tasks embodied in approved project plans in a timely and efficient manner and in accordance with defined policies and procedures.

Success Factors and Evidence

Factor D1: Project has an adequate plan.

Evidence

- There is justification for project
- Educational strategies are described
- There are resource projections and justification
- Logistical schedule requirements are proposed
- Costs per contact hour are estimated
- There is an evaluation plan

Factor D2: Project planning guidelines are followed.

Evidence

- Projected completion dates are documented
- Actual completion dates are timely and documented

Factor D3: Project implemented according to approved plan.

Evidence

- Preproject implementation meeting held
- Any changes to project implementation are approved or justified

- Evaluation data collected and analyzed
- Final report is disseminated

Factor D4: "Official Project File" is created and updated in a timely fashion.

Evidence

- Information is included in file as specified (content and timelines)

Factor D5: Organizational policies are not violated.

Evidence

- Administrative procedures are followed

Factor D6: The competencies required to accomplish projects are present.

Evidence

- Competencies necessary to carry out project tasks are known
- Tasks are assigned to people with appropriate skills
- Supervisor is notified about discrepancies

Factor D7: Project creates a positive image.

Evidence

- Indicated in results of evaluation and needs assessment data
- Negative feedback is minimal
- Informal feedback indicates positive image
- There is documentation of commendation

Factor D8: Evaluation results are reported.

Evidence

- Everyone identified as recipients of evaluation data received results in a timely fashion

References

Ackoff, R. L. "Management Misinformation Systems." *Management Science,* 1967, *14* (4), 1–13.

Anthony, R. N. *Planning and Control Systems: A Framework for Analysis.* Boston: Division of Research, Graduate School of Business Administration, Harvard University, 1965.

Davis, G. B. "Strategies for Information Requirements Determination." *IBM Systems Journal,* 1982, *21* (1), 4–30.

Gorry, G. A., and Scott Morton, M. S. "A Framework for Management Information Systems." *Sloan Management Review,* 1971, *13* (1), 55–70.

Hax, A. C. "Planning a Management Information System for a Distributing and Manufacturing Company." *Sloan Management Review,* 1973, *14* (3), 85–98.

MacKintosh, D. P. *Management by Exception: A Handbook with Forms.* Englewood Cliffs, N.J.: Prentice-Hall, 1978.

Martin, M. P. "The Decision Graph in Systems Analysis." *Journal of Systems Management,* 1980, *31* (1), 29–35.

Mintzberg, H. *The Nature of Managerial Work.* Englewood Cliffs, N.J.: Prentice-Hall, 1980.

Rockart, J. F. "Chief Executives Define Their Own Data Needs." *Harvard Business Review,* 1979, *57* (2), 81–93.

Rockart, J. F., and Treacy, M. E. "The CEO Goes On-Line." *Harvard Business Review,* 1982, *60* (1), 82–88.

Scott Morton, M. S. *Management Decision Systems.* Boston: Division of Research, Graduate School of Business Administration, Harvard University, 1971.

Simon, H. A. *The New Science of Management Decision.* New York: Harper & Row, 1960.

Implementing Educational Quality Assurance Procedures: Self-Study and External Review

David B. Walthall III

This chapter describes an educational quality assurance method that was developed, pilot tested, and implemented by the Regional Medical Education Centers of the Veterans Administration (VA). The

Note: The author gratefully acknowledges the contributions of the following groups and individuals: First, without the help and cooperation of the RMEC Council and its chairman, Francis A. Zacharewicz, the system could not have been developed. Second, the members of the site survey team, Robert Cullen, Ph.D.; R. L. Madkin, D.M.D.; Dorothy Sassenrath, M.S., R.N.; and Richard D. Wilkinson, M.A., made major contributions in the development of organizational criteria and elements. Third, Joseph S. Green, Ph.D., and Cheryl L. Walthall, R.N., contributed significantly to the conceptualization of the system, the development of the criteria and elements, and the preparation of this chapter.

conceptual framework and quality elements described in Chapter One provided the theoretical underpinnings for this approach. This model was developed using concepts from systems engineering, performance analysis, and medical quality assurance. Implementation of the method described has identified outstanding and innovative educational techniques and led to their diffusion throughout the system. It has revealed areas of concern which have been improved and has been considered by those surveyed and the survey team to be an effective learning experience. This chapter is closely related to Chapters One, Seven, Twelve, and Fifteen and should be read in tandem with them.—Editors

The Regional Medical Education Centers (RMECs) are continuing education provider units (CEPUs) within the Department of Medicine and Surgery of the Veterans Administration. They are directly responsible to the Office of Academic Affairs for the delivery of practice-related continuing education to the VA Medical Centers within the geographical boundaries of each RMEC region. Approximately twenty-five medical centers are in each RMEC region. The medical centers within a region have about 25,000 employees, consisting of physicians, nurses, managers, and allied health and support personnel. Each RMEC is staffed with approximately eighteen employees including a physician director, educators, project managers (health care professionals or education specialists), logistics support staff and clerical personnel. The RMECs have access to four major learning resource centers, providing sophisticated audiovisual and television production support. In addition to reporting to the Office of Academic Affairs, the RMECs are governed by a self-governance document, similar to the bylaws of a private organization, and a governing council comprised of two members from each RMEC—the medical director and codirector.

Several events occurring simultaneously led to the development of the self-study and external review process described in this chapter. Staff from some of the Regional Medical Education Centers were heavily involved with the development of the quality elements and the conceptual model described in Chapter One. The RMEC council was asked to formalize its own self-governance procedures in order to be more accountable to the Office of Academic Affairs. In addition, the VA had a commitment to participate in the pilot phase of the Continuing Education Systems Project (CESP). These events led the RMEC Council to develop, pilot test, and operationalize an external review process. A procedure was needed that would allow continuing education (CE) provider units to assess themselves against common criteria and establish comparable performance data over time. The use of concepts from systems engineering (Corrigan and Kaufman, 1966), performance analysis (Mager and Pipe, 1970), and health care quality assurance (Jacobs, Christoffel, and Dixon, 1976; Fox and others, 1974; Williamson, 1977) are the cornerstones for the approach developed. This chapter will describe the rationale, process, and use of this system.

Rationale for CE Quality Assurance

For the purposes of the CE quality assurance system, the word *project* is used to represent the discrete educational interventions of a continuing education provider unit. This includes individual or group activities, educational products, both print and nonprint, and services such as consultation and assistance to individuals or organizations in various aspects of educational development. The word *program* is used to describe the complete set of projects accomplished by the unit or a definitive and discrete aggregation of projects that make up a significant subunit of the entire program. *Quality assurance* describes an activity that compares elements of educational and management practice to explicit criteria, correcting deficiencies that are found and instituting monitoring systems in those areas that have the potential to create negative outcomes.

The self-study and external review process described in this chapter is designed to allow judgments to be made regarding all aspects of the CE provider unit including the strategic management, the general or administrative management of the entire program, the overall educational planning, the management of individual projects, and assistance to self-directed learners. The major reasons for performing this type of quality assurance activity include enhancing unit management, obtaining accreditation status, and engendering public confidence.

Enhancement of Unit Management. The CE provider unit can reap many benefits from such a review system. The review system allows top management of the unit to evaluate its own internal quality assurance program and maintain the activity as a dynamic process. The system provides management with a needs assessment tool for determining knowledge, skill, and attitude deficiencies, as well as developmental opportunities for the entire staff (see Chapter Fifteen). It forces and allows systematic, in-depth troubleshooting of educational projects or management activities when problems arise. Finally, perhaps most importantly, it strengthens each educational project and the entire educational program.

Accreditation. A set of criteria and standards were derived from the quality elements described in Chapter One. They were developed by consensus, using a widely diversified group of recognized educational experts and experts from various health disciplines, then validated both through extensive literature reviews and multiple exposure to health care provider groups (Association of American Medical Colleges, Society of Medical College Directors of Continuing Medical Education (CME), American Association of Dental Schools, and others). Since accrediting groups such as the Accreditation Council for Continuing Medical Education have drawn on the quality elements in the development of their process (see Chapter Sixteen), it would appear that meeting these criteria and standards might satisfy most of the various accrediting organizations. The criteria and standards should, at the very least, prepare a continuing education provider unit to meet any set of standards an accrediting body could require.

Public Confidence. In a world that is becoming more and more accountability-oriented and less willing to accept professional activities on faith, the establishment and use of a quality assurance system by a CE provider unit should go far to promote public confidence in an area that is a major consumer of resources (Miller, 1977). In order to have this effect, the unit must make the public aware that it engages in such a process. Criteria and standards, as well as aggregate data, must be made available to the public while protecting the confidentiality of the CE staff.

Systematic Approach to Quality Assurance

In order to develop a valid and useful self-study and external review process, it is helpful to understand the systems approach used in most quality assurance activities. This section gives an overview of the systems approach, clearly delineating the outcomes of a CE provider unit, while pointing out the difficulty of measuring those outcomes. The establishment of the criteria to be used for the process, the core of the self-study and external review system, is explained.

Systems Approach. There are four key concepts that describe this systems approach: input, process, output, and outcome. *Input* refers to the structure and building blocks on which a program is formed and includes such things as budget, staff, faculty, equipment, and space. *Process* refers to the way things get done. Often there are several acceptable processes for accomplishing the same task. Systematic project design, personnel management, and logistical support are all examples of process. *Output* refers to the product that the organization or unit produces. Ford Motor Company produces cars; a continuing education provider unit produces educational projects. *Outcome* refers to the impact that a project or overall program has on the participants and the health care setting. When health professionals involve themselves in CE, there are a number of potential events that may occur; however, these outcomes are the result of the interaction of a complex set of variables, only one of which is learning (Goldfinger, 1982).

Potential Outcomes of CE Provider Units. Once the CE provider unit has completed an educational project, a series of potential outcomes is possible. After leaving the educational project, the health professionals may:

- have a high degree of *satisfaction* and be motivated to return for more projects and refer projects to their co-workers
- accomplish the output of the project and have the *competencies* (ability to perform) described by the educational objectives
- *perform* the new competencies in the health care setting

- improve their *clinical judgment* in their interaction with patients

As a result of this interaction, the patients may:

- feel *satisfied* about the interaction
- have a new set of *competencies* (knowledge, skills, or attitudes)
- use these competencies to reduce disease or pain (*compliance*)
- *improve their wellness,* which is the ultimate outcome

As one gets further away from the actual educational project, more intervening and uncontrollable variables affect the eventual impact, making it more and more difficult to determine accurately the causes of the outcome.

Measuring Outcomes. The process of developing a model for the quality assurance of a CE provider unit leads to a dilemma. On the one hand, there is a belief in the conceptual model of CE as described in Chapter One. This model places heavy emphasis on problem identification, needs analysis, and evaluation being done in the practice setting. However, in the systems approach discussed in the previous section of this chapter, it was shown that the further one gets from the actual output of the unit (the educational project itself), the more intervening variables one has to contend with and the more difficult it is to attribute the outcomes to the educational project. Therefore, while data from the practice setting would appear to be the most desirable and useful for both needs identification and evaluation, it is apparent that one cannot rely solely on these data for decision making.

It follows that one can defend the fact that the goal of the CE provider unit must be to have a positive impact on the health care setting. It is not unreasonable to insist that the problem identification and needs analysis be derived from the health care setting and that projects be designed to have an impact on that setting. It is also not unreasonable to insist that the CE organization make a positive effort to facilitate the application of learning to practice; however, the educator alone should not and must not be held accountable for what actually occurs after the learning experience is completed as planned. The CE provider unit should conduct impact evaluation whenever feasible. The results should be documented and made available to the public.

Establishing Criteria for Quality. The review process developed by the RMEC system accommodates this dilemma by focusing upon the following major concepts of the quality conceptual framework described in Chapter One.

• importance of data gathering from the entire practice setting— health care providers, institutions, and patients
• ultimate responsibility for the learning process assumed by the health care professional
• importance of applying learning to practice
• importance of strategic management of the CE provider unit
• importance of effective daily administration of the unit
• applying adult learning principles and learning theory to the development and implementation of learning experiences

The process of developing the criteria used in this self-study was based on several ground rules: first, each of the quality elements had to be included, unless there was clear justification for its exclusion (only one of the quality elements was omitted); second, each criterion had to be operationally defined, which in fact strengthened the quality elements and led to a second revision of them in more operational terms.

There are several criterion models of quality assurance that have been developed over the years. The one used in this self-study process is the systems approach defined earlier as including input, process, output, and outcome elements. These criteria may be developed using one or more of the following methods: evidence that has stood the test of rigorous experimental design and referred review, consensus by experts in the discipline involved, and consensus by actual practitioners in the profession.

Any of these methods, if used alone, has major disadvantages or drawbacks. The first method would seem to be the most valid and desirable; however, this evidence is very difficult to obtain in the fields of management and education because the very nature of the profession defies the common use of rigid experimental design. The second method has many merits and is always the most tempting;

however, one must be aware of its major pitfall, the "ivory tower syndrome." Oftentimes the leading experts are carefully shielded from the actual work place and have distorted views of the realities of daily accomplishment. Acceptance of these criteria can easily lead to paralysis precipitated by the quest for perfection. The third approach, while appealing and most easily accomplished, carries with it a real chance of being incomplete and superficial due to the lack of comprehensive, up-to-date expert knowledge in the field. This is very understandable as this group is spending their time "in the trenches" and having their pragmatic approach reinforced daily.

The criterion model developed for this review system (Exhibit 1) consists of the following: a *criterion statement* with a definition and standard (the standard used by the RMEC system is that all elements of a criteria must be met in order to meet that criteria; the leeway allowed in meeting specific elements is described in the instructions); the *elements* of management or education that must be present to meet the criterion; the *evidence* required to demonstrate the presence of the element; the *data* necessary to support the evidence; the *source* of the evidence and data; and *instructions* on how to interpret the data and evidence.

Self-Study and External Review System

The core of this educational quality assurance system consists of twenty-six criteria and their elements that were derived from the quality elements developed by the Continuing Education Systems Project. The criteria are listed in the Appendix at the end of this chapter. The criteria are grouped into five primary review areas, which are listed in the section titled "Primary Review Areas," later in this chapter. Table 1 relates the taxonomy of the self-study and external review process to the CESP taxonomy, and illustrates the terminology.

Instruments. The entire self-study and review process uses the following set of instruments: a self-study and external review manual that includes the purpose and goals, presurvey guide of activities and responsibilities, a set of the criteria, elements, evidence, data, and instructions, the format of the final report, and a typical site visit schedule; a set of surveyor worksheets (Exhibit 2); a set of questionnaires that are sent to a random sample of clients (participants)

Exhibit 1. Criterion Model.

Criterion # _____ Criterion Statement _____

Definition _____

Standard _____ All Elements Must be Met _____

#	Element	Evidence	Data	Source	Instructions
1					
2					
3					
4					
5					

Table 1. Comparison of CESP Taxonomy and Self-Study and Review Taxonomy.

Self-Study Terminology	CESP Terminology	Definition	Example
Primary review area	Major functional category	The highest-order grouping consisting of categories of quality attributes	Overall educational planning
Criterion	Quality attribute	Grouping of related quality elements	Problem analysis
Element	Quality element (QE)	The lowest-order description of those things that define quality	Determine the underlying causes of the identified problems and concerns
Evidence	Not applicable	An entity that shows that a quality element exists	List of suspected causes
Data	Not applicable	The pieces of information that are necessary to provide the evidence	For each problem there should be a list of all suspected causes including educational and noneducational causes
Source	Not applicable	The location of the information and evidence	Project folder

and constituency (managers in the institutions that they serve and managers in the parent organization) and an anonymous questionnaire that is sent to each member of the staff of the CE provider unit; and a set of interview guides for each of the five primary review areas.

Process. There are several distinct steps in the RMEC self-study and external review process. The initial step consists of completing the self-study using the same guidelines and worksheets that the survey team uses. The CE provider unit makes and documents self-judgments on each criterion. The self-study report and required documentation are then sent to the survey team. The survey team concurrently distributes questionnaires to the groups previously identified (clients, constiuency, parent organization, and staff) and analyzes the returns. The survey team makes a site visit, does an in-depth survey in each primary review area, and completes the surveyor worksheets; the chairman of the survey team makes a report to the RMEC council using all the data. The core of the report is a judgment as to whether each criterion was met, partially met, or not met. *Recommendations* are made about the major deficiencies that require correction, and *suggestions* are made for improvements to the operation of the RMEC. *Commendations* focus on the innovative and outstanding aspects of a RMEC. The report is then sent to the RMEC and the council chairman. The RMEC may dispute any of the findings and recommendations at the next meeting of the council. The council makes final recommendations and suggestions and assures the implementation of all recommendations.

Primary Review Areas

One of the most important aspects of this system is the actual review process. In order to accomplish this review with some validity, the twenty-six criteria have been divided into five primary review areas, as follows:

- *Strategic management*
  1. Leadership
  2. Mission and strategic plan

Exhibit 2. Surveyor Worksheet.

Criterion # _____ Statement _____
_____
_____

Definition: _____
_____
_____

Element #	Element	Evidence	Surveyor Comments	Rating	
				Met	Outstanding
1					
2					
3					
4					
5					
6					

Criterion Rating: _____ Outstanding; _____ Met; _____ Partially Met; _____ Not Met.

Narrative Summary:

3. Systematic planning process
4. Organization
5. Policies and procedures
6. Management information system
7. Adequate resources
8. External relations
9. Constituency support
- *Administration of the CE provider unit*
  10. Marketing
  11. Quality assessment and assurance (QAAP)
  12. Information management system
  13. Personnel management
  14. Resource management
  15. Accountability
- *Overall program planning*
  16. Identification of problems and concerns
  17. Problem analysis
  18. Priority listing of proposed educational projects
- *Individual project development and implementation*
  19. Rationale for educational approaches
  20. Appropriate selection of faculty and content
  21. Appropriate selection of educational strategies
  22. Logistical implementation
  23. Application of learning to practice
  24. Planning, conducting, using, and disseminating evaluations
  25. Provision of educational services (consultation) (not self-directed learning)
- *Support to self-directed learner*
  26. Encouraging and assisting individuals in self-directed learning

Each of these primary review areas requires a specific set of knowledge, skills, attitudes, and experience in order to make valid judgments. The members of the survey team must possess this expertise, and each primary review area should be surveyed by someone with skills appropriate to that area. The remainder of this chapter gives an example in each area. These examples consist of a criterion statement, one of the elements that define that criterion, and a sample of the evidence required to assure that the element has been met.

Strategic Management. This primary review area consists of nine criteria that deal with the top management functions of the unit.

Example

Criterion 6. The continuing education provider unit (RMEC) should have a management information system to support planning and control functions.

Definition: Management of any organization depends primarily on planning and control, regardless of the size of the organization. The use of the word *management* implies the planning and control functions necessary to operate an organization. There are four distinct functions: strategic management, CEPU/RMEC administration, project coordination and control, and project development and implementation. Each of these functions requires the manager to make a certain set of decisions critical to the success of the organization. The manager needs to have the appropriate data and information to make informed decisions. The amount of data and information available is usually limitless. The purpose of this system is to have the right information at the right time to facilitate correct decision making.

Element a: The CEPU/RMEC should have a list of factors critical to the success of each function.

Evidence/Data/Examples	*Source*
(1) List of critical success factors for each function.	Documentation
(2) Lists should be limited (usually no more than 7 ± 2 factors).	Documentation
(3) Lists must be individualized to specific unit.	Documentation
(4) Factors must include those things that are critical whether or not they are controllable by that function.	Documentation

(5)   Factors must include those things that are   Documentation
       critical whether or not they are internal or
       external to the unit.

       Instructions: A set of generic critical
       success factors are attached for example (see
       Appendix to Chapter Thirteen). Manage-
       ment must have identified the critical areas
       in which they need to make decisions. The
       method defined by Evidence items 1–5 is the
       recommended way; however, if CEPU/
       RMEC uses another method, this should
       be considered.

       Administration of the CE Provider Unit. This primary review
area consists of six criteria that relate to the day-to-day operational
management of the CE provider unit.

Example

Criterion 11. The continuing education provider unit (RMEC)
should have an effective internal quality assessment and assurance
program.

       Definition: There must be an explicit quality assessment and
assurance plan that includes a defined set of criteria and standards
that at a minimum reflect the criteria elements in these self-study
criteria. This plan may also include standards for staff skills and
provision for impact evaluation. There must be evidence that the
plan has been implemented and that monitoring systems exist
within each appropriate function of management to *assure* compliance with the plan.

       Element a: There should be an explicit set of criteria and
standards that reflect the expectations of management with respect
to quality.

              Evidence/Data/Examples   *Source*

(1)   There should be a quality assessment   Documentation
       and assurance policy and appropriate
       procedures to reflect this element.

(2)   There must be an explicit set of criteria   Documentation
      and standards that reflect at a minimum
      the criteria elements in these self-study
      criteria.

(3)   The criteria and standards must be effective   Documentation
      within the resources of the CEPU/RMEC.   and Interview
      (Survey team must be sure that the
      standards used are appropriate for that
      particular CEPU/RMEC and do not use
      up a disproportionate amount of
      resources.)

Instructions: All three pieces of evidence
must be present.

Overall Program Planning. This primary review area deals
with the overall educational planning function. Problems must be
categorized as either educational or noneducational, and then it can
be determined if they can be solved by educational means. Specifically, this includes: the identification of a listing of the relevant
problems and concerns; the analysis of the causes of the problems,
separated into educational and noneducational needs; and the
development of a priority listing of the proposed educational projects required to address these needs.

Example

Criterion 16. The continuing education provider unit (RMEC)
should have a list of the relevant problems or concerns of the health
providers it serves.

Definition: In order for a CEPU/RMEC to provide quality
educational activities that are responsive to the practice-related
needs of the health professionals it serves, it is essential to identify
the problems or concerns of the potential audience. Various sources
of this information are available including data from the practice
setting, from new developments and technology, and from demographic studies of the target audience. It is highly desirable to cor-

roborate identified problems or concerns from multiple sources and to involve potential learners in this process.

Element a: Sources for identifying health professionals' problems or concerns should provide valid indicators of potential educational needs.

Evidence/Data/Examples	*Source*
(1) Data from the practice setting such as patient or drug profiles, audit information, tissue review committee minutes, administrative audit results, utilization review data, patient charts, and lab studies.	Documentation
(2) Information from technological developments in patient care, new drugs, or different approaches to diagnosis or treatment of specific diseases.	Documentation
(3) Epidemiological data of patients being served by target health professionals, new trends in using physician extenders, or specific health problems in a given geographic area.	Documentation
(4) Parent organization (agency) priorities.	Documentation
(5) Survey of clients and constituency.	Documentation
(6) Previous project evaluations.	Documentation
(7) Data from external reviews.	Documentation

Instructions: Each CEPU/RMEC should demonstrate a list that is current (less than one year old) for its overall program. If the CEPU/RMEC is divided into several "programs" (generic areas), the CEPU/RMEC should be able to demonstrate that it used at least the seven types of data listed to arrive at its list(s). This should be a list of problems and concerns rather than a list of "educational needs" and *could* have practice-related indicators for each.

Individual Project Development and Implementation. This primary review area concerns the systematic program development process for each individual educational project (activity, product, and service).

Example

Criterion 20. The continuing education provider unit should be able to demonstrate that faculty and content experts were selected who could most effectively meet the objectives of the planned educational project.

Definition: Faculty and subject matter experts should be selected for their expertise in the content as well as their experience in teaching health professionals. These experts should be informed of the learning objectives, as well as the nature of the learners and their entry-level knowledge, skills, and attitudes. In addition, the currency and accuracy of the content and its relevance to the learning objectives should be demonstrated.

Element a: Faculty were selected with appropriate content and continuing education teaching expertise for each project.

Evidence/Data/Examples	*Source*
(1) Use content experts to assist planning committee in selecting faculty with appropriate content expertise.	Documentation
(2) Check references and previous evaluation data on faculty to determine quality of their teaching experience with health professionals.	Documentation

Instructions: Both pieces of evidence must be demonstrated.

Assistance to Self-Directed Learners. This primary review area relates to providing educational support and encouragement to self-directed learners. There is only one criterion in this area.

Example

Criterion 26. The continuing education provider unit (RMEC) should encourage and assist the individual in self-directed learning.

Definition: The essence of the whole approach to continuing education suggested by adult learning principles is embodied in this content. This implies that the knowledgeable educator should always be trying to help health professionals assume this responsibility for their learning. In order to do this, the CEPU/RMEC staff should stand ready to aid learners in all phases of the instructional cycle, to improve the learners' educational process skills, and, to this end, both serve as consultants in specific areas and also design and implement specific educational projects that will improve the learners' abilities to assume this responsibility.

Element a: The CEPU/RMEC should encourage and aid the health care professional in accomplishing his/her own practice-related needs assessment.

Evidence/Data/Examples	*Source*
(1) The CEPU/RMEC should encourage the development and acceptance of health care standards as a basis for identifying professional problems and concerns.	
(2) The CEPU/RMEC should encourage health care professionals to compare their own behavior/performance against these standards.	
(3) The CEPU/RMEC should help health care professionals in self-assessment activities including practice profiles, self-assessment examinations, and performance analyses.	

Instructions: There must be evidence that this takes place. The amount should be negotiated with management.

Generalized Use. The usefulness, validity, and reliability of this method to a specific CE provider unit depends on several factors. The first of these is that the CE provider unit leadership has a clear understanding of the purpose for which this method is to be initiated. In addition to the purposes described in the rationale section of this chapter, this method can be used by the parent organization or the CE provider unit leadership in the development of a new, larger, or more sophisticated unit. In conjunction with the major purpose or initial impetus for instituting this self-study and external review system, it provides a method to improve the management and output of the CEPU.

The second major factor concerns feasibility. The system described is both comprehensive and extensive, and it may not be feasible for a smaller CE provider unit with limited resources to implement the entire system to the level of detail described in this chapter. However, to maintain the validity of the approach, there are several suggested ground rules for limiting the amount of resources utilized. First, it is necessary to have a complete understanding of the entire set of criteria, elements, and evidence in order to make informed decisions. Second, no primary review areas should be deleted unless the mission of the CE provider unit clearly excludes them. Third, *all* criteria within each included primary review area *must* be monitored and controlled. It is only at the element and evidence level that compromise should be made. At this level it may be feasible to substitute subjective evidence, such as the opinion of experienced observers, for much of the objective evidence and formal documentation described in this chapter, without sacrificing the validity of the method.

Summary

This chapter has presented a self-study and external review process developed by the RMECs and based on the quality elements presented in Chapter One. Emphasis in the chapter was placed on the extensive criteria development process that used multiple sources and continuous validation. The survey process was described that consists of a self-study; documentation review; client, constituency, and parent body questionnaires; and on-site structured interviews. The criterion model was described and examples were given for each of the five primary review areas. Finally, an approach was suggested for the generalized use of this self-study and external review process.

Appendix: Quality Review Criteria Statements

Criterion 1. The continuing education provider unit (RMEC) should have leaders with the necessary skills and authority to accomplish the mission.

Criterion 2. The continuing education provider unit (RMEC) should have a mission statement and strategic plan.

Criterion 3. The continuing education provider unit (RMEC) should have a systematically developed plan that enables the accomplishment of the mission and strategic plan.

Criterion 4. The continuing education provider unit (RMEC) should be organized to accomplish its goals and objectives efficiently.

Criterion 5. The continuing education provider unit (RMEC) should have policies and procedures that facilitate the accomplishment of the plan.

Criterion 6. The continuing education provider unit (RMEC) should have a management information system to support planning and control functions.

Criterion 7. The continuing education provider unit (RMEC) should have the appropriate resources to ensure implementation of the center's plans.

Criterion 8. The continuing education provider unit (RMEC) should maintain positive relationships with relevant external groups.

Criterion 9. The continuing education provider unit (RMEC) should have support from the facilities in its region (constituency).

Criterion 10. The continuing education provider unit (RMEC) should have a comprehensive marketing program.

Criterion 11. The continuing education provider unit (RMEC) should have an effective internal quality assessment and assurance program.

Criterion 12. The continuing education provider unit (RMEC) should have a functioning information system that provides all functions of management information in a timely, concise, and systematic manner.

Criterion 13. The continuing education provider unit (RMEC) should manage its personnel to maximize their effectiveness in accomplishing its mission.

Criterion 14. The continuing education provider unit (RMEC) should manage its resources to maximize its effectiveness and efficiency.

Criterion 15. The continuing education provider unit (RMEC) should meet its accountability requirements.

Criterion 16. The continuing education provider unit (RMEC) should have a list of the relevant problems or concerns of the health providers it serves.

Criterion 17. The continuing education provider unit (RMEC) should analyze all identified problems and concerns as a basis of developing a list of relevant educational needs.

Criterion 18. The continuing education provider unit (RMEC) should develop a valid listing of proposed educational projects from the analyzed educational needs, which reflect relative priorities.

Criterion 19. The continuing education provider unit (RMEC) should be able to provide a satisfactory rationale for the educational approaches selected for proposed projects.

Criterion 20. The continuing education provider unit (RMEC) should be able to demonstrate that faculty and content experts were selected who could most effectively meet the objectives of the planned educational project.

Criterion 21. The continuing education provider unit (RMEC) should use appropriate educational strategies to facilitate learning within all projects.

Criterion 22. The continuing education provider unit (RMEC) should have an effective logistical support system that facilitates the accomplishment of educational projects.

Criterion 23. The continuing education provider unit (RMEC) should assist learners in the application of learning to the practice setting.

Criterion 24. The continuing education provider unit (RMEC) should plan and conduct evaluations, and use and disseminate evaluation findings.

Criterion 25. The continuing education provider unit (RMEC) should provide appropriate educational services to organizations and individuals.

Criterion 26. The continuing education provider unit (RMEC) should encourage and assist the individual in self-directed learning.

References

Corrigan, R. E., and Kaufman, R. A. *Why System Engineering.* Belmont, Calif.: Fearon, 1966.

Fox, L., and others. "MATS—Medical Audit Team Seminars." In C. M. Jacobs and N. D. Jacobs (Eds.), *The Pep Primer: The Joint Commission on Accreditation of Hospitals' Performance Evaluation Procedure for Auditing and Improving Patient Care.* Chicago: Quality Review Center, Joint Commission on Accreditation of Hospitals, 1974.

Goldfinger, S. E. "Continuing Medical Education: The Case for Contamination." *New England Journal of Medicine,* 1982, *306* (9), 540–541.

Jacobs, C. M., Christoffel, T. H., and Dixon, N. *Measuring the Quality of Patient Care: The Rationale for Outcome Audit.* Cambridge, Mass.: Ballinger, 1976.

Mager, R. F., and Pipe, P. *Analyzing Performance Problems or You Really Oughta Wanna.* Belmont, Calif.: Fearon Pitman, 1970.

Miller, L. A. "The Current Investment in Continuing Medical Education." In R. H. Egdahl and P. M. Gertman (Eds.), *Quality Health Care: The Role of Continuing Medical Education.* Germantown, Md.: Aspen Systems, 1977.

Williamson, J. W. *Improving Medical Practice and Health Care: A Bibliographic Guide to Information Management in Quality Assurance and Continuing Education.* Cambridge, Mass.: Ballinger, 1977.

15

Quality Assurance in the Planning and Developing of Educational Activities

Patrick L. Walsh

Chapter Fourteen presented a comprehensive quality assurance system that looked at both the educational and administrative procedures of an organization. One element of these procedures is the systematic program development process. Chapter Fifteen describes three specific components of a system for assuring the quality of educational development within any size or type of continuing education (CE) provider unit. The three components include a program development competency list, an educational process quality assurance and assessment program, and a program evaluation component. A rationale for using such a system within a CE provider unit and sample forms are provided for the reader.—Editors

This chapter will suggest a process by which managers of CE provider units can assure themselves of the quality of the educational development process discussed in Chapter Seven. It takes a closer look at one of the critical parts of an overall external review system—the educational development process. Because the development of educational projects is the major output of a CE provider unit, it is important to assure that this process is conducted appropriately.

This chapter describes the Educational Quality Assessment and Assurance Program (EQAAP) that was established within the Veterans Administration (VA) InterWest Regional Medical Education Center (IRMEC) at the Salt Lake City VA Medical Center. The IRMEC staff consists of twenty full- and part-time professional educators, administrative, and logistics staff. Although this quality assurance system was designed for a large organization, the principles are equally applicable for any size CE provider unit. CE organizations are encouraged to adapt any part of this system for their own use.

As pointed out in Chapter Fourteen, systems engineering theory and performance analysis provide the foundation for a quality assurance system in health care (Egdahl and Gertman, 1976) and also serve as the basis for the development of a system of educational quality assurance. Irrespective of the target of quality assurance— health care or education—the approach focuses on an analysis of input, process, and output and outcome (Donabedian, 1969). The following sections will offer a rationale for such an educational quality assurance system and describe each of the three components of the system developed by the IRMEC.

Rationale

Continuing education in the health professions should include attempts to assess and assure the input, process, and output and outcome. While CE provider units cannot guarantee that changes in health care provider competence (knowledge, skills, attitudes) will translate to changes in performance or improved patient health status, they can make certain that the individuals responsible for CE are qualified (input), the methods used to develop educational projects are valid (process), and the activities (output) are evaluated to determine the extent to which participants achieved specified objectives and the original needs were met (outcome).

There has been a significant lack of data to document the effectiveness of CE (Lloyd and Abrahamson, 1979). Many explanations may be proposed for this dearth of evidence: the scarcity of scientific evaluation procedures in CE (Abrahamson, 1968), the lack of any attempt to assess learning (Greenburg, Bruegel, and Peskin, 1977), the failure to find significant differences when attempts at evaluation are made (Lloyd and Abrahamson, 1979), the ineffective design of activities (Walsh, 1981), and organizers' lack of knowledge or skills to develop appropriate programs.

One explanation for the apparent lack of significant positive results in CE is that the process for planning activities was haphazard and ineffective. The thesis is that the educational development process is a critical variable in CE effectiveness. Pennington and Green (1976) performed a comparative analysis of educational development processes used in six professions (including medicine and social work) and found that while the steps described a familiar educational model, they were not applied rigorously by programmers. Pennington and Green were particularly surprised by the manner in which their respondents implemented the model they had described as guiding their actions. Some of the discrepancies included little systematic needs assessment, lack of systematic development of objectives, continued reliance on didactic educational techniques, and minimal evaluation effort.

A more recent study by Richardson (1981) reported a literature search of ninety workshops. Richardson discovered that none of the workshop planners utilized all the planning steps described by Pennington and Green, and only a few performed even one or two of the suggested planning steps. For example, only one of the ninety planners reported administering a needs assessment.

If lack of rigor in programming is accepted as a reason for the failure of CE to achieve documentable changes in health care provider performance, it can be argued that those activities that achieve such changes could provide guidance concerning how programs should be developed. Stein (1981) summarized eight studies that reported changes in physician behavior and, in one, improved patient outcomes as a result of CE. In his analysis of the eight studies, Stein deduced that the reason for the effects was that each CE program had been organized on sound educational principles. More specifically, all eight studies reviewed had used the following process components that Stein maintained were essential for any effective learning program: learning needs were identified, audience was specified, clear goals and objectives were stated, relevant learning methods were used, emphasis was given to learner participation, practice-related, hands-on experiences were included, and there was a systematic effort to evaluate.

If CE activities are not developed using sound educational principles, one explanation is that the program developers lack the knowledge or skills to develop activities appropriately. That is, if program developers are unaware of the critical steps in educational development or lack the competencies to perform the steps adequately, the activities would be less likely to reflect the quality attributes desired. Therefore, a process designed to assess and assure the quality of CE interventions should also include a method to assess and assure that program leaders possess skills to develop programs in the appropriate manner.

The belief that the application of a systematic educational development process by qualified staff will result in desired outcomes should not be an act of faith. There should be a mechanism to assess the degree to which use of this process leads to desired results. Therefore, an evaluation mechanism must be built into the functioning of the CE provider unit. This mechanism not only should allow determination of the effects of the systematic planning process but also should provide information to modify and improve the process.

Components of Educational Quality Assessment and Assurance Program

The IRMEC program has three components. *Input* is assessed by use of the Program Developer Competency List; *process* is analyzed by the Educational Process Quality Assessment and Assurance Program; and *output and outcome* are determined within the Program Evaluation Component. Each of these will be described in more detail.

Input—Program Developer Competency List (PDCL). Appraisal of input typically involves the evaluation of the settings and equipment used to develop educational projects. While appraisal of input might include the physical facilities, equipment, organization, and qualifications of staff, the main focus of the Program Developer Competency List is on the qualifications of professional and administrative staff. The first step focuses on defining those competencies required to carry out the educational development process. Authors have described approaches to determining the required competencies (Gale and Pol, 1977), as well as defined specific competencies required to complete a variety of educational processes (Gagné, 1975; Worthen, 1975). The approaches advocated in this chapter to identify the presence of essential competencies may be utilized by other CE provider unit staff to generate their own competency list.

The following listing illustrates those skills a program developer is expected to possess, not only in educational process areas but also in project management.

- Assessment skills
    1. Determine methods to collect data to identify generic areas for programming.
    2. Given a generic area, determine how to identify problem areas.
    3. Develop valid and reliable methods to assess the current status of the field in a problem area.
    4. Develop method to reality test method and include field in development.
    5. Given an assessment method to be applied in the field, determine which analysis strategy is most appropriate to summarize the data.
- Analysis skills
    1. Summarize data collected during needs assessment in terms of practice problems.
    2. Identify standards of desirable performance in problem area.
    3. Compare current performance with desirable performance to identify gaps.
    4. Investigate possible causes of performance gaps: skill/ knowledge, attitude/motivation, environment/opportunity.

    5.   Distinguish between educational and noneducational causes.

    6.   Determine priorities.

    7.   Write instructional objectives.

- Design skills

    1.   Estimate the achievability of a given set of potential activity objectives.

    2.   Given instructional objectives, construct activities that require learners to apply content to their work settings.

    3.   Having determined that sufficient time is available to do so, design the leanest possible set of activities to achieve a given set of objectives.

    4.   Given specific instructional objectives, discriminate between appropriate and inappropriate content for the activities.

    5.   Given a terminal objective and intermediate objectives, sequence the intermediate objectives in an effective manner.

    6.   Given a set of component behaviors, determine whether a logical hierarchy is implied in sequencing these for instruction.

    7.   Given a set of objectives with no predetermined sequence, select an appropriate first-draft sequence when time does not permit further exploration with students.

    8.   Identify specific target group and presenter group.

    9.   Given a lesson/activity plan, specify the minimum prerequisite/entry behaviors required of learners.

  10.   Identify available resources and individuals with previous experience with the problem.

  11.   Include representatives of the target and presenter populations early in planning.

  12.   Specify the relationship of content and format to program objectives.

  13.   Involve program personnel in mutual orientation program (faculty premeeting) at which responsibilities and functions are assigned within the context of program objectives, philosophy, etc.

  14.   Contract personnel, facilities, budget, equipment, and supplies well in advance of planned implementation date.

15.   Develop outreach plans to recruit specific target groups.
- Media selection skills
    1.   Given the demands imposed by the task analysis in inter-action with the available funds, the on-going system, and motivational requirements, select an appropriate medium for each objective.
    2.   Select instructional media that optimize the benefit of all resources—cost of media, cost of instructional staff, cost of student time committed to the instructional effort, longevity (recurrent nature) of instructional task.
    3.   Given specific objective, list the available instructional media capable of presenting the type of stimulus (motion, color, sound, visual) to which the student must attend, as specified by the indicator behavior and conditions of the specific objective and select the most appropriate medium.
    4.   Preview audiovisual aids.
- Evaluation skills
    1.   Specify purpose of evaluation.
    2.   Identify audiences for evaluation.
    3.   State issues for evaluation.
    4.   Define the object of the evaluation.
    5.   Select an appropriate inquiry strategy to address the evalua-tion issues.
    6.   Specify data or evidence necessary to answer the evaluation issues.
    7.   Select appropriate evaluation designs to collect data to re-spond to evaluation issues.
    8.   Apply the evaluation design while recognizing/controlling threats to validity.
    9.   Identify the goals of the program to be evaluated.
    10. Assess the value and feasibility of program goals.
    11. Identify standards/norms for judging the worth of the pro-gram to be evaluated.
    12. Translate broad objectives into specific, measurable ob-jectives.
    13. Identify classes of variables for measurement.
    14. Select or develop techniques of measurement.
    15. Assess the validity and reliability of measurement tech-niques.

16. Use appropriate methods (tests, interviews) to collect data.
17. Monitor the program to detect deviations from design or specified procedures.
18. Choose and employ appropriate techniques of statistical analysis (measure of control, tendency I-test, chi square).
19. Use electronic computers and computer-related equipment (statistical package on minicomputer, design instruments that can be opscanned).
20. Interpret and draw appropriate conclusions from data analysis.
21. Report evaluation findings and implications.
22. Make recommendations as a result of the evaluation.
23. Provide immediate feedback on program performance for use in decisions about program modifications.
24. Obtain and manage resources (material and human) necessary to conduct the evaluation.

- Project management skills
  1. Identify all steps needed to solve a problem in the field.
  2. Develop a plan to eliminate or reduce the needs in the field. Write action plan for the assessment, analysis, design, media selection and evaluation phase of the project. Set timelines for each step in the action plan. Obtain support for the project from all persons involved.
  3. Submit plan to EDQAAP.
  4. Monitor the progress in completing the action plan. Adjust the timelines as needed. Administer contingencies to achieve deadlines.
- Educational process quality assessment and assurance skills
  1. Given data on a peer's progress on phases listed up to this point, identify discrepancies between what was done (is planned to be done) and what should have been done (should be done).
  2. Construct feedback for the peer which identifies the discrepancies and suggests ways in which the discrepancies can be reduced.
  3. Create a supportive atmosphere that does not threaten the peer.
- Communication skills
  1. Utilize active listening techniques.

2. Demonstrate observation skills.
3. Summarize clearly and logically.
4. Problem solve systematically.
5. Utilize group process skills.
6. Use constructive confrontation techniques.
7. Resolve conflicts fairly.
8. Maintain active correspondence with field.
9. Provide quick response to requests.
10. Demonstrate above skills in person, on the telephone, and in writing, where appropriate.

The PDCL has three primary uses: screening candidates for program developer positions during recruitment, appraising program developer performance, and identifying needs for staff development. Prospective program developers can be shown the PDCL to make them aware of the types of activities they are expected to carry out if employed. Candidates might also be appraised on each dimension based on work completed prior to application for the position. The PDCL can be sent to former employers who would be asked to rate the candidate's capabilities related to each competency area. Candidates may also be asked to rate their competency related to each area. During an interview, a performance test might be constructed that requires candidates to demonstrate an example of the desired competencies.

Similarly, the PDCL may be used to appraise present program developer performance. Results of episodes of the Educational Process Quality Assurance and Assessment Program will give administrators a good indication of a program developer's competencies. The PDCL can also serve as self-assessment instruments for program developers. Caution must be taken to ensure a nonthreatening atmosphere when appraising performance so that valid ratings will be obtained from the program developer. If a nonpunitive atmosphere is created, the performance appraisal may be viewed as an opportunity to identify growth areas to improve existing skills. The results of the performance appraisal may be used as a means of assessment to identify staff development skills. The PDCL may require skills or competencies never before demanded of the program developers, and therefore might be used as a needs assessment when the program is originally initiated.

Process—Educational Process Quality Assessment and Assurance Program (EPQAAP). This step requires identifying those aspects of educational development that will be featured as preset quality factors for prospective review of programs. Because proposed activities of the CE provider unit are reviewed with respect to the application of those factors, care should be taken so that the selected factors represent quality program development.

The intent of a prospective, concurrent quality assessment (QA) system is to assure quality programming. The purpose is to influence or regulate the conduct of program development. The criterion to be compared is the degree to which the steps of the educational development process used conform with the standards and expectations of CE experts. A variety of methods may be employed to identify the standards to be applied. One could derive standards and expectations from recognized leaders in the field, infer standards from patterns of program development observed in practice, or establish standards on the basis of research in continuing education.

An approach to educational development may be found in Chapter Seven. However, the primary source of quality factors is the publication by Suter and others (1981). In both instances, the elements of quality were derived by using all three methods just identified for establishing standards.

In the quality elements defined in Chapter One, under the category "Providing CE Activities and Products," there are a number of headings:

- Detecting Problems or Concerns
- Analyzing Problems or Concerns
- Identifying Educational Priorities
- Setting Educational Objectives
- Selecting Educational Approaches
- Selecting Faculty and Content
- Determining Instructional Strategies
- Implementing Educational Projects
- Designing Evaluation
- Planning and Conducting Evaluation
- Using Evaluation Results

Each of these factors (quality attributes) is elaborated in greater detail by the quality elements listed under it. It is the responsibility of the CE provider unit staff to identify those factors and quality elements on which they intend to focus when developing or improving their programs.

The factors or elements identified as standards by a CE provider unit may be stated as "ideal," "good," or "acceptable" practice. It may, however, be desirable to identify minimal standards to be met by all projects. These standards would have to be met in order for the project to be approved for implementation. A CE provider unit may desire to establish one set of standards for its first attempt at prospective assessment, and as program managers become more skilled at meeting those standards, they could be revised to become more demanding. However, this decision and the selection of standards should be made with the staff involved.

The Continuing Education Systems Project (CESP) quality elements will guide the actions of program developers as they go about building educational programs. However, when using the EPQAAP, it is important to recognize that these factors will also be used to review proposed programs to determine their worth prior to implementation. Therefore, it is critical that only those selected factors that can be reviewed prospectively (in terms of documentation of processes completed or plans for their completion) be included in the review process. For example, in "Planning and Conducting Evaluation," one of the guidelines is to "provide succinct, useful, and timely feedback from evaluation data to those who have a need for evaluation information." Clearly, the intent to do this may be documented; however, a plan should be included in the Program Evaluation Component. An example of a form that may be used to document planning is included in Exhibit 1.

Who should be included in the review process? Several options exist. A single reviewer could be designated by the director of the CE provider unit or there could be multiple reviewers, working as a committee or each performing the review independently. To the extent that potential reviewers could learn from committee discussions of other programmers' plans and not perceive it as punitive, the review should be done in committee, with all members having equal input. To the extent that the CE provider unit director

Exhibit 1. Educational Process Quality Assessment and
Assurance Program (EPQAAP).

Documentation Form

A. Program developer: _____

B. Activity title: _____

C. Proposed dates: _____ D. Location (city, facility): _____

E. Need/problem/concern: describe on attachment #1.

F. Indicators of need/problem/concern: describe on attachment #2.

G. Causes of need/problem/concern with educational bases: describe
    on attachment #3.

H. Priority of need: describe method of determination and results on
    attachment #4.

I. Activity planned to eliminate educational causes: justify selection of
    educational approach chosen and describe agenda with time/objec-
    tives/content/activity/faculty on attachment #5.

J. Faculty: identify faculty on attachment #6 with curriculum vitae for
    each.

K. Planning committee: identify on attachment #7.

L. Target audience: identify target audience and selection strategy on
    attachment #8.

M. Evaluation plan: describe evaluation issues/audiences/evaluation
    design/methods/instruments/analysis strategies on attachment #9.

N. Budget: identify resources (people, materials, time, money) needed
    to implement activity on attachment #10.

O. Administrative arrangements: describe logistical and administrative
    plans for activity on attachment #11.

EPQAAP committee participants: _____

_____

Decision of EPQAAP committee: 1. ( ) Proceed with activity as designed.

2. ( ) Do not proceed with activity.

3. ( ) Proceed with modifications described on attachment #12.

Date of EPQAAP meeting: _____

wishes the system to be accepted by all involved, all committee members should be viewed as equally important. Utilizing a committee provides for the necessary involvement of staff members and offers an ideal system for staff development. However, management should not abdicate its ultimate responsibility for assuring quality.

The following are examples of selected factors rated on an EPQAAP form.

- Detect problems or concerns
  a. use data from practice setting
  b. involve learners
  c. corroborate problems by using data from more than one source
- Analyze problems or concerns
  a. identify potential causes of identified problems/concerns
  b. sort causes according to whether educational in nature
- Select educational activities and products for implementation
  a. determine resources available
  b. assure congruence between identified needs and mission of CE provider unit and learners' health care organization
  c. obtain consensus on the relative priority of each identified need
- Set educational objectives
  a. define target audience
  b. involve learner in defining learning outcomes from needs
  c. establish relevant, achievable, and measurable objectives for outcomes
- Select educational approach
  a. consider nature of learning objectives
  b. determine demand characteristics of content of program
  c. review available resources to meet demand characteristics
- Select faculty and content
  a. inform faculty of learning objectives, participants' entry level, and ensure faculty has appropriate content/teaching
  b. assure the currency/accuracy of content to be presented
- Determine instructional strategies
  a. provide learners with opportunities to practice relevant skills

   b.   provide sufficient examples of concepts to be learned
   c.   provide learners with feedback on performance
- Implement educational activities
   a.   administrative arrangements for educational activity (space, materials, equipment, meals) are made
- Determine scope and nature of evaluation
   a.   identify purpose and audiences for evaluation
   b.   specify measurement techniques to be used
   c.   describe data analysis procedures
   d.   focus on participant achievement of objectives
- Conduct evaluation
   a.   address whether learning objectives were met

Several methods can be used for measuring the comparison to each quality standard. Two alternatives are either rating the degree to which the plans meet standards on a five- or seven-point scale or making a yes/no decision concerning whether or not the plan meets the standards. There must be some mechanism for judging the degree to which standards are met; it is at the discretion of the CE provider unit director and staff to determine the most beneficial method.

At the conclusion of the committee meeting, the members tally their EPQAAP sheets and decide to proceed with the planned project or activity as is, to proceed with a modified program, or not to proceed with the project. If the first option is chosen, no further action need be taken. If the third option is chosen, a justification is in order. In the case of the second option, specific modifications should be recommended and an individual identified to review the revised project plan.

Output and Outcome—Program Evaluation Component (PEC). Assessment of output and outcome encompasses the evaluation of end results in terms of health care professional competence, health care professional performance (actual application of competencies in clinical situations), patient health status (Lloyd and Abrahamson, 1979), and learner satisfaction. Evaluation provides evidence of whether the education has been effective and efficient. Further, it is assumed that desirable results are brought about, at least to a significant degree, by sound educational development techniques (process) performed by competent program developers (structure or input).

Evaluation data may answer many questions. The first is whether the prospective assessment system assured the quality of the output. Specifically, was the project, as implemented, of high quality? Assessment of quality may be gathered from judgments of participants, faculty, and planners. A second dimension of that question is whether or not desired outcomes were observed as a function of participation. This aspect seeks to assess the extent to which participants achieved activity objectives and increased competence related to the educational objectives or learner outcomes, the degree to which learners were able to translate new competence into practice in performing their duties, and the extent to which changed performance contributed to desirable outcomes.

It is clear that the extent of investigating any of these dimensions may be dependent on the goals and objectives established for the educational project in question. If the needs assessment indicated a psychomotor deficiency, yet the resultant educational activity is designed merely to provide cognitive information, the likelihood of significant behavior change or change in patient health status is minimal. However, if the objective were to develop new psychomotor skills and the educational activity were designed to provide opportunities to practice those skills, then desirable changes would be expected. For this reason, it is important to establish goals and objectives for educational activities and design the activities to assure their accomplishment. If activities are not planned with such a goal in mind, demonstration of desired outcomes is rarely possible.

If evaluation of end results does not demonstrate desired outcomes, data would be available for tracing back through the entire quality assessment system to determine the reason(s) educational development is not effective, such as faulty needs assessment, faulty design, or inadequate analysis of educational and noneducational causes. As an example, at the end of an educational activity implemented to teach health care personnel the proper use of a ventilator for the treatment of patients in respiratory failure due to chronic obstructive pulmonary disease, the program participants demonstrated mastery of program objectives. However, desired results were not observed in patient health status. An analysis indicated that the reason may have been faulty assessment of the problem. The real problem may have been use of central nervous system depressants rather than use of a ventilator. This information would provide feedback that indicates the necessity to improve the documentation and analysis of need for the EPQAAP system.

Another example might be that an educational activity was developed to train x-ray technicians how to maintain equipment. At the end of the activity, a performance test was administered to determine whether participants could perform the desired behaviors. Unfortunately, they could not. In a review of the project design, it was discovered that most processes used during the activity were didactic transfer of information with little time devoted to actual work with the equipment. Again, data would be available to fine tune the EPQAAP with respect to matching the program objectives with appropriate educational processes.

A final example involves a course instituted to train nursing personnel how to wash their hands, after infection rates had increased on a particular ward in a medical center. The educational program instructed nurses how to wash their hands; a performance test at the end of the activity demonstrated that all participants could perform at the desired level. Subsequent monitoring of the infection rate failed to demonstrate any change. This result may indicate the need to increase program developer skill at discriminating between educational and noneducational problems. The nurses knew how to wash their hands; the problem was that the sinks were a hundred yards away from bed areas. Establishing a new sink area closer to the bed area produced the desired results.

Conclusion

An important consideration in the choice of a method for assessment is the timeliness with which the information becomes available as compared to the uses for which the information is needed. If the purpose is to influence or regulate the conduct of education, the information has to be reasonably current. Otherwise, the opportunity for using the information most effectively may be missed. In this regard, measures of process have an obvious advantage, whereas outcomes, by their very nature, require time to become evident.

Process lends itself to prospective, concurrent, and retrospective assessment for preventive, intervention, and remedial purposes, respectively. Retrospective assessment is ordinarily based on a review of past projects as documented in the educational evaluation reports. The object is to learn from past experience so that education in the future may be improved. Prospective or concurrent assessment is based not on the actual educational projects but on plans for future projects that may be approved or rejected. This form of assessment has a preventive function.

The evaluation component, therefore, will establish whether the desired output and outcomes are occasioned by participation in CE provider unit educational activities, indicate whether the prospective EPQAAP elements contribute to desired effects, and provide data to fine tune the EPQAAP and PDCL mechanisms. Together, this prospective quality assessment and assurance program should enable CE provider units to offer quality continuing education activities that contribute to desired results. The evaluation component provides a mechanism to evaluate whether such a system does, in fact, contribute to the desired results.

The InterWest Regional Medical Education Center is currently in its second stage of developing this quality assurance program, operating under the framework described in this chapter. The IRMEC EPQAAP was under development prior to and concurrently with the development of the quality elements around which this book is based (see Chapter One). Members of the IRMEC staff contributed to the development of the quality elements, which served as a resource for the EPQAAP formulation. The IRMEC quality assurance system has been in operation since 1979, and its outcomes have been documented elsewhere (Walsh, 1982a; 1982b).

References

Abrahamson, S. "Evaluation in Continuing Medical Education." *Journal of the American Medical Association,* 1968, *206,* 625–628.

Donabedian, A. *A Guide to Medical Care Administration.* Vol. 2, *Medical Care Appraisal—Quality and Utilization.* New York: American Public Health Association, 1969.

Egdahl, R. H., and Gertman, P. M. (Eds.). *Quality Assurance in Health Care.* Germantown, Md.: Aspen Systems, 1976.

Gagné, R. M. "Qualifications of Professionals in Educational R & D." *Educational Researcher,* 1975, *4* (2), 7-11.

Gale, L. E., and Pol, G. "Determining Required Competence: A Need Assessment Methodology and Computer Program." *Educational Technology,* 1977, *17* (7), 24-28.

Greenburg, A. G., Bruegel, R. B., and Peskin, G. W. "Surgical Continuing Medical Education: Format and Impact." *Surgery,* 1977, *81* (6), 708-715.

Lloyd, J. S., and Abrahamson, S. "Effectiveness of Continuing Medical Education: A Review of the Evidence." *Evaluation and the Health Professions,* 1979, 2, 251-280.

Pennington, F., and Green, J. "Comparative Analysis of Program Development Processes in Six Professions." *Adult Education,* 1976, *27* (1), 13-23.

Richardson, G. E. "A Sexual Health Workshop for Health Care Professionals." *Evaluation and the Health Professions,* 1981, *4,* 259-274.

Stein, L. S. "The Effectiveness of Continuing Medical Education: Eight Research Reports." *Journal of Medical Education,* 1981, *56,* 103-110.

Suter, E., Green, J. S., Lawrence, K., and Walthall, D. B. III. "Continuing Education of Health Professionals: A Proposal for a Definition of Quality." *Journal of Medical Education,* 1981, *56* (8), 687-707.

Walsh, P. L. "InterWest RMEC Educational Accountability System." *IRMEC Newsletter,* 1981, *3,* 1-3.

Walsh, P. L. "An Assessment of an Operational Accountability System for CE in the Health Professions." *Mobius,* 1982a, *2* (4), 28-38.

Walsh, P. L. "InterWest Regional Medical Education Center Fiscal Year '81 Progress Report." In *Report no. 4, Evaluation Report Series.* Kalamazoo, Mich.: Evaluation Center, Western Michigan University, 1982b.

Worthen, B. R. "Competencies for Educational Research and Evaluation." *Educational Researcher,* 1975, *4* (1), 13-16.

Improving
Continuing Education
in Diverse
Health Care Settings

Sarina J. Grosswald, Emanuel Suter
Gregg R. Seppala, David B. Walthall III

ᴪᴪᴪᴪᴪᴪᴪᴪᴪᴪᴪᴪᴪᴪᴪᴪᴪᴪᴪᴪᴪᴪᴪᴪ

This chapter serves as a complement to Chapter One by describing some of the steps that have been taken to put into practice the concepts of the Continuing Education Systems Project (CESP). The chapter explains how continuing education (CE) provider units can

Note: The authors are grateful to the people, who participated in the pilot test and whose data were used in preparing the section in this chapter called "Applying the Quality Elements": Richard S. Wilbur, M.D. (Accreditation Council for Continuing Medical Education); Richard Adelson, D.D.S., Roy L. Lindahl, D.D.S., Fran Watkins, Ed.D. (American Association of Dental Schools); Mark Cheren, Ph.D. (American Red Cross); Albert J. Finestone, M.D., Salvatore S. Lanzilotti, Ed.D. (Temple University); Henry T. Frierson, Ph.D., Deborah L. Jones, M.Ed., Frank T. Stritter, Ph.D. (University of North Carolina).

use the concepts and quality elements presented in Chapter One to improve the continuing education and management activities within their organization. Several broad uses of quality elements are described, and a five-step approach is presented for applying the relevant quality elements to any CE provider unit. The chapter also describes those organizations that have been involved with the Continuing Education Systems Project in efforts to use the quality elements. The final part of the chapter provides a description of the additional products and materials that have been developed by the CESP.—Editors

This book examines the place of continuing education in the world of health care, the factors that bear upon it, and the roles of the health professional and the CE provider unit. Continuing education in the health professions is a complex collection of components and influences. The model presented in Chapter One represents a system of CE that brings together these components and influences. In the model, continuing education has its genesis in the health care setting, and contributes to improvements in that setting.

The concepts of the model are translated into practical statements of action through the quality elements (QEs) (see Chapter One Appendix). The development of both the model and the quality elements was guided by the theoretical and experiential foundations of learning, particularly adult learning, and the principles of management. Chapters Two, Three, and Twelve describe these foundations, and Chapters Seven through Eleven and Chapters Thirteen through Fifteen describe their application in the CE provider unit. This chapter presents an overview of the broad uses of the quality elements, a process for individualizing and applying the QEs in any setting, the materials available to assist CE providers, and a description of how specific organizations have been using all or selected QEs to enhance the quality of their CE project development and management processes.

Use of the Quality Elements

The comprehensiveness of the quality elements and the reference to a conceptual model may provide a unique means of defining quality. The elements and model are intended to serve purposes at both the conceptual and operational levels. At the conceptual level, they provide a stimulus for consideration and exploration of new approaches to CE. At the operational level, the CE provider unit or those responsible for assuring the quality of CE are able to apply the quality elements to their day-to-day functions to enhance the results.

The quality elements are written as universally applicable principles for quality continuing education. To become meaningful, they must reflect the settings in which they are used. This requires both the acceptance of the quality elements and their underlying principles as valid components of quality and an interpretation and adaptation of the specific meanings of the quality elements for a particular setting. Adaptation takes the form of identifying those aspects of the CE process that might have a particularly significant impact on the outcome of the CE effort in the setting and developing specific examples of actions for the QEs that address those aspects. These examples are referred to as performance indicators. The use of the quality elements can fall into two broad categories—monitoring the quality and operation of a unit and improvement or development of a CE provider unit.

Mechanism for Monitoring a CE Provider Unit. The Continuing Education Systems Project arose from a need for a means to monitor CE offered under institutional sponsorship. Monitoring may be accomplished either through internal self-assessment or external review. Each CE provider unit is responsible for the quality of its educational offerings and for the cost-effectiveness of those offerings. A means of assuring this is by careful monitoring of the process of providing CE and of managing the CE provider unit. Monitoring can be accomplished by a comparison of present practice to agreed-upon standards established by the management of the unit. The quality elements provide a tool for such a self-assessment. The QEs taken as a whole represent a blueprint for quality CE. Through a periodic assessment, strengths and weaknesses can be diagnosed and areas for improvement can be identified. In this way, the QEs serve as the quality criteria. An adaptation of this process, involving ongoing monitoring based on the categories developed by the quality elements, is described in Chapter Fifteen.

External assessment is a means of quality control and assuring accountability to others for all aspects of the CE provider unit. This process usually involves a self-assessment and an outside evaluation of the CE effort, based on standards developed outside the CE provider unit. The quality elements provide a unified, coherent basis for establishing quality criteria for both the educational aspects and the management approaches. Recommendations for improvement, which often accompany this process in some vague form, can truly provide direction for change by being based on specific criteria of quality. A detailed description of such a system is provided in Chapter Fourteen.

Improvement or Development of a CE Provider Unit. The primary result of the CESP was the development of materials that can be used for assisting CE provider units in the provision of their CE offerings. The quality elements allow the CE provider to address all aspects of planning, implementation, and evaluation of educational projects, as well as the management responsibilities associated with these tasks. The QEs provide direction for focusing efforts and developing prescriptions for improvement tailored to the CE provider unit's specific needs. Areas of focus initially may be identified through an internal or external quality assessment process, or a CE provider unit may recognize special areas needing improvement, such as needs assessment. The quality elements provide the guidance for improvement.

By offering guidelines for the functioning of a CE provider unit, the QEs also provide a framework for establishing a new CE organization. The QEs serve as the basis for making decisions about the mission, organization, and functioning of the CE provider unit. This decision process is described in more detail later in this chapter.

These categories demonstrate the broad uses of the quality elements. There are, no doubt, other more specific uses; however, in almost all cases they will intersect with one of the purposes described.

Analysis of the Quality Elements

The quality elements address all aspects of the delivery of CE. As a means of establishing priorities among the QEs, an analysis was undertaken with the assistance of the Sage Institute. The purpose was to identify the most crucial aspects, by asking the question "What would make the CE mission fail?" The analysis, referred to as Sage Analysis (Stephens, 1977), was carried out in three phases.

In the *first phase* a group of experienced CE managers developed a hierarchical listing of factors presumed to cause failure of a CE provider unit's mission. These factors, called failure events, were grouped according to cause and effect. A hierarchical structure, or "fault tree," was then developed. The possible failure events in the fault tree were made to correspond to the structure of the quality elements: the major possible failure events corresponded to the five categories of QEs, the highest-order possible failure events were at the level of the quality attributes, and the lower-order failure events were at the level of the quality elements themselves. Table 1 shows these relationships.

In the *second phase* the same group of experts made the following quantitative judgments on each factor identified in the first phase: rank of the factor in the order to which it contributes to the failure event; percentage contributed by each factor to the failure of the event; level of confidence of the respondent in this percentage figure; frequency of the failure event; and expected difficulty changing, controlling, or eliminating the failure event.

The *third phase* consisted of a computer-based mathematical analysis of the quantitative input resulting in the identification of critical pathways relative to each major failure event and the assignment of a so-called strategic event value (SEV) for each cause of the failure event. This SEV was then normalized so that the most serious event had a value of 1.000. Any value that was greater than 0.8 was considered to be a critical cause for a particular failure event.

The fault tree analysis first established the major categories that appeared important, then traced them down to the quality element level. The analysis provided a statement as to the relative importance of a given quality element in contributing to a possible major failure event. The analysis identified two major critical pathways or possible events that would cause the CE mission to fail (Jones, 1981). The first major critical pathway related to the quality of the CE provider unit's educational output (activities, products, and services). The first-order event on the critical pathway, which

Table 1. Comparison of CESP and Sage Taxonomy.

CESP Terminology	Sage Terminology	Definition	Example
Major functioning category	Grouping by failure logic (cause/effect)	Highest-order grouping consisting of categories of quality elements	Providing CE activities and products
Quality attribute	1st-order events	Primary grouping of related quality elements	Detecting problems and concerns
Quality elements	Root causes of 2nd-order events	The lowest-order descriptor of those things that define quality	Use data from the practice setting and professions as a source for identifying potential problems or concerns

was at the level of quality attributes, was the *failure to determine educational priorities*. Two of the root causes at the quality element level found to be critical were failure to estimate the potential for the educational project to meet the educational need and failure to assess the severity or impact of the health care problems associated with each identified need. The second quality attribute identified in the critical pathway was *failure to determine problems and causes*. The related quality element or root cause was failure to use data from the practice setting and professions as a source of potential problems and concerns.

The second major critical pathway was related to failure of the strategic management process. Two first-order possible causes were identified. The first of these was *failure to elicit support of the parent organization*. Two root causes found to be critical were failure to encourage the parent organization to recognize CE as a specific function in its mission and failure to seek an organizational placement for the CE provider unit within the parent organization that would enable and facilitate the accomplishment of the CE mission. The second quality attribute identified in this critical pathway was *failure to elicit support for the CE provider unit within the health care setting*. The root causes found to be critical were failures to encourage the provision and use of practice data needed for the identification of problems and evaluation of CE impact, promote the provision of resources by the health care setting for the health

Figure 1. Analysis of Quality Elements from a Failure Point of View.

Mission: To describe continuing education (CE) in such a way that CE providers who ascribe to the model will produce relevant, effective and accessible CE.

UE—Failure of the mission because of . . .

C—1.000 Failure in provision of CE programs, materials and services because of

CC—1.000 Failure in determining educational priorities because of

CCB 1.000 Failure to estimate the health care benefits derived from meeting each identified need (QE 76)

CCI 0.898 Failure to determine the priority of each identified need (QE 83)

CCC 0.899 Failure to estimate the potential for educational activities to meet the identified needs (QE 77)

CCA 0.859 Failure to assess the severity or impact of the health care problems associated with each identified need (QE 75)

CAA 1.000 Failure to use data from practice setting and the professions as a source of potential problems or concerns (QE 66)

CA—0.997 Failure in detecting problems or concerns because of

A—0.866 Failure in leadership of the CE unit because of

AC—1.000 Failure in eliciting support for the CE unit from its parent body because of

ACA 1.000 Failure to encourage the parent body to recognize CE as a specific function in its mission (QE 13)

ACD 0.870 Failure to seek authority for the CE unit leader commensurate with the delegated responsibility (QE 16)

ACB 0.809 Failure to seek an organizational placement for the CE unit within the parent body which will enable and facilitate the accomplishment of the CE mission (QE 14)

AD—0.959 Failure in influencing support for CE in the health care setting because of

ADD 1.000 Failure to encourage the provision of practice data needed for the detection of potential problems and the evaluation of CE impact (QE 21)

ADC 0.925 Failure to promote the provision of time, money and other needed resources for health care professionals to engage in CE (QE 20)

ADF 0.895 Failure to influence the health care setting to provide support needed for the application of learning to practice (QE 23)

ADA 0.844 Failure to promote the development of health care quality standards needed for the identification of professional problems or concerns (QE 18)

AA—0.878 Failure in defining the mission for the CE unit because of

AAA 1.000 Failure to determine the general educational needs of the potential audiences (QE 1)

AAE 0.904 Failure to define the mission of the unit considering what is expected of the unit, its capabilities and limitations, and the applicable constraints (QE 5)

to health care professionals in CE because of

care professional in the learning process because of

DBA 1.000 Failure to assist learner(s) in identifying their problems or concerns (QE 123)

DBB 0.867 Failure to assist learner(s) in analyzing their problems or concerns (QE 124)

DCC 1.000 Failure to assist learner(s) in evaluating the impact of learning on their practice (QE 134)

DCB 0.995 Failure to assist learner(s), whenever possible, in applying learning to practice (QE 133)

DCA 0.919 Failure to assist learner(s) in identifying potential reinforcements in the practice setting for application of learning (QE 132)

DAC 1.000 Failure to assist health care professionals to compare their personal and professional behavior against the health care quality standards (QE 119)

DAB 0.935 Failure to encourage the acceptance of health care quality as a basis for the identification of professional problems or concerns (QE 118)

BAB 1.000 Failure to develop a strategic plan which includes long range plans, policies, and procedures to support accomplishing the mission of the CE unit (QE 42)

BAC 0.998 Failure to develop a set of goals and objectives which reflect the mission and the strategic plans of the CE unit (QE 43)

BAD 0.834 Failure to prepare a plan for the CE unit that specifies the sequence of activities to be carried out, the expected progress points, and the desired end points to be achieved (QE 45)

BED 1.000 Failure to set standards for the educational processes and products of the CE unit to assure the use of effective methods consistent with the resources of the unit (QE 65)

EAB 1.000 Failure to assign responsibility and delegate commensurate authority for carrying out the educational and management activities of the CE unit (QE 136)

EAA 0.803 Failure to ensure that the CE unit's plans, policies, procedures and standards are known throughout the unit (QE 135)

DC—0.845 Failure in assisting in the application of learning to practice because of

DA—0.832 Failure in facilitating the assumptions of responsibility for learning because of

BA—1.000 Failure in planning by the CE unit because of

BF—0.913 Failure in setting standards for the CE unit because of

EA—1.000 Failure in managing CE staff and faculty because of

FB—1.000 Failure to use the information obtained from applying the standards to anticipate and/or correct deficiencies in the CE unit (QE 157)

FA—0.988 Failure to implement the standards set for the CE unit, its staff and faculty, management, and educational process and products (QE 156)

FC—0.967 Failure to use the information obtained from applying the standards to provide the feedback necessary to maintain and improve performance (QE 158)

B—0.635 Failure in preparations by the CE unit because of

E—0.517 Failure in administration of the CE unit because of

F—0.372 Failure in monitoring and controlling the CE unit because of

Note: The quality elements listed represent the original version published by Suter and others, *Journal of Medical Education,* vol. 56 supplement, Aug. 1981.

care professional to engage in CE, influence the health care setting to provide support for the application of learning to practice, and promote the development of health care standards needed for the identification of professional problems or concerns.

Although the critical pathways are the most important output of the Sage Analysis, it also allows the consideration of each quality attribute and its quality elements as separate entities, isolating those quality elements within each attribute that have the most potential to lead to its failure. (Figure 1 indicates the relative importance of each quality element and attribute.)

Applying the Quality Elements

The Sage Analysis provided a perspective on the relative importance of the quality elements at a general level. However, to apply the QEs in a specific setting, a more limited approach can be taken. Frequently, a potential user is overwhelmed by the sheer number of quality elements and may become discouraged from using them. Some organizations, on the other hand, may find that the use requires attention to all the elements. An approach for selecting the most relevant QEs was developed when working with various CE organizations. The process can be used to establish long-term goals for improvement, to pinpoint specific areas for in-depth concentration, or to establish a complete quality assessment system. This process provides a starting point, formally or informally, for focusing efforts for improvement in the CE provider unit. The specific steps in this process are described in the following sections.

- *Determining the purpose for using the quality elements.* The first step is to be quite specific in identifying the use of the quality elements, be it improvement of the existing educational development process or establishing a new approach, quality control, or accountability for a CE provider unit, or clarification of management aspects of the unit.
- *Establishing goals and objectives for use of quality elements.* With the purpose clarified, goals and more specific objectives can be established. For example, the goal may be to strengthen the linkage of CE to the health care setting, with such objectives

as to develop a more effective way to identify and assess needs for learning or to enhance the involvement of the health professional in the CE project development process.

- *Selecting appropriate quality elements.* When the objectives have been identified, quality elements that relate to each objective can be selected. Depending on the circumstances, quality elements can be used as stated or may be restated to adapt them to a particular situation. As indicated in Chapter One, there is nothing permanent about these quality elements except their origin and their fit into a conceptual model.
- *Rank ordering the quality elements.* In most situations it will not be possible to work simultaneously with a large number of quality elements. Therefore, the establishment of priorities will help in the process. This should be done on the basis of criteria that allow a rational judgment as to the potential impact of each chosen quality element.
- *Developing performance indicators.* For each selected QE, performance indicators are identified. A performance indicator defines or describes the evidence that the selected quality element has been accomplished. This is the most critical step in the process because the performance indicators are specific examples of what a particular quality element means in the setting. The performance indicator therefore may serve as the guide for improvement as well as the criterion or standard for assessment (see Chapter Fourteen for examples).

Regardless of the ultimate use of the quality elements, in most instances the approach is one of selecting and amplifying each element in greater detail. Both selection and amplification render the quality elements specific and applicable to a particular situation. Thus, a quality element that is originally universally applicable becomes unique in its adaptation to an actual setting.

Examples of Application of Process. Several organizations have adapted the quality elements for application to their unique circumstances. In Chapters Thirteen, Fourteen, and Fifteen applications developed by the Veterans Administration (VA) Regional Medical Education Centers were discussed. The descriptions to follow provide some insight into other approaches to using the QEs.

The hope is that these examples will help readers consider means for incorporating the quality elements in their setting.

Temple University Hospital Consortium. The Temple Consortium for Continuing Medical Education, under the sponsorship of the Temple University School of Medicine, encompasses twenty-seven community hospitals in Pennsylvania. The goal of the consortium is to promote quality continuing medical education offered by the participating hospitals. As part of the consortium activities, a self-assessment program for CME directors was undertaken with fifteen of the twenty-seven member hospitals participating.

The quality elements served as a point of departure for identifying areas of focus. Their objectives were to assess the present level of CE practice with respect to the following: definition and acceptance of the mission of the CE provider unit within the hospitals, overall project development process by the individual CE provider units, evaluation procedures, ability to assist the individual health professionals with their educational needs, and management of the CE provider unit.

In a staged process, quality elements considered relevant to these objectives were selected and assigned priority. Through a committee process, the selected quality elements were then carefully reviewed and reformulated if necessary, and performance indicators were developed. A survey instrument was developed, and each participating CE provider unit was asked to assess its capability of complying with the quality elements and performance indicators.

This survey indicated that the average director of continuing medical education in the participating community hospitals has an active private practice in addition to the CME responsibilities. The formats used for CME are primarily passive approaches including lectures, symposia, and conferences. As a result of the survey, the group identified five areas for improving their skills as CME providers: needs assessment, priority setting, support for self-directed learning, evaluation, and monitoring for quality CME (Lanzilotti, 1982). The consortium then made plans for developing initiatives aimed at assisting the individual CE providers in reaching a higher level of competence in the identified areas.

In addition to identifying areas for improvement, participation in the process had a significant effect on those involved. Simply participating was a learning experience in itself. The members developed a better understanding of the situations in their hospitals that are influencing CME and the options available to them for improvement. They increased their awareness of alternatives for providing CME and recognized approaches that had not been explored. The process also gave the members an opportunity to discuss their situations and share ideas among one another.

American Association of Dental Schools. In an effort to support quality continuing education, the American Dental Association adopted a Sponsor Approval Program as a mechanism for certifying sponsors who can demonstrate their ability to provide effective continuing education. As with most national standards, these were developed for a broad spectrum of CE sponsors and were intended to be appropriate for everyone from local dental societies, specialty organizations, and private entrepreneurs to fully accredited educational institutions.

These standards, while useful for their purpose, specify minimal rather than optimal levels of quality and do not address the contingencies unique to schools of dentistry. Therefore, the American Association of Dental Schools undertook to design a self-study document for the purposes of developing criteria for quality CE specific to dental schools, making available a tool for dental school CE provider units to assess their own performance, and developing a process by which identified deficiencies can be analyzed and corrected. Because the self-assessment is based on optimal levels of quality, CE provider units' efforts toward improvement would correspondingly prepare them for the American Dental Association Sponsor Approval program (National Committee on Dental Education, 1980).

A self-assessment process requires attention to all aspects of the provision of CE. Therefore, through a group process, selected dental school CE directors examined all the quality elements, rewording and regrouping them as appropriate for dental school CE. A task force was then appointed to develop a self-assessment guide to assist the CE director in comparing present practice to ideal practice, establishing priorities for improvement, and identifying resources for more information.

American Red Cross. The Continuing Education Provider Unit of the American Red Cross is composed of representatives from three services within the organization—the Office of Personnel Training and Development, Blood Services Nursing, and Nursing and Health Services. These three services provide the majority of continuing education opportunities for all nurses in the Red Cross. The CE Provider Unit was concerned with the degree to which approved courses and workshops included means for increasing the likelihood that learning was related to participants' job responsibilities and was actually applied on the job.

As a means of improving the efforts in application to practice, the Continuing Education Provider Unit selected the specific quality elements that corresponded to their identified priority (see quality elements 112, 113, 114, Appendix, Chapter One). Goals were established to increase progressively the extent to which courses incorporate support to participants for application of learning to job performance. The goals described the expected percentage of available courses that would include these quality elements in their design.

A survey was conducted of the national courses sponsored by Blood Services Nursing, Nursing and Health Services, Safety Services, and Training and Development, for which accredited continuing education units are awarded to nurses. The purpose of the survey was to assess the current level of practice with respect to the selected quality elements. The results revealed that a higher percentage of courses than expected addressed in some form the quality elements. However, the degree to which there was support for application to practice was quite diverse. It ranged from courses designed and written so that many aspects of the selected quality elements were required or encouraged with strong support from instructors, participants, and the work place supervisors to courses where only mild encouragement was provided. In response to the survey results, efforts for future improvement were shifted to improve the quality of the support for the application of learning to practice and increasing the extent of efforts to assess impact on workers and work unit productivity.

This project addressed only one component of training and development in the Red Cross, continuing education for nurses. On a broader scale, the organization is also exploring the development of a single set of educational standards for all training in the Red Cross in order to bring about some standardization in the various field offices and separate chapters around the country (presently each service has its own policies for educational development). The process of establishing standards, describing expected levels of performance, and assessing the level of adherence will in concept resemble that of the Veterans Administration self-study program (see Chapter Fourteen).

Accreditation Council for Continuing Medical Education. The Accreditation Council for Continuing Medical Education (ACCME) was established as a voluntary organization to assure compliance with basic standards of quality of continuing medical education on a national basis. The council, sponsored by seven national medical organizations (American Board of Medical Specialties, American Hospital Association, American Medical Association, Association of American Medical Colleges, Association for Hospital Medical Education, Council of Medical Specialty Societies, and Federation of State Medical Boards), is aiming for high-quality CE offered to physicians, through the promulgation of essentials of quality for CME. In addition, the ACCME delegates authority to state medical societies for accreditation of institutions and organizations sponsoring CME on a local or state level under the condition that the same standards are met as for national accreditation.

The accreditation program of the ACCME is based on the assumption that the quality of the educational process influences the effectiveness of CE offered to physicians and hence has an impact on the quality of patient care. It is also assumed that there are critical elements or linkages in the CE system that can be identified as having an impact on the quality of the educational experience. Once these linkages have been identified, criteria and standards can be developed that support or prescribe acceptable levels of performance.

Using the quality elements and other sources as a starting point, the ACCME identified seven essentials in the provision of continuing medical education and the criteria pertaining to them. These essentials, approved by all member organizations, are now being used in the accreditation decision-making process. These same essentials form the basis for the procedures established by each state organization for accrediting local CME (Accreditation Council for Continuing Medical Education, 1983).

University of North Carolina. The Office of Research and Development for Education in the Health Professions provides educational support for the University of North Carolina School of Medicine. To explore new ways to support continuing education of the health professionals in the state, the office chose to focus on how it could support health professionals' self-directed learning (SDL). Their objectives were to determine the extent of participation in SDL by the health professionals in the state, to explore their perception of an SDL approach to CE, to study how professionals usually carry out their CE, and to explore methods for stimulating and reinforcing self-directed learning. Ten percent of the practicing pediatricians and physical therapists were randomly selected for telephone interviews to obtain this information. The response to a self-directed approach was overwhelmingly positive. Ninety-five percent of the respondents said they would participate in self-directed learning CE programs. Over 80 percent felt SDL activities should be offered for CE credit. It is expected that the data obtained from this study will help educators identify ways by which university-sponsored programs can facilitate self-directed continuing education for health professionals.

VA Continuing Education Center. Each organization that chose to use the quality elements was faced with the question of how best to incorporate them into their day-to-day activities. The Veterans Administration had a special interest in applying the quality elements to the management of continuing education provider units. One of the ways a CE provider unit of the VA, namely, the Continuing Education Center at the VA medical center in Washington, D.C., chose to apply the elements was to design and implement a unit management information system (see Chapter Thirteen). During the early stages of development, it became apparent that several different information subsystems exist. The first relates to the establishment of a new CE provider unit, the second to the provision of continuing education projects, and the third concerns strategic management, discussed in Chapter Twelve. To address the first and second subsystems, the decision graph approach (Martin, 1980) was used. With this approach, the key to developing a useful management information system is to identify the critical management decision points in a given setting. By selecting the information needed at each of those decision points, one can develop an information system that includes only the necessary information and excludes extraneous information. The remainder of this section will describe the two decision diagrams that were developed.

The decision diagram for *establishing a CE provider unit* assumes that the unit is part of a larger organization (the parent organization) that will have some control over the CE function, the CE provider unit will receive at least some of its resources from this parent organization, and the CE provider unit will embody the quality elements as a basis for its management structure and educational procedures.

A working group of experienced CE managers from the VA and outside organizations identified the critical decision points and the information needed to support those decisions. This resulted in the map of decisions shown in Figure 2. The figure follows the sequence of decisions (indicated as D1, D2, . . . D 21) in establishing a new continuing education provider unit (CEPU) from the initial decision, through planning and staffing, to the point where the organization is ready to function. The decisions are sequenced to show how each one depends on the outcomes of the decisions that came before it. After the CEPU has been established, this sequence of decisions is still important, in that any decision that is revised will affect all that follow.

The information to be provided by the management information system is defined by the specific data or criteria required at each decision point. The first decision in the sequence is a commitment by the parent organization to establish a CE provider unit. This decision point is placed at the head of the diagram to show that all the other decisions depend upon it. Examples of evidence of adequate commitment by the parent organization to the new CE provider unit would include a preliminary mission statement and interim set of policies drafted by the parent organization for the CE provider unit, an initial resource commitment to support the new organization, and a description of the type of person required to

Figure 2. Decision Dependencies Diagram For Establishing a Continuing Education Provider Unit (CEPU).

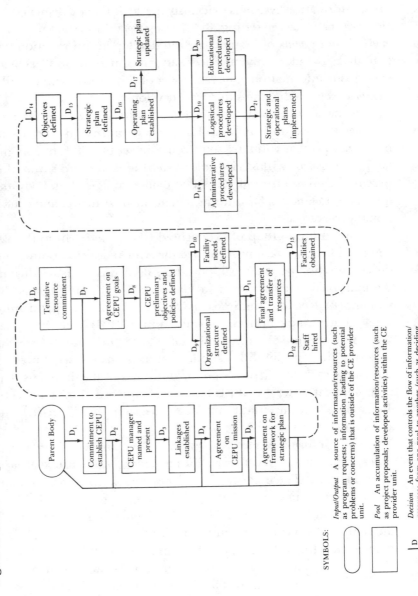

SYMBOLS:

Input/Output A source of information/resources (such as program requests; information leading to potential problems or concerns) that is outside of the CE provider unit.

Pool An accumulation of information/resources (such as project proposals; developed activities) within the CE provider unit.

Decision An event that controls the flow of information/resources from one pool to another (such as deciding which potential undertakings become approved pro-

manage the CE provider unit. In addition, the parent organization would have included the role of continuing education in its own mission statement.

The second decision point is the appointment of the CE provider unit manager. Since CE provider units are usually small, the relationship between the unit and its parent organization often depends on the CE manager's relations with the parent organization. This is reflected in the criteria for this decision, which include agreement between the manager and parent organization on mission, resources, policies, authority, and responsibility, and necessary linkages and incentives the provider unit can offer staff and faculty.

The third decision point is the identification and establishment of linkages between the CE provider unit and groups inside and outside the parent organization that will be important to the life of the CE provider unit. The fourth and fifth decision points are related to setting the general direction for the CE provider unit. This direction should be set in consultation with the parent organization and other important groups with whom linkages were established at the preceding decision point. At the sixth decision point the CE provider unit reaches an agreement with its parent organization and other sponsors on the resources they will provide to it. These resources plus any others that the CE provider unit can reasonably expect to get from other sources must be consistent with the general direction set for the CE provider unit.

At the seventh and eighth decision points, the CE provider unit sets the goals, objectives, and policies that will guide its operations. The criteria ensure that these goals, objectives, and policies contribute to the accomplishment of the CE provider unit's mission. The ninth and tenth decision points represent the transition to a physical reality. These include deciding on the staffing, space, and equipment needs. The criteria stress the importance of carefully designing an organizational structure that will both support the people who work in it and promote productivity.

At the eleventh, twelfth, and thirteenth decision points, the CE provider unit actually acquires the resources it needs to be in operation—money, people, space, and equipment. The criteria identify the kinds of selection criteria and control mechanisms the

manager should have established at this point. The remaining decision points indicate that the current plans and procedures for the
effective operation of the CE provider unit are established and
revised. This planning is done with the participation of the CE
provider unit staff.

This critical decision diagram should help not only with the
original establishment of the CE provider unit but also at each
phase of the organization's maturity and development (Moore,
1982). When organizational changes are imminent, the CE manager
can refer to the diagram to identify those decisions that would be
affected by the changes and can take any necessary action.

The decision diagram for the *provision of CE* (Figure 3)
includes fifteen decisions that relate directly to providing quality CE
activities, products, and services. Although much of this book has
discussed all aspects of systematic project development, this decision
diagram outlines succinctly the nature of the decisions that the CE
provider unit manager has to make to support the process. Decisions
one through six relate to selecting potential CE undertakings. Decisions seven through nine focus on approving internal, collaborative,
or external project proposals. Decisions eleven and twelve relate to
developing or purchasing a CE service. Decision points twelve and
thirteen refer to implementing CE activities, while fourteen and
fifteen complete the cycle by addressing evaluation.

Materials Developed by the Project

One of the objectives of the Continuing Education Systems
Project was to develop materials to assist providers of continuing
education to enhance the quality of the CE offered. This book
represents a major effort in communicating the principles of the
project and providing direction for applying those principles. In
addition to the specifications for a management information system,
described in-depth in Chapter Thirteen, and flowcharts of decisions
made in establishing and managing a CE provider unit, described in
the last section of this chapter, the project created learning packages
describing the design and management of systematic educational
development for CE.

The learning packages are designed to assist those who are responsible for providing continuing education for health professionals but lack the necessary background in the design and development of instruction and in management. The audience includes directors of continuing education in any of the health professions, in-service education directors, and staff of state and national professional societies. The materials include a combination of videotape and print in separate but coordinated packages covering such topics as needs assessment and problem identification, planning educational programs and activities, educational program evaluation, the self-directed learning process, development of an information management system, and implementing a self-study and external review process. The packages explain how to implement the concepts described in Chapters Seven through Eleven and Thirteen and Fourteen. These materials were developed in cooperation with the Learning Resource Services of the Veterans Administration and can be obtained through the National Audiovisual Center in Washington, D.C.

Conclusion

This chapter has looked at the process for adapting and applying the quality elements in an individual setting. The quality elements are universally applicable principles for quality CE. To be operationally meaningful, the appropriate quality elements must become an integral part of the setting through adoption of the principles and adaptation of the products as necessary, including the quality elements.

Throughout the book the point has been made that continuing education can influence health professionals' performance and can serve as the link between potential competence and actual performance within a specific health care setting. The principles and products of the Continuing Education Systems Project are means of enhancing the capabilities and impact made by continuing education. Through a conscious focus on aspects of educational development and management and through the application of criteria for quality, CE in the health professions can match and exceed the expectations placed upon it.

Figure 3. Decision Dependencies in the

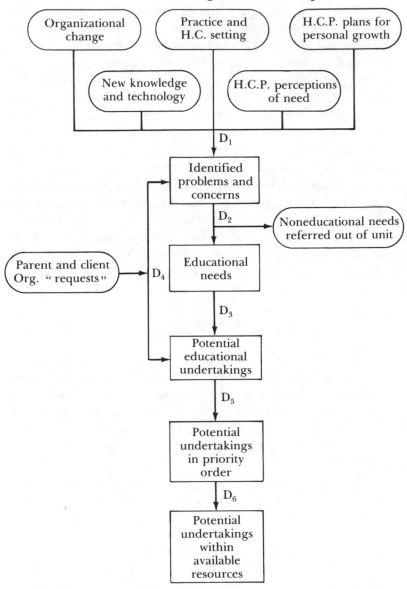

SYMBOLS:

Input/Output A source of information/resources (such as program requests; information leading to potential problems or concerns) that is outside of the CE provider unit.

Pool   An accumulation of information/resources (such as project proposals; developed activities) within the CE provider unit.

Provision of Continuing Education.

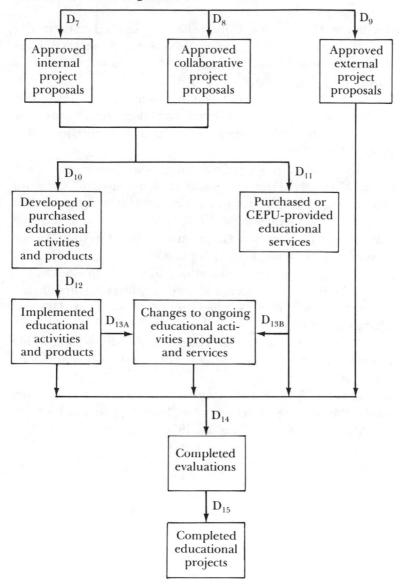

Decision An event that controls the flow of information/
resources from one pool to another (such as deciding
which potential undertakings become approved projects).

Abbreviations:
H.C.   Health Care
H.C.P.   Health Care Professional
Org.   Organization

References

Accreditation Council for Continuing Medical Education. *The Essentials and Guidelines for Accreditation of Sponsors of Continuing Medical Education.* Chicago: Accreditation Council for Continuing Medical Education, 1983.

Jones, R. K. "Sage Analysis of Quality Elements for Continuing Education in the VA-AAMC Continuing Education Systems Project." Unpublished dissertation, Brigham Young University, Provo, Utah, 1981.

Lanzilotti, S. S. *Report of the Continuing Education Systems Project as Needs Assessment.* Unpublished manuscript, Office of Continuing Medical Education, Temple University School of Medicine, Philadelphia, 1982.

Martin, M. P. "The Decision Graph in Systems Analysis." *Journal of Systems Management,* 1980, *31* (1), 29–35.

Moore, D. E., Jr. "The Organization and Administration of Continuing Education in Academic Medical Centers." Unpublished doctoral dissertation, University of Illinois at Urbana-Champaign, 1982.

National Committee on Dental Education. *Guide to Continuing Education Sponsor Approval.* Chicago: American Dental Association, 1980.

Stephens, K. G. "A Fault Tree Approach to Management: An Overview." Presented to conference of Military Operations Research Society, Annapolis, Md., June 29, 1977.

Epilogue: Further Strategies for Strengthening Continuing Education for the Health Professions

Alan B. Knox

Some members of each of the health professions have always provided leadership to encourage and help other members extend their knowledge and improve their practice throughout their careers. Such leadership has included attention to both self-directed learning activities (such as reading and consultation) and group activities (such as meetings and workshops). The accelerating rate of social and technological change during the past century has transformed practice in the health professions and with each passing decade has produced a steady increase in the extent and variety of continuing education. Although recent developments such as quality assurance and mandatory continuing education have increased the visibility of continuing education, they certainly didn't create it.

This growth of continuing education for the health professions has resulted in an expansion of the number of people who plan and conduct the programs. Such continuing education practitioners perform various roles and work for various providers such as educational institutions, professional associations, and health care institutions. In most instances, those who devote all or a major portion of their professional time to continuing education provide coordination or leadership on behalf of many people who help to plan or conduct continuing education activities on a very part-time basis. Those who provide leadership are dedicated to the importance of continuing education but vary greatly in their familiarity with writings and practice elsewhere that could be used to improve the quality of their own continuing education efforts.

This book is for the growing number of health professions continuing education practitioners who want to enrich their understanding of continuing education theory and practice elsewhere in order to strengthen their leadership in their own setting. Thus the book, and the large national project on which it is based, have a very practical purpose—that is, to review theory and practice of continuing education of adults in any setting, to relate the main concepts and procedures to the realities of the health professions, and to provide realistic guidelines that health professions continuing education practitioners can use to strengthen their own programs.

Often an epilogue is provided by someone detached from the action who can comment dispassionately about what has transpired and about implications for the future. As an active participant in the entire project and in related activities, I enjoy no such luxury. Instead, I propose to note major ideas from the book that seem noteworthy and to suggest promising future directions. Because most readers of an epilogue will have read the preceding chapters, it is assumed that brevity is the soul of wit. It is further assumed that most readers who reached an epilogue want to continue their own education about the theory and practice of continuing education. Therefore, this epilogue seeks to connect major examples and suggestions from the book with next steps that readers might take to adapt such ideas to their own use and build on them by further reading and greater familiarity with continuing education practice elsewhere. Each of the three broad sections that follow (on practitioner proficiencies, learner orientations, and coordination strategies) contains two parts: one noting major ideas from the current chapters and another suggesting promising future directions.

Practitioner Proficiencies

The main ideas in the preceding chapters can be viewed in several ways: as a review of pertinent literature and practice, as guidelines for practice, or as standards for monitoring and improving continuing education for the health professions. Another way is as an inventory of major proficiencies required by successful continuing education practitioners.

Current. As indicated early in Chapter One, this book takes a broad view of continuing education and the resultant proficiencies that practitioners need in order to provide it effectively. The intended outcomes for participants include both improved capability to deliver health care and broader aspects of enhanced professional careers. The procedures include both encouraging and assisting self-directed study and conducting more formal continuing education activities such as workshops and miniresidencies. Most people would agree on the central focus on targeted efforts to improve performance. However, the broader approach presented in this book is desirable for several reasons. The disincentives of remedial continuing education aimed at removing deficiencies of people who fail to meet minimal professional standards are replaced with the incentives of developmental continuing education for all members of the profession as an important vehicle for their career development and enhanced service. This broader approach also includes attention to seeking future opportunities as well as solving past problems. It recognizes that in addition to outcomes of continuing education, there are many influences on patient health status that are only partly understood. And the inclusion of self-directed learning accommodates the great variation in learner backgrounds, purposes, and preferred learning styles along with concern about application of what is learned as well as educational achievement.

The scope of the foregoing chapters therefore constitutes a major accomplishment. Chapters One and Six indicate the variety of health professions, providers of continuing education, delivery systems used, and roles involved in planning and conducting programs. When attention to the continuum of preparatory and continuing professional education is added, the complexity becomes almost overwhelming. This is why the broad systems view of the major aspects of continuing professional education and their interrelationships, provided by this book, is so valuable. The heavy emphasis on physicians as continuing education participants reflects the disproportionate attention they receive in continuing education writings and practice and their great influence in many health care delivery systems. Although the project upon which this book is based sought balanced attention to all health professions, most practitioners will need to adapt the examples and guidelines to their distinctive traditions and settings.

  Chapters Two, Three, Four, and Six review characteristics of health professionals as learners, along with some generalizations about learning and information seeking that continuing education practitioners can use to design responsive programs. Part Three contains guidelines for developing and implementing effective continuing education activities, including assistance to individual learners. Chapters Twelve through Fifteen suggest some ways to strengthen the administrative coordination of continuing education activities. This scope is paralleled by the categories of quality elements, presented in the Appendix to Chapter One, which were a major outcome of the project. Because the quality elements are designed for planning, coordination, and accreditation, they emphasize program development and administration. Throughout the book it is assumed that many health professions continuing education practitioners could become far more effective if they would use some of the concepts and overview provided in this book. This is undoubtedly so. It also seems likely that it can help them discover additional ideas and resources in the broader field of continuing education that can enrich their practice. The next part of this section suggests some that seem especially promising.

  Future. As indicated in Chapter One, many health professions continuing educators started in that role with little formal preparation and relevant experience. Especially for them, a useful early way to enhance proficiencies as continuing educators is to obtain some standards of best practice against which to compare their current performance and proficiencies (capability to perform effectively if given the opportunity). This book (especially the quality elements and Part Three on program development and facilitating learning) suggests such standards of desirable proficiencies. A broader view of practitioner proficiencies throughout adult and continuing education generally includes some additional areas of proficiency that might be included (Knox, 1979b). The major areas include a perspective on scope, trends, and issues in the field (types of and relationships among providers, relations with the remainder of the parent organization, major societal influences, resource identification), understanding adult development and learning as a basis for responsiveness to participants, personal qualities (commitment, interpersonal effectiveness, and an innovative approach to practice), program development (needs, context, objectives, activities, evaluation), and administration (attraction and retention of participants, acquisition and allocation of resources, staff selection and development, and leadership including planning and coordination).

Information and assistance to identify and narrow discrepancies between current and desired proficiencies are available to practitioners from several sources. Two broad categories are information from professional literature and from interaction with other continuing education practitioners.

Some pertinent writings are aimed at the health professions. Examples include this book, a personal collection of other books and periodicals related to one's specialty, holdings of a professional library within one's place of employment, and a nearby major library with a satisfactory collection. The broader range of writings on adult and continuing education generally were very useful in the preparation of this book and contain many additional concepts and practices that can be readily adapted.

For example, Jossey-Bass has published *Continuing Learning in the Professions* (Houle, 1980) and quarterly sourcebooks on *New Directions for Continuing Education* (NDCE). The previously mentioned volume on enhancing proficiencies of continuing educators (Knox, 1979b) was the first in the NDCE series. Subsequent volumes include useful suggestions about such topics as staffing (Brown and Copeland, 1979), teaching (Knox, 1980a), attracting external funds (Buskey, 1981), relating education to performance

(Grabowski, 1983) and programs for older adults (Okun, 1982). *Learning How to Learn* (Smith, 1982) contains a rationale and suggestions for assistance to self-directed learners; and *Modern Practice of Adult Education* (Knowles, 1980) is a basic rationale for responsive program development. Outside the health field, there are more than a dozen associations related to various types of provider agencies (such as universities, community colleges, employers, and libraries), each with their own publications. Examples include the *Training and Development Journal* of the American Society for Training and Development and *Continuum* of the National University Continuing Education Association. The most comprehensive umbrella association in the field, with a unit on continuing professional education, is the American Association for Adult and Continuing Education, which publishes books and pamphlets, a monthly magazine for practitioners (*Lifelong Learning*), and a research journal (*Adult Education Quarterly*). In addition, the University of California Press publishes *Möbius*, a journal for continuing education professionals in health sciences and health policy. These few examples illustrate the many sources available to a health professions continuing educator seeking new ideas for an important professional task.

As with administrators in most fields, many continuing education coordinators find conversations with other practitioners especially valuable. One function of reviewing the foregoing publications is to locate other people with kindred interests, to talk with in greater detail. Within the health professions, there are many associations and groups that serve functions such as stimulation, networking, resource identification, and collaboration. Interaction among continuing education practitioners associated with the same provider agency is a starting point for agencies that employ more than one practitioner. Professional associations (with their local, state, and regional affiliates) are a typical means of collegial association. Almost every one of the health-related associations has a committee or division for members interested in continuing education, and there are several associations for continuing education and training practitioners from various health fields.

Some health professions continuing education practitioners are members of broader associations of continuing education practitioners who work in a wide variety of professions. Two with active sections concerned broadly with continuing professional education are the National University Continuing Education Association (for university-affiliated practitioners) and the American Association for Adult and Continuing Education (for interested practitioners in any part of the field). Such contacts help a practitioner discover ideas, opportunities, resources, and strategies that have evolved in other professional fields (such as law, education, engineering, social work, and business) that could enrich continuing education practice in the health professions. In addition, more than eighty universities in North America now offer graduate courses and degrees, as well as noncredit workshops on various aspects of adult and continuing education and training.

Despite the frustration that some old-timers in the field have expressed with the slow progress away from a content model of continuing education, this book contains heartening examples of application of a process model. This emerging model emphasizes active learner roles in both learning and application. As indicated in Chapter One, the project resulted not only in this book but also in learning packages and guidelines for management information systems and program reviews. These products are based on and include examples of a growing number of instances in which continuing education provider units and the practitioners who work there have conducted responsive and effective continuing education activities that have an impact on practice. By enhancing the proficiencies of additional continuing education practitioners, this book can greatly advance the process model of continuing education.

Learner Orientations

The distinctive feature of this book is its emphasis on professional practice and the individual learner. If existing standards of quality for judging and improving formal programs of continuing education have been inadequate in recent years, guidelines for helping individual adults learn have been even less available and satisfactory. This section of the Epilogue reviews the attention the book gives to assisting self-directed learning and suggests desirable future directions based on additional available ideas and resources.

Current. There is substantial attention to the individual health professional as the focus of continuing education. It is assumed throughout that the benefits of continuing education in the form of improved health care and enhanced careers start and end with professional practice. Such practice is the source of information about educational needs and of motivation to improve. Improved practice is the main evidence of continuing education's impact. As indicated earlier in this Epilogue, the definition of continuing education used in the book included both programs provided by educational institutions, professional associations, and health care institutions and assistance for self-directed learning. With the variety of backgrounds that health professionals bring to an intentional learning activity and the variety of specific applications and settings they confront, a high degree of individualization seems essential.

Reviews of writings about learning are contained in Chapters Two and Three. In each instance, highlights of several prominent child-oriented learning theories are followed by more helpful and pertinent characteristics of adults as learners. For example, toward the end of Chapter Two, expectancy-valence theory and systems theory are suggested as ways to gain a more unified view of learning and change. Chapter Three urges that continuing education build on health professionals' motivation to learn and have an impact on their performance by facilitating self-directed learning and improving the conditions of learning.

Chapter Eleven defines self-directed learning and notes that self-directed learners seek to enhance their proficiencies by relating new knowledge and commitment to improved performance to their current capabilities. This problem-solving approach is reflected in Chapter Four. Awareness of discrepancies between current capability and aspirations encourage professionals to seek new ideas. The information actively sought seems to depend on the stage of the problem-solving process, clinical relevance, familiarity and accessibility of sources, and progression and continuity in learning. Together, the repeated attention to self-directed learning throughout the book suggests a more unified way of thinking about and guiding adult learning in which the learner assumes major responsibility for helping to decide what is to be learned, how it will be learned, and ways in which new learnings will be applied.

Future. In recent years a number of ideas have emerged that can be used to enrich and extend current efforts to guide self-directed learning by health professionals. A decade ago the importance of lifelong self-directed education for people engaged in the health professions was recognized, a detailed rationale had evolved, and illustrative self-directed learning practices by learners and teachers were known to people interested in continuing professional education (Knox, 1974).

Underlying many of the efforts to promote self-directed learning have been basic concepts and procedures for the process of problem finding and problem solving. The problem-solving model has been a fundamental ideal of practice in the health professions (Elstein, Shulman, and Sprafka, 1978). Some of the health-related problems that health professionals confront are well defined, very effective solutions are known, and achievable best practice takes on the character of standard operating procedures. However, some of the proficiencies that continuing education practitioners would most like to enhance relate to ill-defined problems (Klein and Weitzenfeld, 1979). During the past decade there have been major advances in cognitive psychology that have clarified differences in the strategies used by expert versus novice problem solvers in many fields (Greeno, 1978). These advances suggest ways to relate educational activities closely to the process of problem solving in relation to needs assessment, learning activities, and encouraging application of new learning (McKeachie, 1980). The basic ingredient is active learning that is self-directing and self-correcting.

Many learning theories that a decade ago appeared to be very separate seem to be converging on problem solving (Bigge, 1982). This emphasis on learning as an active effort to use and extend current proficiencies is consistent with a major personality theory that emphasizes discrepancies between current and desired proficiencies as a basis for growth (Maddi, 1972). But for such change to occur, people have to try, and a sense of being a proficient, effective person is a source of optimism that leads to striving and growth (Bandura, 1982).

This places problem-oriented adult learning and teaching in the context of a transactional view of adult development (Knox, 1977). When people are able to accomplish most of what they and others expect, there is little motivation to learn. When expectations seem excessive, many people feel overwhelmed, do not know where to start, and give up. When the discrepancies between current and desired proficiencies are in a moderate range (challenging but not threatening), many adults are motivated to engage in learning projects (Deci, 1980). Change events (such as a major new work assignment) require some adjustment and often produce a heightened readiness to learn, which triggers participation in an intentional learning project (Aslanian and Brickell, 1980). It has been estimated that more than 80 percent of adult participation in learning projects is triggered by recent, current, or anticipated change events.

Adults who have learned how to learn tend to be more effective in the use of intentional learning activities to deal with such changes, problems, and opportunities (Smith, 1982). There are increasing instances in which continuing education providers have developed procedures to encourage and assist self-directed learning (Knowles, 1975; Knox, 1974; Smith, 1983). Participants in typical group-oriented continuing education activities may benefit from social and emotional support from other participants. Because this may be lacking, continuing education providers may want to emphasize ways to encourage participation and persistence (Darkenwald and Larson, 1980). This may include an informal educational counseling function (DiSilvestro, 1981).

In many instances, continuing education for health professionals aims to produce results beyond personal satisfaction and career enrichment. Quality assurance is concerned with the delivery of health care, and related continuing education activities aim at improving personal performance and organizational productivity. There can be a symbiotic relationship between personal growth and organizational productivity (Schein, 1978). However, this is more likely when continuing education practitioners use effective procedures for both personal and organizational development and have a rationale for doing so. The effectiveness of such programs and of the self-directed learning of the participants can be heightened (especially when the focus is on interpersonal relations) by making the assumptions, reasoning, values, and results (espoused theory) more explicit and comparing them with the theory implicit in people's actions (Argyris, 1982).

A recent rationale for adult learning and teaching, based on analysis of discrepancies between current and desired proficiencies, can be used by health professionals to strengthen their participation in intentional learning projects (Knox, 1980b, 1984). The essential concepts and relationships of proficiency theory are illustrated by the following examples of a fictional internist, Dr. Hart, based on findings from the study by Means (1979) referred to in Chapter Four. When she recently completed her residency and passed her boards in internal medicine, Dr. Hart joined the practice of Dr. Snow, who was approaching retirement as the only physician in a small community served by a regional hospital some miles away. Dr. Hart found that there was much to learn, mostly accomplished through incidental learning and an occasional workshop provided by her medical school or specialty society. However, this example focuses on her participation in self-directed learning projects, including influences, procedures, and results.

The rationale distinguishes between her performance in the practice of medicine and her participation in intentional self-directed learning projects intended to enhance her proficiency (defined as the capability to perform effectively if given the opportunity and composed of some combination of knowledge, attitudes, and sometimes neuromuscular skills). Also, her learning as well as her performance reflect reciprocal interactions with her general environment, so that both personal (abilities, aspirations) and situational (expectations, resources) influences affect her motivation, participation, and enhanced proficiency. Her actual performance as a practicing physician, which also reflects both personal and situational influences, serves to validate current proficiencies, affect aspirations, suggest discrepancies, and utilize enhanced proficiencies. It is a major source of her educational needs and the major setting in which her new occupational learnings are applied.

Adult learning is developmental as well as transactional. Her attitudes toward desired proficiencies (mastering a new clinical procedure) and toward learning projects to enhance proficiencies (reading and consultation) reflect her memories of past experiences in learning (medical school, informal learning projects) and work (solving a difficult practice problem). The informative and incentive values of such memories are a major source of intrinsic motivations to learn. In addition to developmental influences from her past and reciprocal interactions with her current environment, her current proficiencies reflect her aspirations for the future as moderated by her abilities.

Role change events (such as the abrupt retirement of Dr. Snow due to ill health), require adjustments that produce a heightened readiness to learn and often trigger initiation of learning projects. The likelihood that Dr. Hart will engage in a learning project to master an unfamiliar clinical procedure that Dr. Snow formerly performed is associated with how important it is to enhance her proficiency, taking into account how easily she could do so and the benefits to her practice and her patients. Her sense of being a proficient person, which contributes to her willingness to try to become more proficient, also evolves through achievement and interdependence and results from achieving internal standards and from evidence of performance.

The extent and type of Dr. Hart's participation, persistence, and application associated with intentional learning projects reflect multiple personal and situational influences. Many of these influences come together in her perceived discrepancies between current and desired proficiencies. Her extent of motivation to alter such discrepancies is related to perceived costs and benefits to patients, peers, and herself. Her efforts to change are more likely if other people confirm discrepancies that are neither so small as to be trivial nor so large as to be overwhelming. Participation and application are also encouraged by awareness of standards of best practice, resources for learning, expectations of significant others regarding the desirability of learning objectives, receptivity to application of enhanced proficiencies, and similarity and contiguity between action settings and the settings in which learning occurs.

Dr. Hart is also more likely to be an effective self-directed learner if she has a rationale for the types of decisions that teachers sometimes make in more formal educational settings, which she can use to strengthen her understanding and decision making when planning and implementing her learning projects. For example, such a rationale can help her make decisions about including other people in needs assessment, building on current proficiencies, using contextual analysis to take occupational opportunities and educational resources into account, setting cost/beneficial educational objectives, selecting sequences of learning activities that encourage the learner to devote sufficient time to achieve the objectives and apply what is learned, unlearning when past proficiencies interfere with desired performance, and providing for evaluative judgments to redirect efforts and reinforce progress.

Self-directed learning is not solitary learning, and it is not only self-paced learning. It occurs when the learner assumes major responsibility for decisions about learning projects. The foregoing rationale indicates concepts and procedures that health professionals can use to strengthen the process.

Coordination Strategies

Most people in full-time leadership roles in which they might help improve the quality of continuing education for the health professions are in positions in which they supervise or coordinate continuing education programs. There are three types of leadership strategies that such coordinators can use. One is to provide assistance to individual learners, such as by provision of self-assessment inventories, self-study materials, and tutorial assistance. The first third of this Epilogue focused on ways in which continuing education practitioners can strengthen learner orientations to encourage and assist self-directed learning. The other two types are addressed in the remainder of this Epilogue. A second type of leadership strategy deals with program development generally, including both professional development and organizational development. The third has to do with broad administrative concerns such as staffing, resources, marketing, and organizational relations. The two parts in this section review attention to coordination strategies in the preceding chapters and suggest desirable future directions.

Current. Chapter One early on expresses concern about lack of responsiveness by continuing education providers to health professionals both individually and in groups and helpfully notes discrepancies between the high expectations for continuing education practitioners and their limited abilities to deliver. A major reason for this discrepancy is that most practitioners enter continuing education roles with little preparation and mostly learn on the job. As a result, many are unfamiliar with either effective procedures to plan and conduct continuing education programs or standards of continuing education quality against which to judge and improve their efforts. The quality elements at the end of Chapter One constitute the foundation of such a set of standards that was prepared early in the project on which this book was based and that has already proven useful to practitioners in the field.

For example, use of such standards is well illustrated in Chapter Nine, in which practitioners are urged to involve participants actively in planning and conducting learning activities by letting them know what is expected, giving them opportunities to practice new proficiencies, assisting them to apply new learnings to practice, and accommodating various learning style preferences.

Chapters Seven through Ten review major concepts and procedures for continuing education program development. These chapters contain quite a comprehensive set of concepts and procedures for planning and conducting effective programs, along with a rationale for why. Needs assessment is appropriately emphasized as a basis for responsive programming, although there is a tendency in Chapter Eight to emphasize large-scale needs assessment studies to the neglect of cost-effective small-scale procedures. Chapters Seven and Ten include a useful and broad systems perspective in which situational influences (such as occupational trends and agency purposes and resources) and unanticipated as well as anticipated outcomes are included so that program development efforts are focused where they are likely to make a difference. Chapter Nine provides an especially clear overview of program design. The combination of sound program design and program evaluation is the best way to provide evidence of impact, which was noted in Chapter One as much needed (Knox, 1979a).

The pluralistic pattern of multiple providers of continuing education is confusing and frustrating, especially to people seeking to understand the field. This frustration was apparent, especially in Chapter One, as expressed as a lack of focus and system. Health care institutions, professional associations, higher education institutions, and other continuing education providers (such as private consultants) each have a degree of independence and a distinctive contribution they can make. Effective coordinators are able to collaborate with people in their own parent organization (such as a hospital or university) and in external organizations, whose cooperation is important for program success (Knox, 1979b). Chapters Thirteen through Fifteen suggest the types of information about program needs, activities, and outcomes that can be assembled and summarized to monitor and guide both internal and external collaboration. With decentralized arrangements, such information for program coordination is especially important.

Future. The foregoing chapters of this book provide a sound and useful overview of coordination strategies. Fortunately, professional writings from the broad field of continuing education contain books and articles that enable practitioners to pursue topics of interest in greater depth and detail. For instance, the range of proficiencies demonstrated by successful continuing education practitioners include some that received limited attention in this book. Examples include effective interpersonal relations and a sense of direction regarding major trends and issues in the field (Knox, 1979b).

As indicated in the middle section on learning orientation of this Epilogue, an increasing amount has been written during the past decade on self-directed learning and helping people master procedures to guide their own learning (Knox, 1974; Smith, 1982, 1983). Fortunately, there are also efforts to increase attention to individualization and learner responsibility in the preparation of health professionals, which can strengthen the continuum of professional education referred to in Chapter Five (Folk and others, 1976).

One way to use the professional literature on continuing education program development and administration is to specify discrepancies between current and desired efforts (Knox and others, 1980). Discrepancy analysis enables practitioners to compare current practices with desirable practices to which they and others aspire (Argyris, 1982). For example, responsive programming based on needs assessments is widely valued. Familiarity with pertinent needs assessment concepts and procedures that have been used elsewhere helps practitioners identify useful ideas that can be adapted to their situation (Pennington, 1980). In doing so, it is important to use efficient procedures so that the benefits exceed the costs.

The realities of professional practice powerfully influence continuing education efforts. Houle's (1980) rich perspective on continuing professional education (including characteristics of the professionalization process that continuing education activities can address) extend far beyond the aspects of a profession reflected in Chapter Six. The process of helping adults learn during the actual teaching-learning transaction is a dynamic link between the planning that should prepare for it and the application that should flow from it. As noted in Chapter Nine, one way to strengthen this transaction is through use of print and electronic materials (Chamberlain, 1980; Wilson, 1983). Effective strategies for helping adults learn also entail attention to motivation, sequencing, practice, and feedback (Knox, 1980a).

Continuing education coordinators and administrators who provide effective leadership do more than make decisions about individual quality elements. They have broader strategies for sequences of decisions that they and others make to agree upon desirable goals and to contribute to their achievement (Knox, 1982). This provides the framework for the specifics of management information systems and quality assurance procedures described in Chapters Thirteen through Fifteen. Strategies benefit from an understanding of technical procedures that coordinators can use. Examples include financial planning (Shipp, 1982), strengthening internal support (Votruba, 1981), and attracting external funding (Buskey, 1981). Along with mastery of technical procedures, effective coordinators recognize the contributions that beliefs and values make to the decision-making process (Merriam, 1982). Perhaps the greatest contribution of this book is the framework it provides coordinators to ask useful questions to guide their own professional development.

References

Argyris, C. *Reasoning, Learning and Action: Individual and Organizational.* San Francisco: Jossey-Bass, 1982.

Aslanian, C. B., and Brickell, H. N. *Americans in Transition: Life Changes As Reasons for Learning.* New York: College Entrance Examination Board, 1980.

Bandura, A. "Self-Efficacy Mechanism in Human Agency." *American Psychologist* 1982, *37* (2) 122–147.

Bigge, M. L. *Learning Theories for Teachers.* 4th ed. New York: Harper & Row, 1982.

Brown, M. A., and Copeland, H. G. (Eds.). *New Directions for Continuing Education: Attracting Able Instructors of Adults,* no. 4. San Francisco: Jossey-Bass, 1979.

Buskey, J. H. (Ed.). *New Directions for Continuing Education: Attracting External Funds for Continuing Education,* no. 12. San Francisco: Jossey-Bass, 1981.

Chamberlain, M. N. (Ed.). *New Directions for Continuing Education: Providing Continuing Education by Media and Technology,* no. 5. San Francisco: Jossey-Bass, 1980.

Darkenwald, G., and Larson, G. A. (Eds.). *New Directions for Continuing Education: Reaching Hard-to-Reach Adults,* no. 8. San Francisco: Jossey-Bass, 1980.

Deci, E. L. *The Psychology of Self-Determination.* Lexington, Mass.: Lexington Books, 1980.

DiSilvestro, F. R. (Ed.). *New Directions for Continuing Education: Advising and Counseling Adult Learners,* no. 10. San Francisco: Jossey-Bass, 1981.

Elstein, A. S., Shulman, L. S., and Sprafka, S. A. *Medical Problem Solving: An Analysis of Clinical Reasoning.* Cambridge, Mass.: Harvard University Press, 1978.

Folk, R. L., and others. *Individualizing the Study of Medicine.* New York: Westinghouse Learning Corporation, 1976.

Grabowski, S. M. (Ed.). *New Directions for Continuing Education: Strengthening Connections Between Education and Performance,* no. 18. San Francisco: Jossey-Bass, 1983.

Greeno, J. G. "Natures of Problem-Solving Abilities." In W. K. Estes (Ed.), *Handbook of Learning and Cognitive Processes.* Vol. 5. Hillsdale, N.J.: Erlbaum, 1978.

Houle, C. O. *Continuing Learning in the Professions.* San Francisco: Jossey-Bass, 1980.

Klein, G. A. and Weitzenfeld, J. *Improvement of Skills for Solving Ill-Defined Problems.* Technical Report TR 7831. Washington, D.C.: Human Resources Laboratory, U.S. Air Force, 1979.

Knowles, M. S. *Self-Directed Learning*. New York: Association Press, 1975.

Knowles, M. S. *The Modern Practice of Adult Education*. Rev. ed. New York: Association Press, 1980.

Knox, A. B. "Lifelong Self-Directed Education." In Blakely, R. J. (Ed.), *Fostering the Growing Need to Learn*. Rockville, Md.: Division of Regional Medical Programs, Bureau of Health Resources Development, U.S. Department of Health, Education, and Welfare, 1974.

Knox, A. B. *Adult Development and Learning: A Handbook on Individual Growth and Competence in the Adult Years*. San Francisco: Jossey-Bass, 1977.

Knox, A. B. (Ed.). *New Directions for Continuing Education: Assessing the Impact of Continuing Education*, no. 3. San Francisco: Jossey-Bass, 1979a.

Knox, A. B. (Ed.). *New Directions for Continuing Education: Enhancing Proficiencies of Continuing Educators*, no. 1. San Francisco: Jossey-Bass, 1979b.

Knox, A. B. (Ed.). *New Directions for Continuing Education: Teaching Adults Effectively*, no. 6. San Francisco: Jossey-Bass, 1980a.

Knox, A. B. "Proficiency Theory of Adult Learning." *Contemporary Educational Psychology*, 1980b, 5, 378–404.

Knox, A. B. (Ed.). *New Directions for Continuing Education: Leadership Strategies for Meeting New Challenges*, no. 13. San Francisco: Jossey-Bass, 1982.

Knox, A. B. "Adult Learning and Proficiency." In D. Klieber and M. Maehr (Eds.), *Motivation in Adulthood*. Vol. 5, *Advances in Motivation and Achievement*. Greenwich, Conn.: JAI Press, 1984.

Knox, A. B., and others. *Developing, Administering, and Evaluating Adult Education*. San Francisco: Jossey-Bass, 1980.

McKeachie, W. J. (Ed.). *New Directions for Teaching and Learning: Learning, Cognition, and College Teaching*, no. 2. San Francisco: Jossey-Bass, 1980.

Maddi, S. R. *Personality Theories: A Comparative Analysis*. Rev. ed. Homewood, Ill.: Dorsey Press, 1972.

Means, R. P. "Information-Seeking Behaviors of Michigan Family

Physicians." Unpublished doctoral dissertation, University of Illinois at Urbana-Champaign, 1979.

Merriam, S. B. (Ed.). *New Directions for Continuing Education: Linking Philosophy and Practice*, no. 15. San Francisco: Jossey-Bass, 1982.

Okun, M. A. (Ed.). *New Directions for Continuing Education: Programs for Older Adults*, no. 14. San Francisco: Jossey-Bass, 1982.

Pennington, F. C. (Ed.). *New Directions for Continuing Education: Assessing Educational Needs of Adults*, no. 7. San Francisco: Jossey-Bass, 1980.

Schein, E. *Career Dynamics: Matching Individual and Organizational Needs*. Reading, Mass.: Addison-Wesley, 1978.

Shipp, T. (Ed.). *New Directions for Continuing Education: Creative Financing and Budgeting*, no. 16. San Francisco: Jossey-Bass, 1982.

Smith, R. M. *Learning How to Learn*. Chicago: Follett, 1982.

Smith, R. M. (Ed.). *New Directions for Continuing Education: Helping Adults Learn How to Learn*, no. 19. San Francisco: Jossey-Bass, 1983.

Votruba, J. C. (Ed.). *New Directions for Continuing Education: Strengthening Internal Support for Continuing Education*, no. 9. San Francisco: Jossey-Bass, 1981.

Wilson, J. P. (Ed.). *New Directions for Continuing Education: Materials for Teaching Adults: Selection, Development, and Use*, no. 17. San Francisco: Jossey-Bass, 1983.

Appendix:
Definitions of the Quality Elements

)º

Of the total of 141 quality elements (QEs), 73 address the management of continuing education (CE) and 68 address the provision of continuing education. The elements are organized into five major sections (see Chapter One for a discussion of the sections). Within each section, the elements are divided into categories called attributes. In this Appendix, the attributes in each section are described and the quality elements within each attribute are defined.

I. Setting Direction for the CE Provider Unit

A. Defining the Mission

The mission of a CE provider unit is the major end or purpose the unit is established to fulfill. For example, the continuing education office in a hospital may broadly define its mission as meeting the need for continuing education of all health professionals at the hospital. Similarly, the department of continuing education at a college or university may define its mission as meeting the CE needs of all those in specific professional disciplines within the geographical area served by that university.

The defined mission of a CE provider unit is at the topmost level in the unit's hierarchy of goals, plans, and projects. The stated mission of the unit provides the standard of excellence against which all actions and proposals are ultimately judged.

Defining the mission is a more or less continuous process of balancing constituent needs with unit capabilities, parent organization interests, and environmental factors. Six quality elements address defining the CE provider unit mission.

QE 1. Determine the general educational needs of the potential audiences. This quality element suggests that the CE provider unit manager should, as part of the process for deriving a unit mission statement, acquire an understanding of the need for continuing education among the unit's constituency. In a hospital-based CE provider unit the numbers and disciplines of hospital professionals to be served would be essential information; so would other data such as records of any past CE undertakings, information on current and projected practice priorities and problems, and indications of needs gleaned from interviews or surveys of hospital personnel. CE provider units based in professional societies or colleges should collect similar information appropriate to their settings.

QE 2. Identify the relevant expectations of the parent organization and significant external groups and individuals. Few, if any, CE provider units are completely independent as organizational entities. The university-based CE provider unit is a member of the institution as a corporate body; the hospital-based CE provider unit owes allegiance to its parent facility; the CE provider unit in a professional society has a reporting relationship to the society officers. Even the privately held firm that provides CE will probably be a subsidiary or will be accountable to a board of directors, a group supplying capital, or directly to shareholders. This quality element suggests that the parent organization for a given CE provider unit will very likely have specific expectations of that unit and that another essential step in the process of defining the CE provider unit's mission is for the unit manager to determine those expectations. For example, there may be expectations related to cost and revenue. There may be expectations related to the CE provider unit's role in institutional development or change. The parent organization may see the CE provider unit as an instrument for communicating policy, for transfer and infusion of new technology, or for the achievement of other ends and purposes in health care. Some of these expectations may be explicit and others implicit; it is up to the CE provider unit manager to identify any expectations of either kind that may affect the unit's program for the provision of CE. Others besides the parent organization will also have expectations concerning the CE provider unit. Health care professionals who are prominent among the unit's potential constituency, community opinion leaders, and accrediting authorities are all examples of outside individuals and groups whose expectations concerning the CE provider unit may be significant considerations in the formulation of a mission statement for the unit.

QE 3. Identify the present or potential capabilities of the CE provider unit and limitations and constraints affecting it. The CE provider unit manager must carefully examine the current and foreseeable future capabilities of the unit. The manager must be concerned with what could be provided by the unit. To develop this kind of vision of future efforts, it is necessary to learn what faculty, resources, and facilities are or can be available to the unit. In the same way, it is necessary to identify any limiting factors that may apply to the CE provider unit such as laws or regulations that might hinder the unit's development and activities.

QE 4. Define the mission of the CE provider unit, considering what is expected of the unit, its capabilities and limitations, and the applicable constraints. This quality element suggests that the previously listed factors be weighed and that the outcome of the assessment be expressed as a brief statement of the CE provider unit's mission. The statement should name the general purpose that the unit will seek to accomplish. It should contain qualifiers that recognize any applicable constraints or limitations in terms of clientele, area or domain of services, or form of educational offerings.

QE 5. Obtain approval of the mission from external and parent organizations and agreement on the mission within the CE provider unit. The CE provider unit manager is responsible for ensuring that significant external groups do not dissent from the unit's mission, that the parent organization gives explicit assent to it, and that those who will undertake responsibilities for its achievement (faculty, staff) endorse the defined mission.

QE 6. Document and publicize the mission statement of the CE provider unit. The agreed-upon mission of the unit should be accessible to its publics, and the manager should assure that the mission statement is disseminated.

B. Eliciting Support for the CE Provider Unit from its Parent Organization

Quality elements 7 through 11 relate to the responsibility of CE provider unit management to work toward an appropriate valuation of continuing education as a facet of the parent organization's activities. The parent's support for the CE provider unit should be evident in such conditions as the placement of the CE provider unit in the parent organization and the degree to which authority is delegated to the CE manager.

QE 7. Encourage the parent organization to recognize CE as a specific function in its mission. The CE provider unit manager continually should strive to promote and reinforce the view that CE is one of the support components for quality health care. In a specialty society the CE program can help professionals stay abreast of new developments in their field. In a professional school, the CE program can meet educational needs common to those professionals in its geographical area. In a hospital, CE can address solutions to specific problems in care or can support planned enhancements in the standards of care. In any setting, the CE provider unit can help individual health professionals identify educational needs relevant to their practice and provide assistance in their efforts to meet the needs. Senior officials in the parent organization may need to be convinced that CE can and should be treated as a means to such ends. The overall responsibility for this effort falls to the CE provider unit manager.

QE 8. Seek placement for the CE provider unit, within the parent organization, that will enable and facilitate the accomplishment of the CE mission. The CE provider unit manager must strive to obtain a favorable spot for the unit in the parent organization's hierarchy of organizational components. The CE provider unit should have sufficient autonomy to be able to function in partnership with other parent components that support the delivery of care and educational activities.

QE 9. Request designation of a specific person as leader of the CE provider unit based on capabilities for defining and accomplishing the CE mission. Responsibility for general management of the CE provider unit should be given to a particular person, chosen on the basis of competence to function as the chief of the unit.

QE 10. Seek authority for the CE provider unit leader commensurate with the delegated responsibility. The degree of autonomy that the CE provider unit has will be governed by the authority granted by the parent organization to the unit's chief. The principle of parity of authority and responsibility should apply.

QE 11. Negotiate the provision of incentives and rewards for faculty and other experts to become involved with the CE provider unit. It is unlikely that any given CE provider unit will have on its immediate staff all the needed educational and content specialists for every activity it may undertake. Thus, the unit will need to secure such services on an as-required basis. The CE provider unit should be able to offer suitable rewards in exchange for the services, and there should be positive incentives to supply services to the CE provider unit. For example, there should be incentives and rewards for subject experts to provide services as CE faculty, where their content skills and CE skills are appropriate to the need.

C. Developing Support for CE in the Health Care Setting

Quality elements 12 through 18 relate to the CE provider unit manager's responsibility to foster acceptance and support of CE as a means to maintain and enhance the competence of health care professionals and a tool for supporting the provision of quality health care. In these seven quality elements the managerial responsibility to promote this view is specifically addressed.

QE 12. Promote the identification of professional problems or concerns by applying health care quality standards. CE provider unit managers, in their role as spokesmen for CE quality, should support and seek to bring about the formulation of quality care criteria that professionals can use to help define the problems or concerns they may have in maintaining or extending their competence as health care providers.

QE 13. Influence the health care setting to select appropriate individuals to participate in CE activities. To the extent that the wrong people show up at CE activities or use CE materials, the CE provider's effort to assure quality may be wasted. A second type of problem that might occur is when not enough of the right people participate. The CE provider unit manager should urge those in the health care setting to select the right persons or combinations of people to participate in a particular planned activity.

QE 14. Promote the provision of time, money, other needed resources, and incentives and rewards for health care professionals to engage in CE. The CE manager should promote the establishment of policies and procedures in the health care setting that will give specific support to CE, such as tuition payment, release time, furnishing a library, and providing space for journal club meetings. The element also suggests that the CE manager should seek to have a favorable environment for CE in the health care setting so that professionals are given incentives to participate in CE and rewards for their CE accomplishments.

QE 15. Encourage the provision of appropriate practice data and other data to contribute to the detection of potential problems and the evaluation of CE impact. The CE manager should urge health care providers to make practice data readily available to professionals, for use in conjunction with standards of care, as tools to help begin the process of needs identification and also to help verify that CE needs have been met. Other data such as organizational plans may also be appropriate for this purpose.

QE 16. Encourage the designation of individuals responsible for the collaborative analysis of practice problems and concerns and for receipt of referred noneducational problems. The CE provider unit manager should work toward the goal of establishing specific points of contact between education and health management. When such linkages have been made, it will be possible to identify and address specifically and simultaneously those parts of given practice problems that are caused by a lack of knowledge, skills or attitudes, and those parts that may have other causes. This will allow those problems that are not educationally based to be given to those more appropriately placed in the health care setting.

QE 17. Seek coordination of educational activities with any needed noneducational actions or resources. CE provider unit managers should strive to bring about coordination between the use of education and the use of noneducational resources to facilitate needed changes. For example, if new equipment is to be installed, the installation should take place in conjunction with a targeted activity on the use of the equipment. If the solution to a particular patient care problem involves remedial education in the use of given diagnostic tests, then it should be assured that procedures for ordering the tests and making the results available are functioning smoothly so that health professionals seeking to apply the CE can easily do so.

QE 18. Influence the health care setting to provide support for the application of learning to practice. The CE provider unit manager should make those in a position to control the environment in the health care setting aware of and responsive to the possible needs of professionals for specific kinds of support in applying learning to practice. This may include providing practice time, special supervision, or additional personnel or equipment.

D. Relating to Other Parties External to the CE Unit

Quality elements 19 through 21 cover the need for CE provider unit management to tie in to significant influences outside the parent organization and the immediate market setting. Such linkages might include, for example, learned societies, community opinion leaders, or accrediting authorities.

QE 19. Identify individuals and groups, or organizations external to the CE provider unit, whose actions and attitudes can affect the achievement of its mission. The CE provider unit manager should make an assessment of the unit's environment, to find out which individuals and groups will be important to the unit. For example, there are potential learners represented by professional groups, opinion leaders in the health care sector, and contact points in accrediting bodies and other regulatory groups.

QE 20. Establish and maintain appropriate relationships with the identified individuals and groups or organizations. Having identi-

fied the people and organizations important to the CE provider unit,
the manager should form linkages to them.

QE 21. *Determine the goals of the identified individuals and
groups or organizations and consider their implications for the CE
provider unit.* This quality element suggests that the CE provider unit
manager use the linkages that connect the unit to its environment as a
means to obtain information on the goals and attitudes of those people and groups who matter in considerations of the unit's mission,
strategy, policy, and activities.

E. Adapting the CE Provider Unit

Quality elements 22 through 25 address management's role in
changing the CE provider unit to facilitate its growth and development and to respond to outside changes.

QE 22. *Review the CE provider unit's mission, goals, objectives, structure, policies, plans, and procedures periodically and as
needed.* Management should conduct searching reassessments of all
the CE provider unit's managerial responsibilities and techniques on
a regular basis and also whenever special circumstances suggest such
reviews.

QE 23. *Use information from monitoring the CE provider unit
as a source of indicators of potential need for change in the CE provider unit.* The CE provider unit manager continually should be alert
to any signals from inside the unit indicating a need for change. For
example, the results of program evaluations may suggest a need for
improvements in the program. Contradictory evidence between internal evaluations and reports from participants after returning to practice may suggest that evaluation methods themselves could be improved. The manager should keep a constant watch on all the telling
measures of the unit's programs and on the state of its financial,
physical, and human resources.

QE 24. *Use information from monitoring the health care and
societal environments as a source of indicators for potential change
in the CE provider unit.* In addition to monitoring the CE provider
unit itself, the manager must maintain a watch on the unit's environment in order to detect indications of the need for change. The
environment of the unit includes its parent organization, its mar-

ketplace, the health care setting, and all other people and groups capable of exerting influence on the CE program.

QE 25. Promote and foster research in CE and the development of improved methods for CE. Research and development serves as a fountainhead for programs, and CE provider unit managers should take the initiative for this activity. For example, all CE provider units should, according to their means, encourage research in CE that may lead to better approaches to education. Further, any CE provider unit can seek better ways to conduct and manage its programs.

F. Satisfying Accountability

Quality elements 26 through 29 cover the obligation of the CE provider unit manager to render an account of resources, results, or other matters to parent organizations, accrediting authorities, or other people or agencies who impose accountability on the CE provider unit.

QE 26. Identify to whom and in what context the CE provider unit is accountable. The CE provider unit manager should identify to whom the unit is accountable and the context of these accountability expectations.

QE 27. Identify the proposed accountability requirements for the CE provider unit. The manager of the CE provider unit should identify the criteria on which accountability is based and the extant requirements for reporting or other obligations.

QE 28. Negotiate proposed accountability requirements that would cause problems for the CE provider unit. The CE provider unit manager is urged to attempt negotiations toward relief of accountability requirements that would impinge on the quality of CE. For example, if a small CE provider unit is expected to account for its own finances but the time spent on financial bookkeeping and reporting would force less time to be spent on CE program planning, the manager might be able to persuade the parent organization to supply some of the needed accounting services.

QE 29. Provide accountability documentation. There is a need for the CE provider unit to maintain or deliver documents or records to substantiate the proper conduct of accountable activities.

Examples included tax data, personnel files, educational program planning process, or others.

II. Organizing the CE Provider Unit

A. Planning

Quality elements 30 through 37 address the process of creating and documenting the plans that will define the CE provider unit's future targets and mark out the path and timetable for reaching each target. These quality elements deal with planning at both the strategic and operational levels, including market planning as well as planning for activities, products, and services, and for unit management.

QE 30. Define the education and management functions needed to accomplish the mission of the CE provider unit. In the planning for a CE provider unit, each operational and managerial activity necessary for the functioning of the unit should be identified. This process should be repeated periodically or whenever internal or external circumstances make it necessary.

QE 31. Develop a strategic plan, a long-range plan, and policies and procedures to enable the accomplishment of the mission. CE provider management should consider the basic strategies that it will use in accomplishing the unit's mission and incorporate the strategies in a formal plan. For example, a CE provider unit with very few resources might rely heavily on a strategy of promoting and aiding self-directed learning efforts by its clientele professionals in order to accomplish the mission. This would conserve scarce resources of the unit for use in providing learning activities intended to help meet high-priority needs related to present problems or concerns of larger groups of health professionals.

In addition to strategic planning, the quality element asks CE provider unit management to attend to the development of the concomitant policies and procedures the unit will need to perform its various operational and management functions.

QE 32. Develop a set of goals and objectives that reflects the mission and the strategic plan of the CE provider unit. Once the mission and strategic plan have been established, it is important to develop a series of goals. These goals and objectives reflect the mechanisms that the CE provider unit will use to meet its mission and adapt to needed changes as reflected in its strategic plan.

QE 33. Negotiate a resolution whenever requirements and constraints placed on the CE provider unit by its parent organization conflict with the provision of quality CE. It is the responsibility of the CE provider unit manager to seek solutions to any potential problems in CE quality that might stem from impositions of policy, strategy, or procedure on the unit by its parent. For example, a parent organization may intend that the CE provider unit use only members of the parent as faculty for CE. In a given situation, for instance, the persons who would be available under such a policy might not have the necessary level of skills in continuing education to inspire confidence in the participants that they can reach the learning objectives. In such a case, the CE provider unit manager should attempt to negotiate in order to be able to use other faculty when appropriate.

QE 34. Prepare activity plans for the CE provider unit, specifying the tasks to be carried out, sequence of work, time lines, expected progress points, and desired objectives to be achieved. An operational plan for the CE provider unit should be prepared. The plan should incorporate the unit's current objectives compatible with the unit's mission and strategies. It should spell out the resources and schedule for reaching the objectives and should include any intermediate assessments that are appropriate, as well as other measures of progress toward objectives.

QE 35. Select markets according to the capabilities of the CE provider unit. The CE provider unit should identify the segments or portions of the market to be served that should receive particular attention or emphasis. Emphasis is determined by the particular strengths or capabilities of the unit, according to its overall strategies.

QE 36. Develop overall promotional strategies to reach the selected markets. The CE provider unit manager should direct specific attention to mechanisms to reach the unit's markets. For example, a CE provider unit seeking to reach widely dispersed health care professionals might elect to emphasize stand-alone instructional packages or might arrange (perhaps through parent organizations) for the use of teleconferencing or other networking.

QE 37. Obtain concurrence on plans from parent organizations and agreement on them within the CE provider unit. It is important that the CE provider unit manager secure approval by parent organizations of the unit's plans, as well as agreement and support from those within the CE provider unit.

B. Developing the Organization of the CE Provider Unit

Quality elements 38 through 41 address the specific task of creating an ordered set of relationships among the people in the CE provider unit. This task is relatively simple in small units but may be quite complex in larger ones.

QE 38. Delineate the tasks necessary to carry out and manage the provision of CE activities, products, and services. This quality element covers the translation of the basic functions of the CE provider unit (see QE 30) into assignable tasks. For example, the function of providing CE might include the tasks of conducting needs assessments or performing evaluations; similarly, there are the managerial tasks of unit planning or performance appraisal.

QE 39. Organize the CE provider unit to accomplish the tasks with optimal use of resources. The CE provider unit manager should seek to develop an organizational pattern for the unit that facilitates effective work and productive utilization of all resources.

QE 40. Establish lines of communication that facilitate accomplishing the tasks. The manager is responsible for establishing clear lines of communications into the CE provider unit, within the unit, and from the unit to the outside.

QE 41. Develop the organizational arrangements for involving individuals and groups external to the CE provider unit who can facilitate the accomplishment of its mission. The CE provider unit manager should establish ad hoc planning committees, oversight councils, or other groups that will enable the unit to bring the perspectives of learners, parent organizational representatives and others, as necessary, to the educational and managerial processes. For example, a planning committee can assist in the identification of educational needs and in the choice of educational activities to pursue.

C. Developing the Information System

Management's responsibility with regard to developing a system to meet the CE provider unit's information needs is the subject of quality elements 42 through 44.

QE 42. Define the records and documentation essential to support the educational and management functions of the CE provider unit. The information that will be needed to operate and manage the unit must be identified. This should include, for example, unit plans, records of needs assessments, and financial data. All these and other pieces of information will be needed in recorded form.

QE 43. Describe the records and documentation needed by individuals and groups external to the CE provider unit. This quality element addresses identifying the information that will be sent to recipients outside the CE provider unit. Examples would include data for accreditation submittals, budget requests to parent organizations, or evaluation reports to learners or learner groups.

QE 44. Develop a system to collect, store, and retrieve the relevant data. There must be means to obtain, file, and recover the information identified as needed by the CE provider unit. The complexity, organization, and technology of the file should be commensurate with the nature of the information requirement.

D. Obtaining Resources

Quality elements 45 through 49 are directed at the manager's role in getting the resources needed to operate and manage the CE provider unit, including money, facilities and supplies, and staff.

QE 45. Specify the money, people, facilities, materials, and time needed to perform the educational and management functions of the CE provider unit. The total resource requirement for the CE provider unit must be estimated as accurately as possible.

QE 46. Identify the potential sources for obtaining the needed resources. The CE provider unit manager should identify all the sources from which resources might come, such as parent organization, learners, or outside organizations.

QE 47. Seek commitment for timely availability of resources. Agreement should be obtained on the types, amounts, and timing of resources to the CE provider unit. Note that timing may be important in addition to type and amount. For example, resources are needed to be available in time to support preliminary activities like needs assessment and priority setting, as well as to support the actual delivery of an educational activity.

QE 48. Revise activity plans to resolve resource discrepancies without jeopardizing the quality of the CE provider unit's program. The frequent need for readjustment of plans to take fluctuations in resource availability into account should be recognized. It is suggested that preserving quality should be a principal criterion in making needed adjustments.

QE 49. Develop and use criteria for recruiting and hiring staff and selecting faculty based on their ability to contribute to the accomplishment of the CE provider unit's mission. Specific attention should be paid to the unit's CE specialty whenever staff are to be hired or faculty are needed. For example, it is important to ensure that faculty teaching skills embrace CE, in distinction from preparatory education.

E. Setting Standards

Quality elements 50 and 51 address the need to establish standards for the CE provider unit.

QE 50. Set standards to assess the accomplishment of the CE provider unit's plans and the implementation of its policies. It is a basic tenet of management that standards such as standards for policy adherence should be set to cover the unit's entire operation for the accomplishment of organizational objectives and for financial records.

QE 51. Set standards for the educational processes and products of the CE provider unit, to assure the use of effective methods consistent with the resources of the unit. This quality element suggests the need for standards addressing the program planning process including needs assessment, design, and evaluation.

III. Providing CE Activities and Products

This category of quality elements refers to those projects undertaken by a CE provider unit to meet successfully the educational needs of groups of health professionals. The learning projects offered require a series of activities by the organization that assure their quality. These activities include the assessment of a given educational need, development of educational objectives, selection of specific educational approaches, selection of faculty and content, implementation of the educational activities, and their evaluation.

A. Detecting Problems or Concerns

In order for a CE provider unit to develop quality educational activities, it is imperative that the planning process begin with the needs, problems, or concerns of health professionals. This attribute on "Detecting Problems or Concerns" deals with sources of information that can be used to identify or detect problems or concerns of health professionals. It also emphasizes the need to involve the health professionals or a sampling of health professionals in this process.

QE 52. Use data from the practice setting and the professions as a source for identifying potential problems or concerns. The most important source of information that can yield valuable data concerning needs or problems of health professionals is the data found within the practice setting. The charts, the patient-care records, and profiling information are invaluable in detecting the health professional's specific problems that might lend themselves to educational intervention. The CE provider unit should as one of its high-priority activities obtain access to summary data from medical centers, clinics, or private group practices that might suggest areas for educational programming. The professions, in many cases subspecialties within a profession, have also been in the process of developing standards of care against which health professionals can compare their own performance. To the degree that the CE provider units understand the nature of practice undertaken by health professionals and the problems found within those practices, they will better be able to provide quality continuing education.

QE 53. Consider new knowledge and technology and changing attitudes as sources for identifying potential problems or concerns. This quality element deals with another very important source of information relevant to detecting needs, problems, or concerns of health professionals. Because of the explosion of new knowledge and technology, health professionals must make special efforts to stay abreast of new drugs, of new treatment modalities, of new research findings, and of new uses of technology to assist them in their diagnosis and treatment activities. One important function of a CE provider unit is to monitor new knowledge and technology for its implications for health professionals. The CE provider unit should develop CE activities that allow health professionals to synthesize and integrate this new information so that they can constantly improve their practice of health care. In addition, attitudes are constantly changing within the society, directly affecting health professionals' ability to provide quality health care. Attitudes toward death and dying, toward communication and interaction between the patient and the health professional, attitudes of consumerism and of patients' rights all affect the practice of medicine. As new social attitudes and mores develop, CE provider units must remain cognizant of the changes and assist health professionals in determining their implications.

QE 55. Use aggregate data descriptive of populations, health problems, and health-care practices as sources for identifying potential problems and concerns. For the CE provider units with diverse target audiences, data on populations, health problems, and health care practices provide an invaluable source of information that can be used to uncover potential problems or concerns. Gathering these data does not require the additional work necessary to develop questionnaires and secure additional input from individual learners. It should be remembered, however, that these data are only helpful in suggesting possible areas of problems or concerns and not for finalizing specific educational project topics.

QE 56. Corroborate detected problems or concerns by using data from more than one source. This quality element suggests the need to look at multiple sources of data to validate information from one source suggesting problem areas. If data from several sources indicate a given problem area, there is a greater likelihood that the need is valid. It is not always necessary to use more than one data source, but doing so will give the CE provider unit more confidence in the information that they use to plan future educational activities.

QE 57. Involve learner(s) in identifying problems or concerns. The importance of involving the learners in all aspects of the design of educational activities will be seen throughout the list of quality elements dealing with the educational process. This quality element suggests that learners representing the target population be involved in various steps in the identification of problems or concerns that could lead to educational projects for the same audience. Without this involvement there is little likelihood of changing behavior, for awareness is a necessary prerequisite.

B. Analyzing Problems or Concerns

Once specific educational needs, problems, or concerns have been identified, it is necessary to analyze the nature of the suggested problems or concerns prior to subsequent educational planning. This step in the educational process is critical for the further development of educational projects that will be responsive to the needs of the target audience. It requires planners in CE provider units to look beyond the nature of the stated problem or concern to their inherent or possible causes. Furthermore, those causes must be analyzed to determine if some type of educational intervention could solve the suggested problem or concern. Once it is determined that a specific problem can be resolved through an educational project, then the further analysis involves determining what the difference is between current competence (knowledge, skills, or attitudes) and what is considered to be ideal knowledge, skills, or attitudes in the identified problem area.

QE 58. Work with learner(s) and others to identify cause(s) of problems or concerns. It is suggested that CE provider unit planning groups involve samples or all the target audience in suggesting the potential causes behind identified needs, problems, or concerns of health professionals. This involvement may take the form of potential learners represented on the planning group or of survey work done by pencil-and-paper instruments, telephone calls, or in-depth discussion with potential learners. (Depending upon the source of data suggesting the need, there may be additional documentation of the causes of the identified need that would not require additional survey-type of work.) The important point is that for a given educational activity to have the desired impact in terms of behavior, it is imperative that the learner(s) be involved in not only identifying the problem but also helping to explain potential causes and solutions.

QE 58.1. *Classify problems or concerns as educational or non-educational.* When a given need, problem, or concern has been identified and a planning group or individual is working with learners to help explain the causes behind the need, it is suggested that these causes be classified as either educational or noneducational. This is done by determining whether the need is caused by lack of knowledge, skills, or attitudes on the part of individual health professionals or by some other deficiency. If the former seems the case, then the need may be classified as educational. If the latter is more likely, such as a system problem that would require additional manpower, changes in organizational structure, or additional resources, then the need should be classified as noneducational.

QE 59. *Attribute educational needs to a present or potential gap between desirable and actual knowledge, skills, or attitudes.* Once it has been determined that a given need is educational in nature, the next step is to analyze further the cause in terms of possible gaps between desirable and actual knowledge, skills, or attitudes. This is a two-part process. First, the educational need is further broken down into some deficiency of a) knowledge—the information needed to perform, b) skills—the psychomotor requirements of a given performance, or c) attitudes—the psychosocial orientation of health professionals toward quality health delivery. Once this is determined, it is necessary to take each area of knowledge, skills, or attitudes and determine the nature of the gap between present and desirable levels. To do this often requires some educational project assessment activities to determine present knowledge levels or skill levels against which to compare what experts in the field indicate are minimally desired competencies. The difference between the desirable and the actual forms the foundation of the required educational intervention.

QE 60. Refer noneducational needs to those in the health care setting who are responsible for their solution. This quality element suggests that the role of the CE provider unit in improving the quality of health care delivery may require that it work with the health care institution to bring about solutions to the identified problems, even though those solutions are noneducational in nature. This role will probably be limited to suggesting to health care management the nature of findings that indicate specific problems and possible noneducational solutions. The CE provider unit will probably not be involved in making decisions about the implementation of these noneducational solutions.

C. Identifying Educational Priorities

When CE provider units undertake the task of identifying and analyzing specific needs, problems, or concerns of health professionals, it is inevitable that many more needs will emerge than the unit is capable of handling. Because there is a limited amount of resources available and because the number of needs is potentially unlimited, it is essential that the CE organization develop some mechanisms to set priorities. The criteria by which these priorities can be established may include the severity of the identified problem, the potential for meeting the problem, the cost involved, the resources available, factors existing in the environment that could either assist or hinder meeting the needs, and the degree of match between needs of individual health professionals and goals of health care organizations within which they work.

QE 61. Obtain an assessment of the severity or impact of the health care problems associated with the identified need. The degree of severity of the health problem that surrounds the educational need represents an important criterion for deciding about developing educational projects. If a lack of knowledge, skill, or attitude on the part of a health professional or groups of health professionals can lead to a life-threatening situation, the solution to that problem becomes far more important than other identified needs. As with all such criteria, however, it is important to note that none alone can be the sole determinant of whether an educational project is developed to solve a specific identified problem. In the real world it is more likely that a number of these criteria are used to make overall decisions about the development of educational projects.

QE 62. Estimate the health care benefits derived from meeting each identified need. Another important criterion for determining priorities for educational projects might be the magnitude of the health-related benefits that could be derived from providing an educational solution to an identified problem. A CE provider unit may undertake a major educational project, the benefit of which would accrue to increased competence of very few health professionals; however, it may be more cost-effective to meet the needs of multiple health professionals who are dealing with a problem that relates to many patients or potential patients. Again, however, this criterion should be viewed in light of the other criteria described in this section.

QE 63. Estimate the relative potential for meeting the identified needs through education. The focus of this quality element is for the CE provider unit to determine the potential of successfully meeting the needs that have been identified. In some cases needs are detected, the solutions to which are educational in nature. In addition, they deal with severe health care problems; however, there is very little chance that the CE intervention could, within a meaningful time frame, lead to any improvement. For this reason the relative potential for meeting the identified needs through educational activities should be considered.

QE 64. Determine the relative cost of meeting each identified need. In addition to determining the relative potential for impact, the costs to the CE provider unit of meeting the educational need should be determined. There are limited resources, and it may be wiser for a CE provider organization to meet many needs that are of less cost than to focus all the activity on meeting one specific need that is so costly it precludes projects in other important areas.

QE 65. Determine resources available to meet each identified need. All resources required to meet successfully the stated needs must be identified, so that their management can be determined. As the CE provider organization lists the identified needs, it should also determine the potential for impact, the cost, and the exact nature of the resources necessary.

QE 66. Ascertain the potential environmental factors that would assist or hinder meeting each identified need. In some cases identified needs that have been determined to be educational stand very little chance of being met because of certain environmental factors. Co-workers' attitudes, payment and fee schedules, third-party payers, limitations of the work environment, all might work against being able to bring about successfully the desired behavior change of the target health professional audience. In other cases, some of these same environmental concerns may work to facilitate meeting the educational need. The point is that the CE provider unit must be cognizant of the factors that are outside of their control that may assist or hinder in meeting the identified educational needs of health professionals and use this information in deciding about what projects to undertake.

QE 67. Verify the degree of match between learning needs and goals of the learner's health care organization. An identified need may be higher on a CE provider unit's priority list if that particular need is consistent with the documented or recognized goal of the organization within which the health professional works. To the degree that the goals are compatible, the CE provider unit may feel more confident in involving itself in assisting that health professional to meet the identified need.

QE 68. Assure congruence of identified needs with the mission and goals of the CE provider unit. The CE provider unit must not only try to ascertain the degree of match between the learning goals of health professionals and the goals of the organizations within which they work but also to consider the goals and mission of the CE provider unit itself. In some cases certain identified needs would require educational projects that are outside the scope of the agreed-upon mission of the organization. For example, the need may require educational activities for groups of health professionals whom the CE provider unit is not prepared to address.

QE 69. Obtain consensus on the relative priority of each identified need. Once a list of identified needs has been completed, the CE provider unit ought to document the rank order of each identified need. These rankings should be presented by the CE provider unit for ratification by the health professionals they serve. In this way the organization can make more meaningful decisions about which educational needs to attempt to resolve and which needs to ignore temporarily.

QE 70. Select educational needs that will be addressed. In some cases identified needs may be grouped together because the solution of one suggests possible solutions of others. Once critieria have been listed for helping establish the priorities, it is then important to identify and list those educational needs that will be met.

QE 71. Establish a schedule for the timely accomplishment of priority educational projects. A schedule and time line should be prepared to assist the CE provider organization in planning a series or sequence of educational projects based on the priorities established.

D. Setting Educational Objectives

The need exists to define the relevant audiences for each educational project, to obtain further involvement of potential learners in translating identified needs into learning outcomes, and, finally, to state the learning outcomes in such a way that it is possible to determine if they have been met.

QE 72. Define potential audience for educational projects. Once the needs have been identified and ranked according to priorities and a list of educational projects has been established by the CE provider unit, the target audiences for each project must be specified. The audiences should be described in terms of area of specialty, type of hospital, interest, and necessary prerequisite skills or attitudes. The purpose of this activity is to seek a match between the learners and the learning objectives.

QE 73. Obtain involvement of learner(s) to define desirable learning outcomes from identified needs. The learner or samples of learners should participate in translating the needs into desirable learning outcomes. These outcomes when described by learners lead to more relevant learning activities with a greater chance of attaining the desirable impact. Without either the involvement of the learners or the articulation of specific desirable outcomes, it will be difficult to either attain or measure the outcome of the educational project.

QE 74. Establish relevant, achievable, and accessible objectives from identified learning outcomes. The CE provider unit can be most helpful in assisting health professionals on planning groups to take the desired learning outcomes as defined by potential audiences and develop specific educational objectives. These objectives should be relevant to the learning outcomes that emanated from the identified needs. They should also be achievable in that the CE provider unit feels confident in being able to provide the required educational activity. Finally, they should be assessable, for if there is no way to determine whether a given educational objective has been met, it makes little sense to spend the time developing learning projects. It should also be remembered that educational objectives are not an end in themselves; they are merely a means to link identified needs of health professionals with relevant learning activities to satisfy needs.

E. Selecting Educational Approaches

Needs, problems, or concerns of health professionals have been identified, causes have been analyzed, and educational objectives have been described. The next set of activities deals with decisions about what type of educational approach should be used to meet the agreed-upon objectives. Within this quality attribute are such activities as determining availability of resources, ascertaining learning style preferences, and determining where and when educational activities, materials, and services would best meet the needs. All these activities should ideally occur prior to making final decisions about a given educational project.

QE 75. Determine resources available for educational activity. For any CE provider unit it is imperative to make decisions early in the planning process about the amount and nature of the resources to be made available for a given educational activity. After educational objectives have been defined, the exact amount and type of resources available to meet those objectives must be made known to the CE planners. It is important to base decisions about the resources required on the nature of the objectives and decisions about the educational approach designed to meet the needs based on the resources available.

QE 76. Ascertain learning style preferences of learner(s) for consideration in selecting educational approaches. All learners have different ways of learning. In making decisions about what educa-

tional approach a CE provider might use to meet a given set of
educational objectives, it is helpful to obtain some input from the
target audiences as to their preferences for educational formats, methods, and media. This input can help the planning committee design
activities that have a greater chance of having the desired impact.

*QE 77. Consider the nature of the learning objectives in
selecting educational approaches.* Learning objectives that deal with
the development of psychomotor skills obviously require different
kinds of educational approaches than are typical for a large conference made up of several lecturers. This quality element suggests
that, whenever possible, a match should be made between the type of
learning objective—bringing about cognitive gain, developing a certain skill, or changing a specific attitude—and the educational approach selected to meet that objective. If a psychomotor skill is the
primary focus of the need, then opportunities ought to be made available for individual learners not only to understand the specifics of that
skill but also to practice the desired behaviors with appropriate feedback from experts.

*QE 78. Determine when and where instruction should take
place.* The planning committee or planners should obtain suggestions
from learners regarding the most convenient time and location for any
educational project aimed at meeting their identified, practice-related
needs. This consideration will increase the chances of meeting the
identified needs in a way that is most convenient for the learners.

*QE 79.1. Determine what educational activities, products, and
services would be best to meet the identified objectives.* A decision
regarding educational activities, products, or consulting services must
be made at this point in the planning process. Information gathered
and analyzed concerning the need, the nature of the educational objective, the resources available, and the learning style of the learners will
facilitate that decision.

*QE 79.2. Determine whether educational activities or products
can be selected from available resources or must be developed.* Once
the decision has been reached concerning the educational approach,
it needs to be determined whether additional development is needed
or whether activities and materials previously developed can be used
to meet the identified objective(s). All too often CE provider units

are reinventing the wheel instead of using existing information or courses and materials to meet the specified objectives. Some systematic way of searching available educational resources can uncover many quality programs and materials that can save staff development time and will be equally relevant and effective.

F. Selecting Faculty and Content

After educational objectives have been established and the approaches selected, the next series of tasks relates to the selection of faculty and the determination of currency and accuracy of the content to meet the stated objectives. It is suggested for faculty and planners to assess or assist learners to assess their present knowledge, skills, or attitudes as they relate to the specified objectives. This enables the planner to relate objectives, content, and target audience.

QE 80. Select faculty with appropriate content and CE teaching expertise. Frequently, the planning of continuing education activities begins with the selection of faculty, followed by content development based upon the expertise of the faculty. The quality elements suggest the reverse, a more logical process beginning with an up-front analysis of educational needs, followed by an analysis of the content necessary to meet the needs. With the content firmly in mind, the selection of faculty is easier and will yield a more valuable contribution toward meeting the needs of the learners. It is also suggested that in selecting faculty the CE provider unit consider the level of teaching experience and specific expertise in teaching adult health professional colleagues.

QE 81. Assess or assist learners to assess present knowledge, skills, or attitudes related to established learning objectives. CE provider units ought to develop mechanisms to allow learners who will be attending conferences to compare their knowledge with stated objectives. In this way learners will be better able to focus their learning within the structured activities to assure the desired outcome.

QE 82. Inform faculty of learning objectives, the nature of learners, and their entry-level knowledge, skills, and attitudes. The faculty should be informed about any data relative to the level of knowledge and skills of the potential audience relative to the educational objectives. In this fashion faculty are cognizant of not only what is desired in terms of the objective but also who the learners are and what their entry-level skills, knowledge, or attitudes appear to be. When so informed, the instructors are better able to provide content to learners in a way that has a much greater chance of meeting the learning objectives for the project.

QE 83. Assure the currency and accuracy of content and its relevance to the learning objectives. It is desirable that the planning group select content and validate its currency and accuracy in regard to the stated objectives. This helps to avoid the situation where faculty decide on their own what is relevant content. For this purpose the planning committee should have available content outlines from faculty prior to the actual activity. The importance of a dialogue among the faculty members of a given project cannot be overemphasized.

G. Determining Instructional Strategies

There is an entire body of knowledge on instructional psychology that is relevant to designing instruction to meet prespecified objectives. From that body of knowledge several concepts exist that could assist CE provider units in the design of educational activities to meet the needs of learners. These concepts relate to sequencing of content, providing examples and practice opportunities, and providing the learners with feedback on their performance.

QE 84. Sequence content in a manner to assist learner(s) in meeting learning objectives. There are a number of algorithms suggested for sequencing content that can assist learners in meeting their own learning objectives. Some of these include sequencing the material from simple to complex, from the more general to the more specific concepts, from the central point outward to peripheral ideas. Each of these methods of sequencing has its strengths and weaknesses. The main point, however, is to develop content in an organized, systematic fashion that assists learners to learn and to validate the sequence of the CE organization to determine whether its sequencing strategies seem to facilitate learning.

QE 85. Assure that instruction incorporates sufficient examples of concepts to be learned. Instruction should be enriched by examples to facilitate the comprehension and learning of concepts. In some cases it is also helpful to provide what has been termed nonexamples to contrast with the examples provided. This will further increase the learner's ability to discriminate between the desired concept and other notions or ideas.

QE 86. Provide opportunities for involvement if content is related to changing attitudes. If the objectives relate to changing attitudes, one of the more effective ways of accomplishing these is to provide opportunities for the learner to discuss and, perhaps, personally experience the significance and consequence of specific attitudes in particular situations. Experiential learning as supported by role playing can often be the most powerful form of incentive for behavior change, while attendance at a lecture on the subject may not be very effective.

QE 87. Provide opportunities for practice if content is related to the development or maintenance of skills. If one is to learn a concept that provides information necessary to perform a certain skill, it is not only important to provide examples of that skill but also to design opportunities into the learning experience for the learner to practice what is being taught. A combination of comprehending the concept, being given examples of what kind of skill is desirable, and being allowed to practice that particular skill seems to be most effective in bringing about the desired learning.

QE 88. Provide learner(s) with feedback on performance. Feedback on performance should link with the development of examples and opportunities for practice. Learning a new skill, provision of sufficient examples, opportunities for practice, and receiving feedback on the practice by an expert enhance the learning of the new skill(s) necessary to maintain or improve professional competence.

H. Implementing Educational Projects

Once the educational project has been designed, it is then necessary for the CE provider unit to implement the activity in a way that is consistent with the purpose and design of the activity. The CE provider unit must make every effort to meet the needs of the participants. This includes assuring that the learning activity occurs in a manner, time, and place convenient for the learner and that all relevant resources are made available to learners.

QE 89. Implement educational projects as designed. This quality element suggests that the design of the educational activity is the guideline for its implementation. Provided an activity is designed according to established principles, care must be taken that those involved in the implementation—the logistics staff, the faculty, the evaluators, and the learners—are proceeding according to design and introduce modifications only to improve the chances of meeting the stated objectives. Often a workshop is planned based on information received from potential participants. Should, however, the needs of the audience appear different from what was anticipated, modifications are needed to assure that the activity assist the actual learners in meeting their educational objectives.

QE 90. Assure that instruction occurs in a manner, time, and place convenient to the learner. All the logistical activities that are so critical to the success of an educational activity should be guided by the idea that the learner needs to feel as comfortable as possible in the learning environment. This requires obtaining input as to the time and place most convenient for them, given what is to be learned and how long the learning is going to take. Looking at learning styles is also helpful in assuring that the instruction occurs in a manner that seems to be appropriate not only to the objectives and the content but also to the individual participant.

QE 91. Make relevant resources available to learner(s) to assist in meeting objectives. The CE provider unit must bring together all the suggested resources that could support the learners in their attempts at meeting their learning objectives. This might include audiovisual support, paper-and-pencil tests, additional journal articles, magazines, books, or anything else that would facilitate meeting the objectives.

I. Designing Evaluations

In evaluating continuing education projects it is important to start with an analysis of the individuals and organizations with a need for evaluation data. It is then important to determine what the nature of these evaluation data are and what resources are required to obtain them. This information will guide decisions about the extent of the evaluation plan for a given CE activity.

QE 92.1. Identify the individual(s) or organization(s) having an interest in or need for evaluation. For any given educational activity there are many aspects that can be evaluated. The first step in designing an evaluation plan includes making a more systematic determination of who the audiences are for the evaluation data and the relative importance of these audiences, be they individuals or organizations. Typical audiences include upper-level management of the health care setting, funding organizations for the CE projects, the learners, and the CE provider unit.

QE 92.2. Determine evaluation needs. Once the specific audience or audiences have been identified, it is important to ascertain what information they need to make decisions regarding the educational activity. A consideration of the importance to the CE provider unit of the identified audiences and of the relative significance of the specified information will assist the CE provider unit in narrowing the focus of the evaluation effort to avoid unnecessary expenditure of resources.

QE 92.3. Determine the focus of the evaluation. Based upon the audiences for evaluation data, the information needs of those audiences, and the nature of the learning project, the CE provider unit must make a decision concerning the focus of the evaluation efforts. This focus, among others, might be the potential impact of the CE activity, the amount of resources expended to meet the educational needs, the learner satisfaction with the learning activity, the cognitive gain, attitudinal shift, or skill development attained by learners. Of all the variables that can be evaluated, the specification of the focus sets the parameters within which the evaluator makes determinations as to the relative worth of the educational project.

QE 93.1. Estimate resources required for the evaluation and compare with resources actually available. Once the focus has been identified, it is important to determine the amount of resources available for evaluation. The CE provider unit that controls the resources must make the decision as to the extent of resources going toward evaluation of a given project. The evaluator brings to that decision the information about the audience, their information needs, and the focus of the evaluation. The CE provider must match that information with the amount of resources available so that a final allocation of resources can be made.

QE 93.2 Determine the scope of the evaluation. On the basis of actual resources allocated to evaluation, the CE provider unit (and evaluator) will determine the extent of the proposed evaluation. This should include scope and depth at which the success of the educational project will be evaluated. As an example, if cognitive gain score is one of the focuses of the evaluation, the amount of resources still may limit this kind of determination to a simple multiple-choice cognitive pre- and posttest; on the other hand, more resources would allow for use of standardized testing and scoring.

J. Planning and Conducting Evaluations

The development of an evaluation plan is a critical step in the evaluator's tasks and serves the purpose of clearly delineating what will be evaluated and how it will be done. The selection of the evaluation methods flows from the focus and extent of the evaluation as determined mutually by the CE provider unit and the evaluator. Once an evaluation plan is developed and implemented, it is necessary to analyze the data obtained. This section deals with planning and conducting evaluations by CE provider units.

QE 94. Choose evaluation methods that will best meet the identified information needs within the available resources. The evaluation methods are dictated by two major considerations: the information needs of the identified target audiences and the resources available to meet the identified information needs. Some evaluation methods require extensive use of resources, expertise, and time, while others are simpler, obtain data much quicker, and require less extensive use of resources and expertise. There are payoffs for these types of decisions in terms of validity and reliability of the data gathered, and these must be taken into consideration in selecting the methods. In the final analysis, the CE provider unit desires the least expensive way to obtain the most valid data that allow determinations as to the relative value of a given educational project and the methods used to obtain the desired learning outcomes. This information can then be used by the provider unit to increase the quality of its activities and increase the chances of meeting learning objectives.

QE 95. Develop an evaluation plan. The evaluation plan should clearly state the audiences, the objectives of the learning activity, the information needs of the audiences, the evaluation methods to be used, the instruments to be developed, the responsible party or parties to collect the data, the analyses to be used, and time lines that can be agreed upon by all concerned. This will prevent problems within the CE provider unit that can develop when the evaluation plan is not clearly articulated and agreed upon by all involved. This evaluation plan then serves as the foundation for evaluative decisions throughout the learning experience and can be changed upon mutual agreement of those involved.

QE 96. Implement the evaluation plan. The evaluator is the individual within the CE provider unit who is responsible for implementing the plan as agreed upon by those involved. If changes are to be made in the evaluation plan, they should be documented and approved by all who are involved with the implementation of the plan. As an example, if a given evaluation methodology that was suggested in the plan turns out to be much more costly, time-consuming, or impractical, then it should be clearly known by all concerned that a cheaper but perhaps less valid instrument will have to be used in its place.

QE 97. Analyze the evaluation data. Data collection by the CE provider unit is prescribed by the evaluation plan, using the instruments developed by the educational evaluator. Once the data are collected and summarized, it is up to the evaluator to make a determination as to the best way to analyze these data. That decision is often guided by the information needs of the target audiences. What is desired is the least costly and most robust analysis, given the major purposes and information needs of the target audiences.

K. Using Evaluation Results

The purpose of evaluation is to determine the worth of the educational project. Once evaluation results and data are obtained, summarized, and analyzed, the information must be made available to the audiences identified in order to meet the information needs that have been expressed.

QE 98. Provide reports according to the evaluation plan. Reports and journal articles are two typical ways that evaluation results can be shared with a larger audience. Depending upon the information needs of those audiences, reports should be made available in a timely fashion, written in a way that clearly communicates the outcomes of the educational activity.

QE 99. Use evaluation results to make decisions concerning issues on which the evaluation was focused. For the CE provider unit, it is imperative to use the results of the evaluation efforts to improve the educational process used by the unit. In this way the evaluation serves an information-gathering function within the CE provider unit, allowing decisions to be made that help improve the processes and the chances of future educational activities having the desired impact. CE provider management must work closely with the evaluator to assure that it is obtaining the kind of information that allows it to make appropriate decisions.

IV. Providing Educational Assistance and Services

This section of quality elements addresses a function of CE provider units that has little tradition. As presented in the model in Chapter One, one of the primary purposes of the CE provider unit is to assist individual health professionals in improving their learning skills so that they may become more focused and independent in their educational endeavors. Providing such assistance is not commonly considered a function of CE provider units. When these activities are combined with the more traditional role of developing educational projects for groups of learners, a more comprehensive view of the potential of CE provider units is possible.

A. Facilitating the Assumption of Responsibility for Learning

The quality elements found within this section deal with the role of the CE provider unit in assisting learners to take responsibility for maintaining or improving their competence. This involves helping learners develop learning skills necessary to become focused, efficient learners whose learning activities result in better patient care. In addition, one quality element relates to the role CE provider units can play in encouraging the use of and acceptance for health care quality standards as a basis for determining individually perceived needs.

QE 100. Promote and facilitate the individual's acceptance of responsibility for maintaining and extending professional performance. Inherent in the role of professionals is the concept of taking responsibility for one's own performance and for the maintenance and enhancement of that professional performance. This quality element deals with the role the CE provider units play in promoting that concept among the professionals that it serves. Without the acceptance of the responsibility for learning on the part of individuals, nothing a CE provider can do educationally will have any impact on that professional. For changes to occur in behavior, a potential learner must perceive that a problem, need, or concern exists, in order to be willing to resolve it.

QE 101. Encourage the acceptance of health care quality standards as a basis for identifying professional problems or concerns. Professionals who have developed mechanisms for understanding their practice should have an opportunity to compare their performance with the performance of their peers or with accepted standards for health care. Without these standards or basis of comparison, the health professional has no mechanism for identifying gaps in performance and competence. Without such standards the ability to evaluate health care is limited. The CE provider unit's role is to encourage the development of quality standards for health care and to promote their application.

QE 102. Assist health care professionals to compare their personal and professional behavior to the health care quality standards. Once standards have been identified on a local, regional, or national basis, the CE provider unit can assist health professionals to use them for making judgments about their own professional behavior in comparison to what is considered standard by a group of peers, as a first step in identifying educational needs.

QE 103. Assist health care professionals to use learning as a mechanism for maintaining and extending professional performance. This quality element suggests that one of the roles of CE provider units is to promote among health professionals the recognition of the value of learning as one of the primary mechanisms for maintaining and enhancing competence. Learning should be perceived as an integral part of practice, not something that is separate and only occurs in isolated, formalized educational settings. It is this ability to learn from and within one's own practice that is the mark of professionals. Learning is a means to an end, not an end in itself and should be encouraged to be perceived this way by health professional learners.

QE 104. Support the development, maintenance, and improvement of individual learning skills. To use learning effectively as a means for resolving practice-related needs, problems, or concerns, it is important that the health professional develop the skills of self-directed learning. These skills include, for example, developing practice profiles, using systems to identify potential problems in the practice setting, using mechanisms to link into data bases to provide answers to practice problems, setting up individual filing systems for reprints that relate to specific, frequently encountered patient problems, and knowing how to access other educational resources.

QE 105. Assist learner(s) in identifying their resources for CE. Another role that should be assumed by the CE provider unit is to assist individual health care professionals in accessing available resources. This could be a simplified literature search system, special learning packages, or other information sources such as consultation.

B. Assisting the Health Care Professional in the Learning Process

The quality elements of this attribute deal with assisting health care professionals in pursuing their continuing education, including analyzing their own problems to arrive at educational priorities, setting objectives, determining their learning style, choosing activities and materials that will best meet their needs, and evaluating learning activities. This role of the CE provider unit is novel as it requires from the CE provider unit a concern for the learning process rather than, as usual, predominantly for content. The importance of this activity of assisting health professionals to be better self-directed learners cannot be overemphasized.

QE 106. Assist learner(s) in identifying and analyzing their problems or concerns. The CE provider unit can help learners set up systems that will allow them to identify and analyze specific practice-related problems or concerns. Such data will help the learners develop their learning plan, but they also provide the CE provider units with a cross section of needs of learners. When the same problems surface repeatedly, CE provider units will probably plan projects addressing problems identified by multiple health professionals. (QEs 61–71).

QE 107. Assist learner(s) in determining their educational priorities. Using the same approach as suggested in Attribute C, the CE provider unit can assist health professionals in determining their educational priorities. This allows the professional to approach first those problems that are of greatest importance to them and their patients.

QE 108. Assist learner(s) in setting their educational objectives. Individual health professionals may require help from the CE provider unit in translating identified needs, problems, or concerns into objectives that have a clearly stated outcome so that the learner will know whether or not they have resolved the stated need.

QE 109. Assist learner(s) in determining their learning style preferences, for consideration in choosing educational approaches. After having set learning objectives, the learners may need assistance in understanding the ways by which they best learn. They may use that insight as they select learning approaches that best suit their style.

QE 110. Assist learner(s) in choosing which educational activities, products, or services would best meet their objectives. Given the learners' educational objectives and learning style preferences, the CE provider unit can assist them in matching those realities to available activities, products, and services that will most likely lead to the resolution of their identified problems.

QE 111. Assist learner(s) in choosing educational activities, products, or services. The CE provider unit can assist health professionals in surveying available activities, products, or services and evaluating the relative strengths and weaknesses of each potential educational resource for meeting stated objectives.

QE 112. Assist learners in evaluating their activities, including the impact of learning on practice. The key to successful completion of a CE effort is the feedback as to what extent the stated objectives have been reached and the original problem or concern has been resolved. The CE provider unit can give guidance to the learners on how to evaluate the degree of success of their own CE efforts. In the case of limited success, the CE provider unit will attempt to show the learner how alternative approaches may have greater success.

C. Assisting in Applying Learning to Practice

This attribute addresses the role of a CE provider unit in helping learners apply to the practice setting what they have learned.

QE 113. Assist learner(s) in identifying potential reinforcements in the practice setting for application of learning. A given learning activity frequently may not lead to successful application of that learning to practice unless the practice setting is analyzed for aspects that can be manipulated to reinforce the new desired behavior. This need for reinforcement of a given learning activity can be discussed with the learner by a CE provider unit. Reinforcements can then be incorporated in a given learning plan that would take health care realities into consideration, build upon them, and use them for successful application of the learning activity to the practice setting.

QE 114. Assist learner(s) whenever possible in applying learning to practice. In some cases the individual learners will need assistance from the CE provider unit in being able to apply to practice what they have learned. It may be that the CE provider unit would need to talk with the management of a hospital to secure time that learners require to practice the newly acquired skill. In another case, different equipment might need to be purchased by that hospital to allow a learner to implement what has been taught. A CE provider unit can play a significant part in increasing the chances of learning having the desired impact on health care outcomes.

D. Providing Assistance and Services to Other CE Provider Units

QE 114.1 Provide educational consultation services to other CE provider units. This attribute and quality element address the responsibility that a CE provider unit has in assisting other CE provider units to improve their own educational and management functions so that more health professionals will be able to benefit from the improved services of the CE provider units.

V. Administering the CE Provider Unit

A. Managing Staff and Faculty

Quality elements 115 through 121 address the manager's responsibility to guide, conserve, and develop the CE provider unit's human resources.

QE 115. Ensure that the CE provider unit's plans, policies, procedures, and standards are known throughout the unit. It is mandatory that the CE provider unit manager communicate all essential information about intentions, requirements, and guidelines throughout the unit.

QE 116. Assign responsibility and delegate commensurate authority for carrying out the educational and management activities of the CE provider unit. This quality element relates to the allocation of tasks to the people who occupy jobs in the CE provider unit. It is suggested that parity of responsibility and authority apply in delegating work. Task allocation should be reviewed periodically on the basis of performance and activity reports.

QE 117. Negotiate work obligations, clearly define what is expected, and communicate the relevant standards. In the day-to-day oversight of activities, the CE provider unit manager should consider the strengths, limits, and development needs of the staff in assigning work and should assure that each person who accepts work assignments knows what is to be done, when and how it should be accomplished, and what conditions of quality have been agreed upon.

QE 119. Create and maintain a supportive environment in the work place. The issue of working conditions within the unit should be addressed. There should be a positive, sustaining set of relationships among members of the CE provider unit.

QE 120. Provide incentives for quality performance. An important aspect of management is a system of adequate compensation, benefits, and other rewards for membership in the unit and performance of its work.

QE 121. Promote staff and faculty growth and development as a means to fulfill individual goals and those of the CE provider unit. Continued satisfaction and strengthening of the unit's human resources through opportunities for development can serve as an important stimulus for quality performance. For example, continuing education for the unit's staff can help in building staff morale and cooperation.

B. Managing Other Resources

While the quality elements just described relate to the CE provider unit's human resources, QEs 122 through 125 cover the unit's financial, physical, and temporal resources.

QE 122. Allocate money, time, facilities, and materials to assure cost-beneficial and timely accomplishment of assigned activities. A proper share of the unit's resources should be assigned to each activity in the unit by the CE manager.

QE 123. Make resource allocations consistent with the CE priorities. The share and quality of resources accorded to a given project should reflect the importance and priority attached to the project.

QE 124. Monitor resource status and expenditures. The CE provider unit manager should determine the use of resources within the unit. Any discrepancy of resource utilization from the original plan should be noted, and if necessary, corrective action should be taken.

QE 125. Provide resource maintenance and upkeep as needed. This quality element suggests attending to the need for periodic refurbishment, repair, or service in the case of equipment and facilities.

C. Marketing

Quality elements 126 through 129 address the need to sell the CE provider unit and its products. The QEs are intended broadly to cover not only entrepreneurial CE ventures but also in-house or "captive" CE provider units, such as a hospital CE office. This broad approach recognizes that the need for some form of marketing applies in all CE settings.

QE 126. Implement the CE provider unit's overall promotional strategies to develop specific approaches for each educational project. The CE provider unit manager should implement the unit's plans for marketing. This applies to internal and external marketing.

QE 127. Develop a realistic fee structure. In cases where CE is provided on a fee basis, the fee should be related to the value the CE contributes to the health care professional's capability to serve the patient.

QE 128. Provide sufficient information in promotional materials for potential learners to make sound decisions about participation in educational projects of the CE provider unit. This quality element suggests a "truth-in-advertising" policy for the CE provider unit.

QE 129. Emphasize the quality aspects of CE activities, products, and services in promotional efforts. A quality-oriented institutional approach should be taken to the selling of CE to participants, as well as to parent organizations and others.

D. Managing Information

Quality elements 130 through 132 address the operation of the CE provider unit's information system. (The development of the information system is covered in QEs 42 through 44.)

QE 130. Implement the CE provider unit's information system. This quality element asks the CE provider unit manager to set into motion the processes of information management. The CE provider unit manager should be familiar with the legal requirements of this provision.

QE 131. Implement mechanisms for timely analysis and reporting of essential information. Reports or other means for getting information to people who need it must be prepared at the required time and in a format useful to the recipients.

QE 132. Protect confidentiality of data and information as required. In the course of getting and using information for the purposes of providing CE, the privacy of the individual must be respected.

E. Coordinating Functions

Quality elements 133 through 135 address the managerial task of coordination. Three dimensions of coordination are covered in the elements: coordination within the CE provider unit, between the CE provider unit and its parent organization, and coordination with potential participants in CE and with other CE provider units.

QE 133. Coordinate the educational with the management functions within the CE provider unit. Management functions are subordinate to the goals and objectives of the educational functions of the unit. To assure that management serves the attainment of quality in the educational process, the support or oversight activities should be synchronized with the conduct of CE.

QE 134. Coordinate the education and management functions of the CE provider unit with those of its parent organization. For smooth operation and to avoid friction within the institution, the management of the CE provider unit should be integrated with that of the parent institution. Exception should be sought if such integration interferes with the quality of the CE activities.

QE 135. Accommodate the educational activities of the CE provider unit to the requirements of potential learners and the plans of other CE provider units. The CE provider unit manager should see to the need for conforming the schedule of CE activities offered by the unit to the needs of its clients and the health care professionals. This includes working out a fit between the schedules of various CE provider units, whenever possible, for the benefit of potential participants.

F. Monitoring and Controlling

Quality elements 136 and 137 address the oversight responsibility of the CE provider unit manager. As the unit operates, standards are applied to produce the needed signals for guidance and necessary adjustments.

QE 136. Implement the standards set for the CE provider unit. It is an important management task to develop policies and procedures that enforce adherence to standards set for the operation and management of the CE provider unit.

QE 137. Use the information obtained from applying the standards to provide the feedback necessary to maintain and improve performance and to anticipate and correct deficiencies in the CE provider unit. Application of standards toward assessing the operational functioning of the CE provider unit should yield feedback for the evaluation of the unit. If found deficient, the data should provide directives for corrective action.

Name Index

Subject Index

A

Accountability: defined, 134; and program development, 134; and quality assurance, 300; quality elements for, 21, 389–390

Accreditation: for continuing medical education, 97; and quality assurance, 300

Accreditation Council for Continuing Medical Education (ACCME), xiv, 9, 260, 300; and quality elements, 351–352

Activities, quality elements for providing, 17, 23–26, 395–412

Ad Hoc Committee on Continuing Medical Education, 7, 9, 29

Adapting provider unit, quality elements for, 21, 388–389

Administration: and quality assur-

ance, 309, 311–312; quality elements for, 17, 27–29, 417–421

Adults: development of, and self-directed learning, 370, 376; and experience, 43; as learners, 40–44, 223; learning styles of, 43–44; physiological characteristics of, 41–42; and psychological factors, 42–43

Advisory committee, for needs assessment, 168

Albany Medical College, and continuing medical education, 92

American Association for Adult and Continuing Education, 366, 367

American Association of Dental Schools, 300; Sponsor Approval Program of, 349

American Board of Medical Specialties, xiv, 351

American Board of Pediatrics, 200–
201, 215, 229, 239
American Heart Association, 125
American Hospital Association, xiv,
351
American Medical Association, 82,
84, 91, 94, 95, 98n, 99, 102,
104, 109–110; and Accreditation
Council for Continuing Medi-
cal Education, xiv, 351; and
computer-assisted instruction,
183–184; Council on Medical
Education and Hospitals of, 90,
91, 92, 93, 97, 110; Division of
Medical Education of, 88, 110
American Nurse's Association, 229,
240
American Red Cross, 125; and qual-
ity elements, 350–351
American Society for Training and
Development, 366
Analysis skills, 324–325
Androgogy, and program develop-
ment, 137
Application assistance, quality ele-
ments for, 27, 416
Area Health Education Centers
(AHECs), 125
Arthritis Foundation, 125
Assessment skills, 324
Association for Hospital Medical
Education, xiv, 105–106, 110, 351
Association of American Medical
Colleges (AAMC), 6, 7, 9, 29, 94,
300, 351; and Continuing Educa-
tion Systems Project, xiv, xviii,
xxi
Autonomy, of health care profes-
sionals, 118–119

B

Behaviorism: and learning, 33–35;
and motivation, 55
Bi-cycle model, for continuing med-
ical education, 100, 101, 137
Birmingham, University of, MIST
(Medical Information Service via
Telephone) System of, 235

Brainstorm technique, for needs assessment, 167

C

California Press, University of, 366
Canada, patient care evaluation in,
102
Change: and continuity, 252–253;
openness to, by health care professionals, 120–121
Cognitive dissonance, for family
physicians, 78
Cognitive testing, for needs assessment, 166
Cognitivists: and learning, 36–37;
and motivation, 56–58
Colleagues: as information sources,
76, 79, 80; review by, for needs
assessment, 166, 229–230; and
self-directed learning, 234–235
Communication skills, 327–328
Community hospital, and continuing medical education, 104–106
Computer-assisted instruction
(CAI), as educational method,
183–184, 185
Conference, as delivery approach,
189
Continuing education: analysis of
strategies for strengthening, 361–
379; conceptual model for, 11–16;
context for, 2–9; and coordination strategies, 373–376; defined,
1–2; defining quality for, 1–31;
demand increasing for, 5, 361–
362; as educational continuum,
3–4, educational process in, 12,
14; expectations high for, 6; impact of, 5, 135; implications of
model for, 15–16; improving,
338–360; as information source,
76–77, 79, 80, 81–82; issues in, 4–
7; and learner orientations, 367–
373; and learning process, 12, 13;
and learning theory, 32–71; medical, 87–114; multiple factors affecting, 7–9; and new knowledge
and technology, 12, 13; for prac-